CONDUCTING & READING RESEARCH
in Kinesiology

Fifth Edition

Ted A. Baumgartner
University of Georgia

Larry D. Hensley
University of Northern Iowa

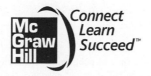

The McGraw-Hill Companies

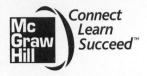

Mc Graw Hill

Connect
Learn
Succeed™

CONDUCTING & READING RESEARCH IN KINESIOLOGY, FIFTH EDITION

Published by McGraw-Hill, a business unit of The McGraw-Hill Companies, Inc., 1221 Avenue of the Americas, New York, NY, 10020. Copyright © 2013 by The McGraw-Hill Companies, Inc. All rights reserved. Printed in the United States of America. Previous editions © 2006, 2002, and 1998. No part of this publication may be reproduced or distributed in any form or by any means, or stored in a database or retrieval system, without the prior written consent of The McGraw-Hill Companies, Inc., including, but not limited to, in any network or other electronic storage or transmission, or broadcast for distance learning.

Some ancillaries, including electronic and print components, may not be available to customers outside the United States.

This book is printed on acid-free paper.

1 2 3 4 5 6 7 8 9 0 DOC/DOC 1 0 9 8 7 6 5 4 3 2

ISBN: 978-0-07-802255-5
MHID: 0-07-802255-X

Vice President and Editor-in-Chief: *Michael Ryan*
Publisher: *David Patterson*
Sr. Sponsoring Editor: *William J. Minick*
Developmental Editor: *Darlene M. Schueller*
Marketing Coordinator: *Colleen Havens*
Project Manager: *Jolynn Kilburg*
Buyer: *Nicole Baumgartner*
Design Coordinator: *Margarite Reynolds*
Cover Design: *Studio Montage, St. Louis, Missouri*
Cover Image Credit: *Design Pics / Tim Antoniuk*
Media Project Manager: *Sridevi Palani*
Compositor: *Aptara®, Inc.*
Typeface: *10/12 Times LT Std*
Printer: *RR Donnelley*

Library of Congress Cataloging-in-Publication Data

Baumgartner, Ted A.
    Conducting & reading research in kinesiology / Ted A. Baumgartner, Larry
D. Hensley.—5th ed.
        p.; cm.
    Rev. ed. of: Conducting & reading research in health and human performance / Ted A. Baumgartner, Larry
D. Hensley. 4th ed. c2006.
    Includes bibliographical references and index.
    ISBN 978-0-07-802255-5 (alk. paper)—ISBN 0-07-802255-X (alk. paper)
    I. Hensley, Larry D. (Larry Duncan), 1948- II. Baumgartner, Ted A.
Conducting and reading research in health and human performance. III. Title.
[DNLM: 1. Research. W 20.5]
610'.72—dc23   2012005930

The Internet addresses listed in the text were accurate at the time of publication. The inclusion of a website does not indicate an endorsement by the authors or McGraw-Hill, and McGraw-Hill does not guarantee the accuracy of the information presented at these sites.

www.mhhe.com

About the Authors

Ted A. Baumgartner earned his undergraduate degree in physical education from Oklahoma State University, his master's degree in physical education from Southern Illinois University–Carbondale, and his doctorate from the University of Iowa. He was on the faculty at Indiana University from 1967 to 1977, teaching measurement courses and statistics courses. Since 1977 he has been a professor at the University of Georgia teaching measurement courses, statistics courses, and introduction to research courses. Dr. Baumgartner is a co-author of the book *Measurement for Evaluation in Physical Education and Exercise Science,* 8th edition. He started the journal *Measurement in Physical Education and Exercise Science* and was the first editor of the journal. Dr. Baumgartner is a member of the National Academy of Kinesiology.

Larry D. Hensley earned his undergraduate degree in physical education from Southern Methodist University, his master's degree from Indiana University, and his doctorate from the University of Georgia. Dr. Hensley is an Emeritus Professor in the School of Health, Physical Education, and Leisure Services (HPELS) at the University of Northern Iowa. He was a Distinguished Visiting Professor at the U.S. Military Academy at West Point from 1999 to 2000 and served as an Advisory Professor at the Hong Kong Institute of Education in 2004. Dr. Hensley has authored numerous articles, chapters, and monographs in the areas of applied measurement and exercise science and has taught research methods, measurement, and statistics courses for more than 30 years.

Dedication

This edition of the book is dedicated to Dr. Clint Strong. He taught Introduction to Research Techniques in the School of Health, Physical Education, Recreation, and Dance at Indiana University for many years. His lecture notes and course packet were the basis for the first edition of this book (Baumgartner and Strong 1994). Dr. Strong edited the chapters of the book he wrote when the book was revised for the second edition (Baumgartner and Strong 1998). Larry Hensley, one of Dr. Strong's former master's students, was added as a co-author for the third edition of the book (Baumgartner, Strong, and Hensley 2002). There is still a sizable amount of material in the present edition of the book that originated with Dr. Clint Strong.

Contents in Brief

Contents

Part Three   *Data Analysis   248*

13   *Descriptive Data Analysis   250*

Part Four   *Writing and Reporting   342*

Preface

This book was developed based on the methods its authors have used to teach the master's-level introduction to research course for many years. One author has taught an upper-level undergraduate course numerous times. It is assumed that students come to this course with varied backgrounds in areas related to kinesiology. This book is specifically designed for students studying exercise science, physical education, sport management, and related areas. The two major objectives of our courses are to teach students how to conduct their own research and how to read with understanding the research that others have done. The book is comprehensive yet practical and understandable. Many examples of the application of various research methods and techniques commonly used in kinesiology are presented in an attempt to increase students' grasp of the research process.

Many students begin the introduction to research course with little research background, little interest in research, and considerable fear about their ability to succeed in the course. These students may not write a master's thesis. However, it is still important that they develop an appreciation for research and an understanding of how different types of research are conducted so they will become good consumers and readers of the research of others. The book is written with this type of student in mind.

Other students begin the introduction to research course knowing they will write a master's thesis or complete a master's project. These students need to be aware of the many possible research approaches and the procedures that are basic to many types of research. This book will also serve the needs of this type of student.

Doctoral students and beginning researchers who want an overview of the research process should find this book helpful. However, the procedures and techniques specific to a certain type of research in a specialized area are generally not covered in this book.

In Chapter 2 we suggest that a research project begins with the identification of a research topic and progresses through a series of steps until the research is conducted and a report describing the research project is written. The book's chapters are organized in this manner. The first seven chapters are essential to cover. Portions of Chapters 8 through 12 may be covered quickly if only certain types of research are of interest to the student. Likewise, some of the content in Chapters 13 through 17 could be omitted depending on the particular interests and needs of the students.

The three chapters on experimental research, descriptive research, and qualitative research cover the common research approaches in kinesiology. The two statistics chapters are inclusive but are presented with an orientation toward practical use and without emphasis on calculational ability. The computer programs accompanying the statistics chapters are presented with considerable explanation and use of examples. Even the emphasis on doing and understanding research is somewhat unique in this book.

CHANGES TO THE FIFTH EDITION

The fifth edition of *Conducting & Reading Research in Kinesiology* builds upon the strengths of previous editions, with updated material and pedagogical changes designed to increase accuracy in content and clarity in presentation.

Changed Title

The title of the book has been changed from *Conducting & Reading Research in Health and Human Performance* to *Conducting & Reading Research in Kinesiology*. This change was made in recognition of the growing acceptance of the term *kinesiology* to reflect the discipline that serves as the foundation for a number of professional and academic fields of study, such as physical education, exercise and sport science, human performance, and sport management, in particular. The change in title enables the authors to more specifically focus the fifth edition toward research practices and studies that are commonplace in kinesiology and to provide examples that are more meaningful for kinesiology students.

Revised Organization

In order to better reflect the sequence of steps in the research process, the chapter "Reading and Evaluating Research Reports" (now Chapter 4) has been moved nearer the beginning of the book and now follows immediately the chapter "Reviewing the Literature." This reflects the authors' belief that students should begin reading the scientific literature in their chosen area early in the research process and be able to make an informed judgment about the quality of the research being reported. A revised Chapter 3, "Reviewing the Literature," emphasizes the process involved in searching the scientific literature and offers a detailed sequence of steps for conducting a database search. In keeping with the changed title and the focus on research in kinesiology, Chapter 12 now includes sections specifically on historical research and action research.

Updated and Expanded Content

Throughout the fifth edition, the authors have retained pedagogical features, such as *chapter objectives, chapter-ending summaries, marginal glossary,* and *integrated examples,* that characterized previous editions of the book. The authors have replaced examples of many dated studies with newer, up-to-date studies. All chapters have been revised and modernized, discussions have been updated, and examples now focus exclusively on research in kinesiology.

In Chapter 1, a figure is added that is designed to help the reader conceptualize how research may build the body of knowledge for a field of study. A brief historical perspective on research in the kinesiology field is included.

In order to better reflect published research in the field and provide clarity on the topic, Chapter 2 includes a revised discussion on the purpose of a research study and how to frame the purpose statement in a research report.

Chapter 3, "Reviewing the Literature," has been completely rewritten to emphasize the process involved in searching, reading, and documenting the scientific literature. Particular attention has been given to conducting a database search and using the Internet.

In order to better reflect the actual steps in the research process and to provide students with a framework for reading scholarly articles, "Reading and Evaluating Research Reports" has been relocated as Chapter 4. Many new examples taken from published research studies are included.

Chapter 5, "Developing the Research Plan," builds upon the basic framework for conducting a research study by including detailed information concerning data collection. A completely updated and revised section on measurement techniques, including new examples of various scales commonly used in kinesiology research, is provided.

Chapter 6, "Ethical Concerns in Research," provides a historical perspective on misconduct in scientific research that led to the establishment of ethical principles and regulations related to research practices. Current regulatory guidelines for the protection of research participants as well as detailed information about obtaining informed consent, complete with an informed consent template, are included.

Guest author Jennifer Waldron has completely rewritten Chapter 10, "Qualitative Research." The author emphasizes the interpretive or constructivist paradigm in qualitative research and explains the six traditions of qualitative research. Numerous new examples of qualitative studies found in kinesiology research are presented throughout the chapter. Methods of data collection are emphasized and the author provides many helpful hints based on her own research.

Chapter 12, "Historical Research and Action Research," has been substantially revised. The chapter now includes sections on Historical Research and Action Research, while dropping information on epidemiological research, single participant research, and creative research. The Action Research section is new and reflects the growing trend toward practitioner research in kinesiology.

Data analysis discussions in Chapters 13 and 14 have been updated to match the newest version of SPSS software. A revised Appendix A offers updated instructions for using the newest version of SPSS.

Chapters 16 and 17, "Developing the Research Proposal" and "Writing the Research Report," have been updated with more recent examples from student theses or published articles.

ANCILLARIES

SPSS

Sites where the most recent version of SPSS can be leased for a modest fee are identified in Chapter 13. SPSS empowers students to reach the in-depth answers that come only from using advanced analytical techniques.

McGraw-Hill Create™

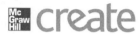

Craft your teaching resources to match the way you teach! With McGraw-Hill Create, you can easily rearrange chapters, combine material from other content sources, and quickly upload content you have written like your course syllabus or teaching notes. Find the content you need in Create by searching through thousands of leading McGraw-Hill textbooks. Arrange your book to fit your teaching style. Create even allows you to personalize your book's appearance by selecting the cover and adding your name, school, and course information. Order a Create book and you'll receive a complimentary print review copy in 3–5 business days or a complimentary electronic review copy (eComp) via email in minutes. Go to www.mcgrawhillcreate.com today and register to experience how McGraw-Hill Create empowers you to teach *your* students *your* way.

Electronic Textbook Option

This text is offered through CourseSmart for both instructors and students. CourseSmart is an online resource where students can purchase the complete text online at almost half the cost of a traditional text. Purchasing the eTextbook allows students to take advantage of CourseSmart's web tools for learning, which include full text search, notes and highlighting, and email tools for sharing notes between classmates. To learn more about CourseSmart options, contact your sales representative or visit www.CourseSmart.com.

Instructor's Resources

Instructors's resources to accompany the fifth edition of the book include an Instructor's Manual, a test question bank, and PowerPoint slides. These resources may be downloaded from the Instructor's Resource website at www.mhhe.com/baumgartner5e.

ACKNOWLEDGMENTS

This book is the product of the influence of many people and occurrences. First, the professors who trained and educated the authors must be recognized. Second, the research experiences of the authors have been influential. Third, the experience of teaching the introduction to research course at both the undergraduate and graduate level and the feedback from students in the course are reflected in the book.

Thanks must be expressed to the people in the profession who have reviewed this book and suggested improvements:

FOR THE FIFTH EDITION

Charles D. Sands III
Samford University

John T. Foley
State University of New York, Cortland

Joseph Kwame Mintah
Azusa Pacific University

Katherine M. Polasek
State University of New York, Cortland

Megan Babkes Stellino
University of Northern Colorado

FOR PREVIOUS EDITIONS

Stan Bassin
California State University, Pomona

Thomas Chandler
Marshall University

Mary L. Dawson
Western Michigan University, Kalamazoo

James M. DiNucci
Stephen F. Austin State University

Mark Huntington
Manchester College

Mark Kelley
Southeastern Louisiana University

Beverly Mitchell
Kennesaw State College

Greg Payne
San Jose State University

Steve Sanders
Tennessee Technological University

Kurt A. Stahura
Arkansas State University

Donna J. Terbizan
North Dakota State University

Kesia Walker
Dillard University

Reuben L. Wright
Prairie View A&M University

Special appreciation goes to Jennifer Waldron, Ph.D., of the University of Northern Iowa, who wrote Chapter 10, "Qualitative Research."

In addition, thanks go to the editors at McGraw-Hill Higher Education, who improved the manuscript considerably.

Finally, the authors must thank their wives and families for allowing them the time to write the book. Adjustments and sacrifices were necessary by all in order for the book to be completed.

T.A.B.
L.D.H.

CONDUCTING & READING RESEARCH

in Kinesiology

Part One

The Research Process

A professional in exercise science, physical education, sport pedagogy, or any one of the fields within kinesiology is constantly faced with challenging situations or problems that require new and innovative solutions. We often turn to the scientific method in search for these solutions. While not everyone will receive a Nobel Prize for his or her research, we can all benefit from a better understanding of the research process. Although the research process may be unfamiliar to many beginning graduate students, the exhilaration and satisfaction of completing a research study is often the highlight of their academic experience. This textbook, and a good course in research methods and statistics, can lay the groundwork for attaining the knowledge and skills necessary to be a competent researcher and an informed kinesiology professional.

In Part One of this textbook, the foundation for the research process is described in seven chapters. Chapter 1, "The Nature and Purpose of Research," describes (1) the importance of research in the acquisition of knowledge by kinesiology professions, (2) how the scientific method of solving problems fits into the research process, (3) various types of research, and (4) the significance of research in kinesiology. Chapter 2, "Understanding the Research Process," discusses (1) the various steps in the research process, (2) how research questions are initiated, selected, and defined, and (3) the concept of variables. Chapter 3, "Reviewing the Literature," details (1) the importance of the literature review in the research process, (2) methods for reviewing and evaluating the literature, and (3) sources of literature pertinent to kinesiology. Chapter 4, "Reading and Evaluating Research Reports," describes (1) the typical format for a research report and (2) evaluative criteria for reading and judging the quality of research reports. Chapter 5, "Developing the Research Plan," describes (1) the various research approaches common in kinesiology, (2) the role of hypotheses in research, (3) techniques for collecting data, and (4) criteria for selecting or developing data collection instruments. Chapter 6, "Ethical Concerns in Research," addresses (1) the history of research involving human participants that led to the formation of ethical standards for the conduct of research, and (2) those standards and guidelines most applicable to research in kinesiology. Chapter 7, "Selection of Research Participants: Sampling Procedures," discusses (1) the importance of selecting research appropriate for the research, (2) the concepts of population and sample, (3) various methods for selecting research participants, and (4) sample size.

1

The Nature and Purpose of Research

OBJECTIVES

Members of the kinesiology profession have a wealth of information upon which they make decisions. Quite frequently, this information is passed down to us, as opposed to our discovering it through direct observation of our experiences. Many times we don't bother to examine the source of the information prior to using it. However, when members of a profession engage in various aspects of the research process, current information can be checked out—and new information acquired.

After reading Chapter 1, you should be able to

1. Explain the relationship between research and a profession.
2. Describe the nature of research.
3. Explain the scientific method.
4. Understand the various types of research classifications and how they are applied.

Why take a research methods course? For most of you, the answer is that it is probably required in your program of study. Maybe the more appropriate question is why is research methods a required course? The simple answer is that the knowledge learned and skills developed in a research methods course are considered essential qualities of being well-educated. Each of us is a consumer of research on a daily basis. We cannot read the daily paper, watch television, explore the Internet, or even read signs along the highway without being exposed to the results of research. But what are we to do with this information? The choices we make and products we buy are frequently based upon the results of product research and the marketing of the results. For example, we choose one brand of toothpaste over another because it is more effective in preventing cavities, tastes better, or whitens our teeth better. The sunscreen we select is based on the fact that research has shown it to be effective in reducing the harmful effects of the sun's rays. Professionals in all disciplines, including kinesiology, rely on research to build the body of knowledge upon which the profession is based. Likewise, as professionals in the various kinesiology fields, our practices as a coach, a teacher, an exercise technician, or a physical activity professional are greatly influenced by the results of research in our field. Since the publication of the landmark report *Physical Activity and Health: A Report of the Surgeon General* (U.S. Department of Health and Human Services 1996), numerous research studies have sought to explain why one chooses to be physically active. A better understanding of the factors associated with a physically active lifestyle will undoubtedly lead to the development of better and more effective programs designed to promote physical activity. The growing epidemic of obesity in the United States, as well as other countries, has led to a plethora of research studies by kinesiology professionals that are designed to identify causes, as well as solutions, to the problem. In effect, almost everything we do is influenced by research in one way or another. As professionals, many of you will also be producers of research, either as part of your formal educational experience or as an expectation of your employment. A research methods course will provide you the basic knowledge and skills required to actually conduct a research study. All of you will be consumers of research information in one way or another. The information presented in this book and taught in a research methods course will help you become a wiser consumer of research information and help you make educated decisions about research claims you encounter in both your daily life as well as professional life.

THE ESSENCE OF A PROFESSION: KNOWLEDGE

An essential quality that differentiates a profession from other vocations is the continuous pursuit and dissemination of new knowledge. All professions produce a variety of monthly, quarterly, and annual publications. The creation, reading, and interpretation of articles, books, theses, and dissertations are integral parts of the formal education and in-service education of the members of a profession. Moreover, the quality and quantity of such publications are an index of the vitality and soundness of a profession as a whole. The publications, and their use, also identify the professional stature of individual members. The information contained in the publications contributes greatly to the body of knowledge of a profession. A continuous flow of new facts and ideas must come from the laboratory and classroom, and this new information must be passed along. A profession's body of knowledge must grow and professional practices must adapt to new findings. If new knowledge suggests that an accepted practice is unsatisfactory, obsolete, or hazardous, then that practice must be modified or eliminated. Research tells us, for example, that the use of straight-leg sit-ups poses problems for the lower back and therefore is not recommended as an exercise. The body of knowledge that characterizes a profession can be advanced, and must be for a profession to continue to contribute to the constituency it serves. The major vehicle by which a

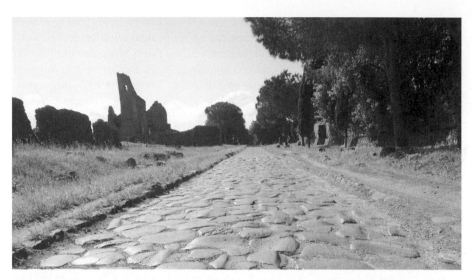

This portion of a cobblestone street symbolizes building the "road of knowledge."

profession advances its knowledge base is the process of research. Building a profession's body of knowledge can be likened to building a cobblestone road, where the road grows incrementally as stone after stone is laid. The stones represent individual pieces of knowledge that may be produced through research. The road is of infinite length and does not follow a linear path, thus depicting the unlimited nature and uneven manner of building a body of knowledge. The stones are irregular in shape and do not contribute equally to the complete road. This illustrates that pieces of knowledge are not of uniform importance to the body of knowledge being built.

Research is exciting and challenging, and it makes an essential contribution to the development of those who engage in it. Research accomplished by professionals in kinesiology is exciting because the results frequently contribute to and guide professional practice. It is challenging because the exploration of research ideas demands critical thinking and requires that judgment be exercised on both procedural and conceptual questions. Research contributes to the professional's development because the process builds a new set of skills that can be used to better comprehend the research literature and to recognize new questions that need to be researched.

RESEARCH: THE KNOWLEDGE PIPELINE

Research is a greatly misunderstood activity. For many people, the term conjures up the image of a person in a white laboratory coat, wearing black-framed glasses, and pouring the contents of one beaker into another. Others see a person sifting through volumes and volumes of numbers or statistics. And yet others may think of a person holding a clipboard and standing in a shopping mall, poised to interview an unsuspecting shopper. The perception is that this person, the researcher, is cold, shy, disinterested in people as individuals, interested in people only as research participants, and concerned primarily with test tubes, stopwatches, figures, and published articles. In effect, as soon as the word "research" is spoken, a barrier is raised as one's preconceived and misguided image of a researcher comes to mind.

In its simplest context, research is nothing more or less than finding answers to a question in a logical, orderly, and systematic fashion. Although there is not a single, universally accepted definition of research, the myriad of definitions that we see contain many similarities. Foremost, perhaps, is the fact that research is usually *systematic* in nature and focuses on a *question* of interest. Consider the following descriptions of research:

- Research is a structured way of solving problems (Thomas, Nelson, and Silverman 2005, 17).
- Research is a systematic attempt to provide answers to questions (Tuckman 1999, 4).
- Research may be defined as the systematic and objective analysis and recording of controlled observations that may lead to the development of generalizations, principles, or theories, resulting in prediction and possible control of events (Best and Kahn 2005, 18).
- Research is a systematic, controlled, empirical, and critical investigation of hypothetical propositions about the presumed relationships among natural phenomena (Kerlinger 1973, 11).
- Research is a systematic way of asking questions, a systematic method of inquiry (Drew, Hardman, and Hosp 2008, 4.)

Our definition of **research** is very similiar; research is a systematic attempt to find solutions to a problem or to answer a question. Virtually all definitions of research speak to its systematic nature and to the fact that it represents a process for acquiring information that may be used to posit answers to questions and to generally advance a body of knowledge. Professional practice in virtually every field, including kinesiology, involves many problems and questions that can be investigated through the research process. Answers to these research questions should be based on evidence that is as objective and free of bias as possible. Objectivity is a key element of research, which is why researchers employ the scientific method in their quest for knowledge. In effect, research is the application of the scientific method to the study of a question. The scientific method offers researchers a structured means of finding the answers to research questions. Scientific solutions shape the body of knowledge for a profession, which, in turn, can be used to help synthesize,

Research
A systematic way of finding solutions to a problem or an answer to a question.

validate, or change the philosophy, theoretical relationships, and, ultimately, the practices of a profession.

THE SEARCH FOR KNOWLEDGE

Men and women have been searching for knowledge since the beginning of time. In doing so they have relied, in general, upon five sources of evidence: (1) tenacity, more commonly referred to as custom or tradition, (2) authority, (3) personal experience, (4) deductive reasoning, and (5) scientific inquiry. The earliest search for knowledge was characterized by the first three sources, and each provided a modicum of truth. Tradition or custom involves believing something because it has always been believed or accepted. While there is something secure, serene, and peaceful about customs and traditions, the information acquired might not be accurate. For example, there is really no credibility to the notion that breaking a mirror will result in seven years of bad luck. Reliance on an authority served people well in the past, but fell short as a complete source of truth. Many authorities have been wrong. There was a time when the word of a coach, a teacher, or even the president was considered unimpeachable, but we now are reluctant to accept the word of authorities merely because of the position they hold. There is also value in personal experience, but it, too, has limitations as a source of truth. First of all, one's experiences are limited. Moreover, one's response to a given situation is likely to be quite different from the response of another, depending upon previous experience, and personal values and beliefs. Brothers and sisters in a family grow up differently because they are affected differently and have different experiences in the same situation. Nevertheless, the use of personal experience is relatively high on the continuum of methods of acquiring knowledge. As humans have thought about problems over the ages, each of these sources of evidence has played an important role. The shortcomings of each source, however, dictated inadequacies in the search for truth. Thus arose the appeal of other sources for new knowledge.

Deductive reasoning
Thinking that proceeds from a general assumption to a specific logical conclusion.

Deductive reasoning (logic) was the first major contribution to the process of seeking truth systematically. In deductive reasoning, thinking proceeds from a general assumption to a specific application. We begin with a set of known facts or assumptions and then use logic to answer a question or reach a conclusion. Phrases such as "It figures" or "That figures" also imply a conclusion based on deductive reasoning. Early philosophers ushered in the era of logic through statements referred to as a categorical **syllogism.** Here is such a statement:

Syllogism
A process of logical reasoning in which conclusions are based on a series of propositions or assumptions.

> All presidents are mortal. Barrack Obama is a president. Therefore, Barrack Obama is mortal.

Two ideas, or premises, form the basis for the conclusion. If the relationship between the two is true, then the conclusion is true. However, if either premise is false, the conclusion is also false. This represents the major weakness of deductive reasoning; that is, we have to accept the information contained in the premises as being true without really knowing that it is true.

> All heavy cigarette smokers die from cancer. John smokes six packages of cigarettes a day. Therefore, John will die of cancer.

The ultimate truth or falsity of the conclusion concerning John's demise depends upon the truth of the first two statements. Do all heavy smokers die of cancer? Are six packs of cigarettes a day enough to cause John to develop cancer?

Deduction is valuable and is a part of almost every research project. Reasoning of this kind enables the researcher to organize the information already known to exist concerning the research problem of current interest, to theorize about the relationship of this information to the problem, and then deduce various hypotheses to be tested by the research. Deduction moves backward from the general to the specific. Despite the value of deductive reasoning as a source of knowledge, the information acquired should not be accepted as true without some verification that the premises are accurate.

The human thought process then turns to inductive reasoning in an attempt to get at the elusive truth. **Induction,** in which thinking proceeds from the specific to the general, is considered to be the basic principle of scientific inquiry. Conclusions about events are based on information generated through many individual and direct observations. In the inductive process, the researcher observes an individual or group of individuals from a larger population of similar individuals. Then, based upon these observations of the smaller group, inferences, conclusions, or generalizations are made back to the larger population. Hence, thinking moves forward from the specific to the general. Ary, Jacobs, and Sorensen (2010) have clearly illustrated the difference between deductive and inductive processes.

> *Deductive.* Every mammal has lungs. All rabbits are mammals. Therefore, every rabbit has lungs.
>
> *Inductive.* Every rabbit that has been observed has lungs. Therefore, every rabbit has lungs.

Induction, then, is based on seeking facts, which is a primary goal of science. There are two kinds of induction, *perfect* and *imperfect.* **Perfect induction** results in conclusions based on observations of selected characteristics of all members of a group or population. This is frequently not possible, especially when groups are large. **Imperfect induction** results in conclusions based on the observations of a small, specific number of members of a population. Most research is based on imperfect induction. The information obtained may not be absolutely perfect, or true, but is sufficient to make fairly reliable generalizations. It is generally conceded that Charles Darwin was responsible for integrating deduction and induction in his research on evolution in the nineteenth century. This integrated process became known as the scientific method.

Induction
Thinking method that proceeds from the specific to the general; basic principle of scientific inquiry in which information gained through observations of a small number of cases lead to generalized conclusions.

Perfect induction
Conclusion derived through inductive reasoning based on the observations of all members of a population.

Imperfect induction
Conclusion derived through inductive reasoning based on the observations of a small number of members of a population.

THE SCIENTIFIC METHOD

Scientific method
A way of solving problems and acquiring knowledge that involves both deductive and inductive reasoning in a systematic approach to obtaining data.

The **scientific method** of solving problems and acquiring knowledge has been delineated in many different ways in the past. It is an approach, however, that is usually thought of as being accomplished in a series of logical stages that define a pathway for the acquisition of knowledge. Although the number of stages may vary, authorities are in general agreement as to the overall process and the type and progression of activities undertaken. This is not to suggest, however, that the scientific method is governed by a strict adherence to a set of prescribed actions that must be followed faithfully during each stage in the process. Whereas the specific actions or steps undertaken within each stage may vary depending upon the research approach taken, participants, and techniques used, the general method for acquiring knowledge remains much the same and the logical progression from one stage to another reflects the systematic nature of the scientific method. Figure 1.1 shows the various stages of the scientific method and illustrates the cyclic nature of the process. A brief summary of the stages involved in the scientific method follows. In subsequent chapters, a more thorough discussion of each stage is presented.

1. **Identifying the Question**
    The first, and arguably the most important, stage in the scientific method is the identification of the **research question.** This is really an acknowledgment that a question needs to be answered and that at this time there is an insufficient knowledge base to answer the question. The research question may arise from several sources. It may have a theoretical underpinning, it may derive from professional practice or personal experience, or it may simply be based on the curiosity of the researcher. While the choice of a suitable question may be difficult, particularly for the beginning researcher,

Research question
The central focus of the research effort that serves as the basis for the research problem and provides direction for the entire process.

FIGURE 1.1
Conceptualization of the research cycle.

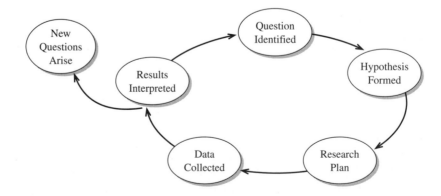

once identified and properly delineated, the research question becomes the central focus of the research effort. Consequently, considerable thought and serious reflection should go into the identification of the research question. One should also recognize that the research question is inevitably broad in nature and must be narrowed or distilled into a potentially researchable problem. This will lead to the specification of the problem statement that should provide direction for the research process.

2. **Formulating a Hypothesis**

   A **hypothesis** is a belief, hunch, or prediction of the eventual outcome of the research. It is a concrete, specific statement about the relationships between phenomena and is based upon deductive reasoning, following a thorough review of previous research related to the problem and considering the researcher's own past experience. Suppose a researcher wanted to study the effects of two different diets on selected physiological indices. Evidence from previous research suggests that a vegetarian diet provides a stronger and healthier person than does a nonvegetarian diet. If this theory holds true, what observable consequences could be expected? The deduced hypotheses, presented in a series of separate statements, would predict that the individuals on the vegetarian diet would show (a) lower cholesterol levels, (b) lower blood pressure, (c) greater energy, (d) a higher strength index, (e) less body fat, and so on, depending on the number of physiological indices observed. Not all studies have hypotheses, however. If a study is exploratory or simply descriptive in nature and not making comparisons between groups, no formal hypothesis is required. In such instances the researcher would carefully delineate the research questions that serve to provide focus for the study. In addition, qualitative research is not guided by hypotheses; rather the outcome of a qualitative study is often the specification of a hypothesis that may, in turn, guide subsequent research efforts.

   Hypothesis
   A tentative explanation or prediction of the eventual outcome of a research problem.

3. **Developing the Research Plan**

   In this stage, the strategy is developed for gathering and analyzing the information that is required to test the hypotheses or answer the research questions. Essentially, this becomes the "blueprint" or a "step-by-step plan" for conducting the research. The researcher will design a plan to test, measure, weigh, experiment, or observe the phenomena of interest in order to be able to answer the research questions. Typically, this plan consists of four parts: selection of a relevant research methodology, identification of the subjects or participants, description of the data-gathering procedures, and specification of the data analysis techniques. The choice of the research method is largely influenced by the questions being investigated. Certain types of questions require strategies that use quantitative methods, while others lend themselves to qualitative methods. Moreover, the research method selected then influences the specific details of the study, such as the participants, the instrumentation, and the actual procedures undertaken. In the diet study example, the researcher might select two groups of people and place one group on a vegetarian diet and the other on a nonvegetarian diet. The plan calls for each group to be tested on the selected physiological indices, then proceed with their respective diets for a preset period of time, and then be tested again on the same indices at the end of the experimental period. Lastly, the plan describes how the collected data will be analyzed in order to confirm or refute the stated hypotheses.

4. **Collecting and Analyzing the Data**

At this point, the research plan is actually implemented and the data collected. Assuming that the research plan was carefully developed, this stage of the scientific method requires the investigator to systematically follow the prescribed procedures. This may include the management of an experimental treatment, or it may consist of actually testing or observing the participants, conducting an interview, or administering a questionnaire. Although it is critical to focus attention on the operational details of gathering the data, arguably the most important aspect of data collection is the preplanning—the development of a sound research plan. Once the data are collected, appropriate techniques are used to analyze the data. In quantitative studies, numerical data are typically analyzed statistically, first to simply describe the data and then, if appropriate, to determine if the evidence supports the hypotheses being tested. Inasmuch as qualitative studies generally result in non-numerical data, such as interview records or detailed descriptions of events, data analysis becomes inductive in nature, relying on coding and categorization processes.

5. **Interpreting Results and Forming Conclusions**

While data analysis is an important step in the overall process, it is not an end in itself. At this point the researcher attempts to interpret the results of the data analysis and formulate meaningful conclusions. Does the evidence support or refute the hypotheses? Depending upon the nature of the research study and keeping in mind that not all studies have hypotheses, a decision to accept or reject each hypothesis is made. And most importantly, what does this mean? Conclusions should not be simply restatements of the results or findings of the study. Rather, conclusions attempt to provide an explanation of the results. It is important to recognize that the conclusions relate back to the question that prompted the study in the first place, yet inferences are typically made to situations beyond the specific study. Ultimately, researchers will report the details of their study to interested persons, describing the underlying basis for the study, the participants and procedures used, and the results and conclusions. In so doing, a researcher is thereby submitting his or her work for open and public review, a feature that distinguishes scientific inquiry from the other sources of knowledge.

The stages described above provide the framework of the scientific method. The research process, then, is the application of the scientific method to solve a problem or answer a question. It is important to note that the research process is cyclic in nature, whereby the first stage in the process begins with the identification of a problem or question. The process then proceeds through a number of other stages, ending with the researcher affirming or rejecting the research hypothesis and drawing conclusions that enable the question to be answered. In effect, the process begins and ends with a focus on the question of interest. Inevitably, however, the results of a single research study will give rise to other questions that warrant further investigation as the whole process starts anew and the body of knowledge continues to grow. Drew, Hardman, and Hosp (2008) refer to this model as the closed-loop conceptualization of the research process.

The essence of the scientific method is the structure, objectivity, and marked control it can provide the researcher. The structure and rigor imposed by the scientific method has served the natural sciences very well as investigations focus on physical and biological phenomena. But in the social sciences, including education, health, and much of kinesiology, the strict application of the scientific method has proven to be more challenging. The use of human research participants diminishes our ability to administer some treatment conditions as well to control all factors that could affect an experiment.

For example, the use of performance-enhancing drugs in sports has received considerable attention in recent years. To truly determine the effect of these drugs, a sample of athletes should be drawn from the population of interest, these individuals should be given drugs over a period of time, and then the effects on various body organs should be observed. Yet medical research and individual case studies suggest that performance-enhancing drugs may be harmful to the body. There are considerable moral, ethical, and legal reasons that would preclude studies designed in the manner described. Research participants have a right to expect researchers to prevent or minimize harm from coming to them and to pay attention to their safety and human dignity. Researchers cannot hope to know all the potential risks and hazards to the participants, but must inform them of all those that *are* known. There is much current evidence that indicates that performance-enhancing drugs are harmful. A study requiring research participants to use performance enhancing drugs in order to see what happens to body organs five to ten years after they are ingested is highly questionable on ethical grounds.

Also, many research studies in kinesiology involve attitudes and personal opinions. While it is possible to determine the prevalence of one opinion or another, to fully explain the basis for such opinions is problematic because they are so subjective in nature and are influenced by many factors. A major limitation associated with research involving human subjects is the inability of the researcher to exercise the degree of control often needed. Not only are there moral and ethical issues that should be considered, but practicality also becomes a major factor when dealing with human behavior. Yet the scientific method as previously described has provided the basic framework for research in the social and behavioral sciences and has led to the accumulation of a vast amount of knowledge. Despite the use of the scientific method, the social sciences have generally not attained the scientific stature of the natural sciences (Ary, Jacobs, and Sorensen 2010).

Since the social scientist is typically dealing with human research participants and their behaviors, problems of control, accuracy of measurement, and complexity of function are considerably greater than would be expected in the natural sciences. Control over the research situation will be more difficult in studies done in gymnasia, swimming pools, camps, and playing fields. The major concern is that, whatever the problem, researchers try to adhere to the scientific method as much as possible.

SCIENCE, RESEARCH, AND THEORY

Theory
A belief or assumption about the causal relationship between variables that serves to explain phenomena.

The ultimate goal of science is the formation of theory based upon the synthesis and interpretation of facts and information. Through scientific research efforts, facts are discovered. As these facts grow, there is a need to organize and synthesize this information in order to make meaningful interpretations. Theories are formulated to bring order to the facts and to provide meaningful generalizations about the phenomenon being studied. The word "theory" is often misunderstood. A **theory** is simply a belief or assumption about how things relate to each other. According to Best and Kahn (2005), "a theory establishes a cause-and-effect relationship between variables with the purpose of explaining and predicting phenomena."

Not only does theory summarize and organize existing knowledge, it also enables scientists to predict and, ultimately, control phenomena. Theories abound concerning the relationship between human behavior and the environment. Moreover, as these relationships are delineated and explained, predictions are offered as to what will happen if certain human behaviors are either changed or not changed, depending upon the circumstances. For instance, a growing body of scientific evidence clearly establishes the relationship between physical activity and one's health. The Surgeon General's Report on Physical Activity and Health concludes that people of all ages, both male and female, benefit from regular physical activity. The human body responds to physical activity in ways that have important positive effects on the musculoskeletal, cardiovascular, respiratory, and endocrine systems. These changes are consistent with a number of health benefits, including a reduced risk of premature death and reduced risks of coronary heart disease, hypertension, colon cancer, and diabetes mellitus (U. S. Department of Health and Human Services 1996). Based on this evidence and our increasing ability to predict the consequences of specific health behaviors, various national organizations such as the American Heart Association (AHA) and the American College of Sports Medicine (ACSM), to name a few, have issued physical activity recommendations to the public.

Various theories have been advanced by researchers in different fields that purport to explain various aspects of human behavior. Many of these theories have important applications in kinesiology and related areas. For example, the Social Cognitive Theory (Bandura 1986) is often cited as the basis for adopting various health behaviors. In this theory, it is proposed that behavior change is influenced by factors in three domains: environmental, biological, and psychosocial. Consequently, intervention programs designed to change one's health-related behaviors— such as commencing an exercise program or stopping smoking—would focus on elements in one or more of these domains.

The Transtheoretical Model is another theory that is often cited by researchers to explain the various stages that one goes through when adopting a certain behavior. Originally utilized in areas of smoking, weight control, and psychotherapy, it has recently been applied to other health behaviors, including exercise (Prochaska and DiClemente 1983; Marcus and Simkin 1994). Comprehensive in nature, this theory proposes that individuals move through five stages of readiness in health behavior change: precontemplation, contemplation, preparation, action, and maintenance. Moreover, movement through the various stages is not necessarily linear, as individuals may move back and forth through the stages. Understanding an individual's readiness for change may assist health professionals in designing programs to meet the specific needs and motivation level of the individual.

Theory is also a vehicle for obtaining new knowledge by providing hypotheses for additional research in a particular area. Frequently, scientists investigate theory under a different set of circumstances to determine if valid generalizations are possible. In effect, the theory is being tested. Theory, then, provides a framework for explaining phenomena and may serve as the basis for further research as well as practical application. For example, as obesity rates continue to rise throughout the world, considerable attention has been directed toward developing a better understanding of contributing factors, namely dietary and physical activity behaviors. Interest in physical activity among children has resulted in numerous research studies in recent years that have sought to identify and explain the various factors influencing a child's physical activity behavior. In an attempt to synthesize the research on determinants and activity promotion in youth, Welk (1999) proposed the Youth Physical Activity Promotion Model. This model presents a theoretical framework which connects the known determinants and influences on youth physical activity. The resultant social-ecological model now is used to guide new research in the area.

As previously mentioned, the strict application of the scientific method to research investigations in the social and behavioral sciences has proved challenging. Moreover, research efforts in physical education, exercise science, athletic training and other areas in kinesiology, have not always emphasized theory. Consequently, theory development has occurred less than in the physical sciences. The continued development of kinesiology as a field of study is dependent upon greater attention being given to theory development and the explanation of observed facts and relationships. In the quest for theory development, the veracity of the knowledge is paramount. As a result, it is generally agreed that the scientific method represents the best means of acquiring knowledge.

TYPES OF RESEARCH

While the underlying framework of research is founded upon the scientific method, there are various types of research that have differing purposes and approaches to the process. Virtually every research methods textbook provides some system for classifying research. It is also noted that the various research categories are not mutually exclusive, meaning that a given research study could be identified in several different classification systems. For instance, a study to determine the physiological characteristics of elite distance swimmers could be classified as applied research, quantitative research, or descriptive research, among others. Virtually every research study could be identified in multiple categories. The ability to classify research is not important in itself, but has value in making the research processes more understandable, particularly for the beginning researcher. Moreover, by developing knowledge of the various types of research, you will acquire an understanding and appreciation of the goals, methodologies, and activities that guide the research efforts. It is important to understand, however, that how a given research problem is attacked depends largely on the nature of the problem being investigated and the question being asked.

Basic and Applied Research

Basic research
Research whose primary aim is the discovery of new knowledge through theory development or evaluation.

Generally, **basic research,** which is sometimes referred to as pure or fundamental research, is theoretical in nature: its primary purpose is the discovery of new knowledge and the development of theory. It is largely motivated by intellectual curiosity and interest in a specific problem area. Fundamental knowledge about such phenomena as the environment, space, human behavior, exercise, and the human gene makeup is sought. Broad generalizations and principles, such as the overload and cross-transference principles and laws of learning, frequently result from basic research. The results of this type of research may have no immediate practical application or utility since such an approach often leads to knowledge for knowledge's sake. It may take years before the results from basic research find some practical utility. The majority of this research is done in highly controlled experimental settings, often using animal subjects, in which selected variables are formally manipulated by the researcher in order to test causal relationships. Some examples of what might be considered basic research studies include the following:

1. Research on operant conditioning undertaken by psychologist B. F. Skinner in which he observed the effects of reinforcement on behaviors of rats.
2. A study to identify the specific genetic code of the fruit fly.
3. A neurologist who studies the brain to learn about its general workings.

Applied research, on the other hand, has as its central purpose the solution of an immediate practical problem, yet seeks to make inferences beyond the group or situation studied. Much applied research is guided by and builds on theories and findings of basic research. Most research in kinesiology is applied research in which professionals in the field are confronted with real-world problems and are interested in solving them. A conditioning coach may be interested in determining the effectiveness of a new weight-lifting technique or a youth sports coach may seek to compare different motivational strategies for boys and girls. A new theory of motor skill acquisition may be tested by the physical education teacher. The idea is to improve products and processes and to test theoretical concepts. We are interested in improving our professional practices and services. The results of this type of research are intended to be generalized and to extend to the target population and setting. An adapted physical education researcher who finds that a particular motor activity is successful in improving the social skills of a sample of individuals with mental retardation is likely to want to apply those results to all similar individuals with mental retardation. Some examples of what might be considered applied research studies include the following:

Applied research
Research whose primary aim is toward the solution of practical problems, yet seeks to make inferences beyond the study setting.

1. A study to determine the relationship between children's physical activity behaviors and that of their parents.
2. A study comparing two models of heart rate monitors on their accuracy measuring heart rate response to exercise among children.
3. A study to investigate the attitudes of pre-service physical education candidates toward working with diverse populations.

Although sometimes presented as a distinct type of research, **action research,** in our view, represents a special form of applied research in which the interest is in local, not universal, applicability. This research is typically very pragmatic in nature, albeit objective, but the problem exists in a local setting. For instance, in an effort to increase the distance of goal kicks, a soccer coach may experiment with having the goalee utilize a new kicking technique. Although the approach is scientific in nature, the coach is interested only in this local situation. Methods, techniques, and practices are tried out which may promise better results and provide the basis for improved decisions. Behavioral modification, intervention, and in-service training skills are frequently employed in action research studies. To be

Action research
A distinct type of applied, practical research often seen in education in which the focus is on local needs, problems, or issues.

successful, the researcher must adhere to sound research procedures. The approach should be as scientific as possible given the less-controlled, local setting in which it takes place. Action research is discussed in more detail in Chapter 12.

Quantitative and Qualitative Research

Another way of classifying research is based largely upon the philosophical assumptions the researcher brings to the study and the approach taken to collect and analyze the data. At the practical level, quantitative research tends to focus on specific behaviors that can be measured and quantified (expressed as numbers), and lends itself to testing theories; qualitative research tends to focus on describing the meaning of behaviors occurring in natural settings by gathering in-depth information (usually expressed in words) on a relatively small number of individuals. It may be useful to think of these approaches to research as existing along a continuum. At one end of the continuum is quantitative research and at the opposite end is qualitative research. The terms quantitative and qualitative are conveniently used to differentiate one research approach from the other, but the terms themselves are generic in nature and refer to a family of research methods that fall under these broad categories. In fact, specific family members of each research approach fall at various points along the quantitative-qualitative continuum, suggesting that some methods more fully embrace the principles of quantitative or qualitative research than others.

Quantitative research
Research involving the collection of numerical data in order to describe phenomena, investigate relationships between variables, and explore cause-and-effect relationships of phenomena of interest.

Quantitative research uses an approach that is designed for the collection and analysis of numerical data that are usually obtained through direct testing, questionnaires, or a multitude of paper-and-pencil instruments. This approach to research, which is also referred to as the traditional or positivist approach, has been and continues to be the predominant method used in kinesiology. Quantitative approaches are commonly used to describe existing conditions or phenomena, investigate relationships between two or more variables, and explore cause-and-effect relationships between phenomena. The general procedures for carrying out the research activities, analyzing the resultant data, and deriving the conclusions have been widely accepted. Although the nature of the data collected serves as an easy and useful means of regarding quantitative research, a quantitative approach involves more than simply the use of numerical data. First of all, a quantitative approach is based on a paradigm adopted from the natural sciences that subscribes to the assumption that reality is relatively stable, uniform, measurable, and governed by rational laws that enable generalizations to be made. Moreover, a quantitative approach follows a linear research path and involves (1) clearly stated questions, (2) rationally conceived hypotheses, (3) fully developed research procedures, (4) controlling extraneous factors that might interfere with the data collected, (5) using relatively large samples of participants in order to provide meaningful data, and (6) employing data analysis techniques based upon statistical procedures (Drew, Hardman, and Hosp 2008).

Although long used in anthropology and sociology, and more recently educational research, **qualitative research** methodologies are relatively new to kinesiology, gaining popularity only during the past 20 to 25 years. Most authorities would agree that qualitative research generally includes research methods that rely heavily upon extensive observations and in-depth interviews that result in nonnumerical data. Furthermore, qualitative research is often conducted in natural settings and does not attempt to control the context or conditions surrounding the research setting, thus prompting the use of the term "naturalistic research" to describe this approach. Founded upon beliefs and assumptions different from those of quantitative research, qualitative research does not subscribe to the viewpoint that the world is stable and uniform and can be explained by laws that govern phenomena. Rather, qualitative research takes on a constructionist perspective, suggesting that meaning and reality is situational specific, thus allowing for many different meanings, none of which is necessarily more valid than another. Thus, there may not be an attempt to generalize the results of qualitative research since the context of the study is situational specific. In qualitative research, the researcher tends to not state hypotheses before the collection of data. Moreover, qualitative research tends to follow a nonlinear research path as the research procedures are not fully articulated prior to conducting the study since the methods tend to evolve as the research proceeds. Analysis and interpretation of data collected using a qualitative research approach is mainly interpretative and descriptive in nature, resulting in a categorization of the information gathered to identify trends and patterns. Statistical procedures are rarely used. Further discussion of qualitative research methods is presented in chapter 10.

An overview of the distinguishing characteristics of quantitative and qualitative approaches to research is shown in Table 1.1. Although some researchers perceive qualitative and quantitative approaches as oppositional and incompatible, a more prudent view is to consider them as complementary methods in the pursuit of truth and knowledge. Each has its advantages and disadvantages, and taken together, they allow us to know and understand different things about the world in which we live. In fact, we are seeing both approaches being utilized in the same studies. For instance, a study to investigate the nature of authentic assessment techniques in school physical education first administered a questionnaire to a randomly selected group of teachers (quantitative) and then followed up with a small number of detailed interviews and classroom observations (qualitative) in order to obtain a deeper understanding (Mintah 2000). Authorities have used the term mixed methods research to describe a research approach that combines both quantitative and qualitative methods of data collection and analysis (Creswell 2009). However, according to Locke, Silverman, and Spirduso (2010), a true mixed methods approach involves more than merely mixing data collection methods from the two research strategies; it involves merging the underlying philosophical perspectives as well. The nature of the question or the problem to be investigated will usually determine the preferred research approach, whether it is

Qualitative research
Research based upon nonnumerical data obtained in natural settings through extensive observations and interviews whose primary aim is the interpretation of phenomena and the discovery of meaning.

TABLE 1.1 Characteristics of Quantitative and Qualitative Research

QUANTITATIVE RESEARCH	QUALITATIVE RESEARCH
Positivist philosophy	Constructivist philosophy
Objective social reality	Social reality is constructed by the participants in it
Social reality is relatively constant across time and settings	Social reality is continuously constructed in local situations
Objective relationship with research participants	Collaborates with research participants
Predetermined methods	Emerging methods
Study samples that represent populations	Study cases
Study behavior and other observable phenomena	Study the meanings that individuals create
Study behaviors in natural or contrived settings	Study behaviors in natural settings
Use theories to guide research	Theory generation
Numerical data	Verbal and pictorial data
Statistical methods to analyze data	Analytic induction to analyze data
Seeks generalizability from sample to defined population	Little generalizability from cases to other cases or settings

Source: Adapted from Gall, Gall, and Borg (2003).

quantitative, qualitative, or both. (See Table 1.1 for descriptions of qualitative and quantitative research.)

Experimental Research and Nonexperimental Research

A major distinction is generally made between experimental and nonexperimental research. While the general purpose of research is to increase our understanding and the body of knowledge within a given field, there are substantial differences in the approach one may take in pursuit of this end. While the previous introduction to quantitative and qualitative research methodologies characterizes the nature of research activities using each respective approach, understanding the distinction between experimental and nonexperimental research adds yet another perspective to fully understanding the research process and the wealth of methodologies available.

The following sections briefly discuss experimental research and the most prevalent forms of nonexperimental research in kinesiology.

Experimental Research.   In **experimental research,** the researcher explores the cause-and-effect relationship between variables by manipulating certain variables (referred to as independent variables) to determine their effect on another variable (referred to as the dependent variable). Furthermore, the researcher attempts to control all other factors that could possibly influence the dependent variable. Consider, for example, a situation in which a researcher is interested in investigating two different methods of training (free-weights and weight machines) on strength development. In this case, the method of training represents the independent variable and is being manipulated by the researcher. Ideally, the researcher would be able to randomly assign research participants to either a treatment group that utilizes free-weights or a treatment group that utilizes weight machines, have the participants train for a specified length of time, and then determine if there were differences between the two groups in terms of strength development. One could also add a control group to the study that did not perform any training. In such a study the researcher would attempt to ensure that both groups trained for the same length of time, for the same duration, and at the same intensity. Moreover, the researcher would attempt to control other factors that could reasonably affect the outcome, factors like diet, physical activity, and even motivation, to name a few. The researcher would compare the two groups based on the research participants' strength scores (dependent variable) at the end of the training period. Assuming that there were no differences in strength when the study commenced, if the final strength scores were significantly higher for the group using free-weights, the researcher would be able to conclude with some confidence that training with free-weights was more effective than training using weight machines.

Experimental research is designed to answer the question "What if . . .?" by systematically manipulating one or more variables and observing the consequences on another variable. The researcher is interested in the future. Experimental research methods are quantitative in nature, typically begin with clearly stated hypotheses to fit the research questions, and are commonly associated with a laboratory setting. It is the most formally structured of all the various types of research. According to Ary, Jacobs, and Sorensen (2010), in its simplest form, experimental research has three characteristics: (1) an independent variable that is manipulated by the researcher, (2) control of other relevant variables, and (3) observation of the effect of the manipulation of the independent variable on the dependent variable. A more thorough discussion of experimental research is presented in Chapter 8.

Causal-Comparative Research.   **Causal-comparative research** is similar to experimental research in that it seeks to investigate possible cause-and-effect relationships. However, in causal-comparative research the independent variable is not

Experimental research
Type of research in which an independent variable is manipulated to observe the effect on a dependent variable for the purpose of determining a cause-and-effect relationship.

Causal-comparative research
Research that seeks to investigate cause-and-effect relationships that explain differences that already exist in groups or individuals; also called *ex post facto research*.

manipulated by the researcher, either because it cannot be manipulated or because it would be unethical to do so. With causal-comparative research, the independent variable is often referred to as an attribute or organismic variable because frequently it is some attribute or characteristic that the research participant already possesses due to the natural course of actions (e.g., gender, ethnicity, medical condition, family background, employment status). As a result, the participants are already members of a particular class or group of individuals that possess the same attribute. The researcher then compares groups that differ on the attribute (independent variable) to determine if there are differences on some dependent variable of interest. Since the researcher has no control over the independent variable, which is either innate or has already occurred, this type of research is also called *ex post facto* (after the fact) research.

A good example of causal-comparative research is represented by many studies that have investigated the effect of smoking (independent variable) on lung cancer (dependent variable). Because of the potential harm to subjects, it would be unethical to assign some subjects to a group and force them to become heavy smokers and other subjects to a group that is forbidden to smoke; researchers would instead compare the incidence of lung cancer in a group of nonsmokers to a group of longtime smokers. Clearly, the researcher did not have control over the independent variable in this example, or in causal-comparative research in general. The group membership, either smoker or nonsmoker, was determined before the study commenced; the researcher merely selected research participants from each of the preexisting groups and compared them on the dependent variable—in this case, lung cancer. Because of the lack of control, especially the capability to manipulate the independent variable, the ability of the researcher to draw cause-and-effect conclusions is limited compared to experimental research. This has been one of the arguments used by the tobacco industry in refuting the findings of most research pointing to a linkage between smoking and lung cancer, although a preponderance of the evidence today clearly shows such an association. Another example of causal-comparative research is Eisenmann and colleagues' (2010) study investigating whether prepregnancy obesity of the mother affects the physical activity and blood pressure of young children. The participants included 144 mother-child pairs in which prepregnancy BMI was used to divide the mothers into normal weight and overweight groups. Measures of physical activity, blood pressure, and body fatness were obtained on the children. Since the researchers were not able to manipulate the independent variable (prepregnancy weight of the mother), this study represents causal-comparative research. Consequently, conclusions regarding the causal relationship between maternal prepregnancy obesity and the various child measures were limited. Causal-comparative research generally functions to identify group differences and discover relationships among variables, but stops short of establishing causality. Although there are limitations associated with causal-comparative research, it nevertheless is frequently used in kinesiological research.

Descriptive Research.   **Descriptive research,** as the name suggests, attempts to gather information from groups of research participants in order to describe systematically, factually, and accurately specific characteristics of interest or conditions that presently exist. Quite simply, a descriptive study first determines and then describes the way things are. Nonexperimental in nature, a descriptive study is concerned with the present and describes *what is.* It typically precedes experimental research. There is no manipulation of an independent variable in descriptive research since there is no intent to explore a cause-and-effect relationship. Descriptive research utilizes a wide variety of methodologies to collect data—surveys, interviews, direct measurement, and observational techniques being the most prevalent. Frequently, descriptive research is interested in comparing relevant subgroups (for example, groups based on gender, age, grade level, socioeconomic status, or ethnicity) with the results being reported according to each subgroup as well as for the total sample. An example of such a comparative study is a recent investigation by Columna, Foley, and Lytle (2010) in which survey methodology was used to investigate physical education teachers' attitudes toward cultural pluralism. They compared the attitudes of male and female physical education teachers, adapted physical education specialists, and teacher education candidates toward cultural pluralism and diversity. Although descriptive research is similar to qualitative research in some regards, there are important distinctions: (1) methodology for descriptive research is more structured and standardized; (2) variables of interest are predetermined in descriptive research; (3) descriptive research inevitably uses more research participants, often selected through randomization procedures; (4) data are analyzed predominately through the use of statistical procedures in descriptive research; and (5) there is typically less in-depth researcher interaction with the participants in descriptive research.

Descriptive studies have been commonplace in kinesiology as well as in education and the social and behavioral sciences. Best and Kahn (2005) indicate that descriptive research is the predominant research method used in the behavioral sciences. Furthermore, many doctoral dissertations and master's theses involve descriptive research. Descriptive research methodology is particularly suited to studies that seek to identify the attitudes or opinions of various groups of individuals or to those that purport to detail behaviors that may naturally occur in the classroom, gymnasium, workplace, playing field, or home, for example. Since descriptive research commonly seeks to generalize the information collected from a sample (e.g., opinions, attitudes, abilities, behaviors) to a target population, researchers often employ randomization procedures in an attempt to obtain a sample that is representative of the population of interest.

Some of the best examples of descriptive research are represented by public opinion surveys in which the respondents are asked their opinion or attitude on a multitude of topics ranging from presidential preference, to physical activity and exercise, to abortion. The Centers for Disease Control and Prevention (CDC) regularly conduct a number of national probability studies aimed at describing health

Descriptive research
Research that attempts to systematically describe specific characteristics or conditions related to a subject group.

behaviors of Americans (e.g., Youth Risk Behavior Survey [YRBS], National Health Interview Survey [NHIS], and Behavioral Risk Factor Surveillance System [BRFSS]). In addition, a study to identify the physiological characteristics of elite women distance runners or a study to ascertain the physical activity behaviors of adolescent males and females are additional examples of descriptive research in kinesiology.

Correlational research
Type of research that seeks to investigate the extent of the relationship between two or more variables.

Correlational Research.   Nonexperimental in nature, **correlational research** is closely related to both descriptive and causal-comparative research. It is similar to descriptive research in that it describes currently existing phenomena; it is similar to causal-comparative research in that it explores relationships between or among variables. According to Gay, Mills, and Airasian (2008), the purpose of correlational research is to either determine whether, and to what extent, a relationship exists between two or more variables or to use these relationships to make predictions. That is, it may be either relational or predictive in nature. If a relationship exists, the degree of relationship is usually expressed as some type of correlation coefficient. A good example of a relationship study in kinesiology would be an investigation to determine how self-esteem corresponds (relates) to physical fitness among adolescent females. Measures of self-esteem and physical fitness would be collected on a representative group of adolescent girls and the association between the variables measured as a correlation coefficient.

  Contrasted to experimental research, there is no manipulation of variables in correlational research, therefore it is important to recognize that correlational studies never establish cause-and-effect relationships between variables, even in the presence of a high correlation. Therefore, even if we found a high correlation between self-esteem and physical fitness in the example above, this does not mean that self-esteem causes physical fitness or that physical fitness causes self-esteem. It simply means that adolescent girls who have high levels of self-esteem tend to have high levels of physical fitness and those who have lower self-esteem tend to have lower levels of physical fitness. Although similar to causal-comparative studies in the fact that causal relationships cannot be definitively established, correlational research methodology differs in that usually there is only a single group of subjects from which data on two or more variables are collected for each participant, while causal-comparative research methodology takes into consideration scores from two distinct groups of subjects (e.g., smokers and nonsmokers). It is noted, however, that the existence of a high correlation does permit more accurate predictions based on the relationship. For example, correlational research has established that there is a relationship between one's grades in high school and college grade-point average (GPA). As a result, we can now establish a prediction model (equation) whereby we can predict, with a certain degree of accuracy, a student's college GPA on the basis of the student's high school GPA. In fact, other variables, such as performance on the Scholastic Aptitude Test (SAT), could be added to the prediction model to improve the accuracy. As this example illustrates, often the results of prediction studies are used to facilitate decision-making or selection processes, as in the case of admission to college.

Historical Research. Authorities differ as to whether the activities undertaken in historical inquiry can be considered scientific or not (Best and Kahn 2005). Moreover, it is not easy to classify historical research into a particular category, although it seems obvious that it is nonexperimental. Most historical research can be regarded as qualitative and descriptive in nature, yet relationships can be explored and hypotheses tested in certain types of well-designed and well-executed historical studies. In the historical approach, the researcher endeavors to record and understand events of the past in order to provide a better understanding of the present and suggest possible directions for the future. For instance, a researcher might be interested in investigating the "evolution of football in Texas public schools." Such a study would likely be based upon official records and reports of state education agencies, school officials, and local school boards, as well as newspaper and magazine articles, school yearbooks, and interviews with selected individuals who had some involvement with Texas school football programs in past years.

The historical approach is oriented toward the past as the researcher seeks to provide a new perspective on a question of current interest by conducting an intensive study of material that already exists. Yet historical research differs from other forms of research because its subject matter, the past, is difficult to capture and the researcher cannot generate new data, but can only synthesize and interpret data that already exist. Moreover, locating all the relevant data and information concerning a particular question from many, widely scattered sources is typically a difficult and tedious process. Sources of data, or the evidence, for historical research can generally be classified into two main categories, primary sources and secondary sources. Primary sources of data consist of original materials prepared by individuals who were participants or a direct eyewitness of an event under investigation. On the other hand, secondary sources of data are one step removed from the historical happenings of interest and consist of materials based upon secondhand accounts of events, accounts that are prepared by individuals who were not present or witness to the events. In Chapter 12 we provide a more extensive description of historical research methods.

THE SIGNIFICANCE OF RESEARCH IN KINESIOLOGY

The body of knowledge in the various kinesiology fields is currently expanding at a rapid rate. Tremendous progress has been made because scholars in these fields have focused on all aspects of the human being—the physical, mental, and emotional.

The whole person is studied in relation to movement, attitude, and lifestyle. The research has been both theoretical and practical and has reflected a sharp increase in quality, range, and depth.

Research in the kinesiology field, or what some would refer to as physical education or perhaps sport and exercise science, has a relatively short lifespan compared to other disciplines. Most authorities agree that systematic research in physical education in the United States originated in the mid-1800s. Although the Association for the Advancement of Physical Education (the predecessor of the American Alliance for Health, Physical Education, Recreation, and Dance) was established in 1885 to serve as the professional organization for the fledging field, the disciplinary knowledge base was just being shaped. In the 75th anniversary issue of the *Research Quarterly for Exercise and Sport,* Roberta Park (2005) traces the historical development of research and building the body of knowledge we know today as kinesiology. This is an interesting read as Park describes the difficulty early scholars and professional leaders had in reconciling the diverse interests often expressed under the "physical education" name. It was not until the publication of the *Research Quarterly* (now the *Research Quarterly for Exercise and Sport*) in 1930 that a professional journal devoted exclusively to reporting scholarly research in physical education existed.

As the *Research Quarterly* matured as a professional journal for reporting research findings, subdisciplines of physical education (e.g., sport psychology, sport sociology, biomechanics, exercise physiology, pedagogy, sport history, motor behavior) began to emerge and create their own knowledge base. Park described the 1960s as a time of rapid growth in scientific and scholarly endeavors, leading to the creation of several specialized journals associated with the various subdisciplines (e.g., *Medicine and Science in Sport,* 1969; *Journal of Motor Behavior,* 1969; *Journal of Sport History,* 1974; *Journal of Sport Psychology,* 1979). In 1986, leading scientists representing several of the subdisciplines gathered at Arizona State University for a symposium on Future Directions in Exercise/Sport Research. An edited monograph of the symposium proceedings provides a historical perspective of exercise and sport science research and provides recommendations for future research needs in the various subdisciplines (Skinner, Corbin, Landers, Martin, and Wells 1989). Similarly, a conference held in Pittsburgh, Pennsylvania, in 2007 brought together researchers to reflect on research about teaching and teacher education in physical education. The resulting conference proceedings, *Historic Traditions and Future Directions of Research on Teaching and Teacher Education in Physical Education* (Housner, Metzler, Schempp, and Templin 2009), provide a valuable resource for students and young professionals in physical education pedagogy, curriculum, and teacher preparation.

Much has been written about the advantages and disadvantages of the various types of research and the ways to interpret their results. Although quantitative methods have historically been the preferred approach by most researchers in kinesiology, the use of qualitative research methodologies has become much more commonplace. The body of knowledge in kinesiology continues to expand at a rapid rate. This is partly due to the fact that the scope of research activities within the kinesiology discipline is very broad, including biomedical research, social and behavioral research, educational research, as well as marketing research. Researchers are becoming more adept at using better research designs, improved instrumentation, and sophisticated analysis techniques. The tremendous progress in the volume of research has led to the creation of a number of new professional journals in recent years, including the *Journal of Physical Activity and Health, Pediatric Exercise Science, Journal of Clinical Sport Psychology,* and *Measurement in Physical Education and Exercise Science,* among others, all created within the last 20 years. This does not even consider the new e-journals, such as the *International Journal of Exercise Science, Athletic Insight: The Online Journal of Sport Psychology,* and the *International Journal of Behavioral Nutrition and Physical Activity,* which are popping up all the time.

The demand for research to provide answers to many of the questions and problems facing society continues to grow. More and more we hear the call, *show me the evidence*! Leaders and professionals in many fields often demand empirical evidence to help guide decision making and professional practice. It is not uncommon to hear of evidence-based medicine, evidence-based education, evidence-based therapy, and so forth. The kinesiology practitioner has become more active in research in recent years, while the focus of the professional researcher appears to have become more fixed on research having utilitarian value. The so-called gap between the researcher and the practitioner appears to be narrowing. We are seeing more and more cooperative efforts between the researcher and practitioner, a trend that promises to help solve practical kinds of problems as well as to validate theoretical concepts.

In its simplest form, research is just another way of looking at the problems which permeate the fields of kinesiology. Research is for everyone, and everyone can and should engage in that process. Deep knowledge of statistics and research design is not necessary to carry out creditable research. All that is needed is someone who is interested and willing to undertake the activity and who has some background knowledge of the problem to be studied. Research should not be relegated to just a few "name" people in the profession, but rather it is the responsibility of many people. Larger numbers of people engaging in research are needed to guarantee that the problems, questions, and interests of all fields of kinesiology are represented in research investigations. Research can help broaden the knowledge and improve the practices that have long been associated with kinesiology. It is, and should continue to be, an active and continuing ingredient of the scholarly efforts of those fields. It is a tool that professionals cannot do without. It is the lifeblood of a profession and must be pursued vigorously.

Summary of Objectives

1. **Explain the relationship between research and a profession.** Research is the lifeblood of a profession because it produces information that adds to the profession's body of knowledge. In kinesiology professions, research is a growing field that has produced a variety of conceptual and methodological approaches for dealing with all aspects of human health.

2. **Describe the nature of research.** The research process is a formal, systematic, and logical attack on a problem using the scientific method as the mode of inquiry. An organized endeavor to obtain facts about some subject and ultimately answers to a specific question, research attempts to discover truth.

3. **Explain the scientific method.** The scientific method is a systematic approach to solving problems and acquiring knowledge that involves a series of stages: identification of the problem, formulation of a hypothesis, development of a research plan, collection and analysis of data, and interpretation of results.

4. **Understand the various types of research classifications and how they are applied.** Research that is theoretical in nature and intended for the fundamental purpose of discovering new knowledge is called basic research. In kinesiology, research is usually done for the purpose of addressing a specific problem or issue, and as such is considered applied research. The methodology should always follow the research question: which type of research appropriate for a given study depends upon the nature of the question being asked.

Understanding the Research Process

2

OBJECTIVES

Beginning researchers often have a misconception of what research entails. Through no fault of their own, they simply do not understand the nature of research and the concepts underlying the scientific method. A basic understanding of the types of research questions and the different types of variables associated with research is requisite to designing a research study. The emphasis of this chapter is on developing an understanding of the research process and the various steps involved.

After reading Chapter 2, you should be able to

1. Understand the various steps of the research process.
2. Recognize the different types of research questions.
3. Understand those factors that must be considered when selecting a research question.
4. Recognize the different types of variables.

Careful planning is a critical ingredient in being able to design a worthwhile study. As we have previously shown, the research process consists of several distinct stages. With a holistic view of the research process as a backdrop, it is now incumbent for the researcher to embark on a series of smaller steps that will lead toward the design and implementation of the research plan. First, and arguably the most important step, is the identification of the research question. Once the question has been identified and properly narrowed to a researchable problem, the researcher must select the best approach for investigating the problem and then proceed to develop a plan of attack accordingly.

STEPS IN THE RESEARCH PROCESS

The **research process** is founded upon the scientific method and operates in several stages: (1) identifying the question, (2) formulating hypotheses, (3) developing the research plan, (4) collecting and analyzing the data, and (5) forming

Research process
Procedure founded upon the scientific method for investigating research problems that involve systematic progression through a series of necessary steps.

conclusions. Each stage is undergirded by certain necessary steps, and from each step definite results can be expected. Many of these steps combine mental activity, such as reflective thinking, and the physical activities of searching, evaluating, interpreting, and writing. In reality, there is no universally applicable order in which these steps are incorporated in a given research project. The order and importance of these steps will vary according to the type of research being conducted, the purpose for doing the study, and the whims of the researcher. In many instances, various steps will be combined or accomplished concurrently. For example, the steps of identifying the research question and definition of the problem for a research investigation involve, simultaneously, a literature search, an estimation of the success potential of the study, and consideration of the way in which the research will be approached. The authors of this text believe that the following steps apply to most types of research in kinesiology. The content embodied in these steps is discussed in appropriate sections of the book. The steps, outlined in Figure 2.1 are as follows:

1. **Identifying the research question:** Becoming aware of research questions, where to look for them, and how to select and define them.

2. **Initial review of literature:** Reading sources that will provide an understanding of the basic body of knowledge surrounding the question.

3. **Distilling the question to a specific research problem:** Judging the potential of the research and narrowing the research question to a specific researchable problem statement.

4. **Continued review of literature:** Becoming thoroughly knowledgeable in the problem area and obtaining ideas about methods, techniques, and instrumentation needed to attack the problem of interest.

5. **Formulation of hypotheses:** Based upon the literature reviewed and the researcher's experience, establishing the expected outcomes of the research.

6. **Determining the basic research approach:** Depending upon the type of question being asked, determining the preferred research approach (e.g., experimental, nonexperimental, quantitative, qualitative) and basic plan of attack.

7. **Identifying the population and sample:** Determining the type of participants who will produce the needed data to answer the research question. Are the participants available? How many participants are needed? How will they be selected?

8. **Designing data collection plan:** Determining the techniques for experimental protocols, if required, as well as the methodological approach for gathering research data.

9. **Selecting or developing specific data collection instruments or procedures:** Considering the data collection plan as well as the availability and

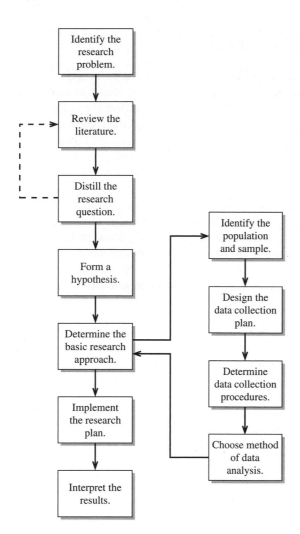

FIGURE 2.1
Steps in the research process.

adequacy of available instruments; deciding what specific instrument(s) is (are) needed to procure the needed data.

10. **Choosing the method of data analysis:** Depending upon the nature of the variables and the types of data collected in the research, identifying what statistical procedure(s) will be applied.

11. **Implementing the research plan:** Conducting the research as planned.

12. **Interpreting the results:** Analyzing the data, drawing conclusions regarding the research question, and providing meaningful recommendations based upon the results.

SELECTING THE QUESTION

Research question
The central focus of the research effort that serves as the basis for the research problem and provides direction for the entire process.

A researcher necessarily begins any study with a question. The selection of a **research question,** however, is often a major source of anxiety and frustration for graduate students. We have observed that students typically fall into one of three categories when it comes to selecting a research question: (1) those who know precisely what they want to do and have a well-conceived problem, (2) those who have many interest areas and are having difficulty deciding exactly what they want to study, and finally, and (3) those students who do not have any idea about a worthwhile research question. While the source of research questions will vary according to the experience of the person contemplating an investigation, it is generally agreed that the process begins with an idea or question in the mind of the researcher. The initial question is typically broad in nature, lacking the specificity required of a researchable problem. The beginning researcher, most frequently graduate students with no previous research experience, will often identify a problem area of interest but will not have selected a researchable question. For instance, if asked, "What are you interested in researching?" they may reply sport psychology, athletic training, strength training, coaching, exercise physiology, or some other problem area, but are vague to a specific researchable question. Each of these problem areas contains innumerable research questions. The challenge for the researcher is to identify a specific question within the problem area that is amenable to research.

There are many reasons why people engage in research. Questions often arise from issues, controversies, concerns, or problems that need to solved. Curiosity is as good a motivational factor as any. A former graduate student was interested in the broad problem area of dietary disorders, specifically, anorexia nervosa and bulimia. This student was curious about where the attitude began that led to the development of these disorders in teenagers and young adults. Is it possible that the dietary problems are rooted in childhood? Such curiosity led to an excellent study in which an attempt was made to determine and compare body image perception and preferences among male and female preadolescent children (Collins 1989). So, from this initial curiosity, a definitive problem was identified.

Many methods for finding worthwhile research questions have been suggested to graduate students by their professors over the years. The following list represents some of the methods which have been helpful in the past:

1. Write out your philosophy of the kinesiology field in which you are studying. Divide the field into its several parts and study them. When you come to something you would like to know, but do not know, write it down for your research "hope chest."

2. In reading, in discussions, at lectures, and at all times, write down at once any hunches or ideas that come to you. Many times reading or philosophizing

will reveal gaps in your present field of knowledge. Write these down. Read the best studies in your interest area. Think about a problem, and note the questions which arise. Criticize and challenge statements made in current professional periodicals, in books and research studies, and in your own and allied fields. Hundreds of research problems exist in those sources.

3. Prepare a paper on some subject that interests you and extend it into unknown realms. When you meet an obstacle in your thinking, analyze it for the problem it suggests.

4. With what in your field are you dissatisfied? What problems does it suggest? Investigate these.

5. Analyze, challenge, and criticize the popular beliefs and practices in your field of interest. You will be appalled by their unquestioned acceptance. Again, note your hunches.

6. What procedures or practices in your field interest you? Observe the problems inherent in those procedures and practices that could be researched. What problems have you observed during your work experiences? Could these be the source of a research question?

7. Browse reference and bibliographical lists in books, journals, magazines, and theses. Just running down a list of titles frequently sparks a viable idea for a research problem. Examine the lists of master's and doctoral studies done at your institution. Then, move on to the lists from other institutions or research centers.

8. Talk to your professors or other professionals that work in your interest area. You will find that most professors have an abundance of ideas about potential research problems and are eager to share them with interested students.

Several of the suggestions listed above involve the utilization of hunches. Becoming sensitive to such ideas can become a valuable mental habit. Upon inspection, most of them will not be viable research problems or will already have been studied. Occasionally, though, a hunch will lead to an important research question that, when solved, will make a major contribution.

TYPES OF RESEARCH QUESTIONS

The foundation of scientific inquiry and the first stage of the research process is the identification of the *research question*. While the research question will inevitably be refined and transformed into a specific statement of the problem that is amenable to investigation, it is especially useful for the beginning researcher to develop an understanding of what constitutes an appropriate research question. Obviously, there is a great variety of research questions that may be investigated.

It is possible, however, to group research questions into three basic categories: descriptive, relationship, and difference (Drew, Hardman, and Hosp 2008). Being able to identify the basic type of question being asked helps in understanding the very nature of the research, the preferred research design and methodology, and the appropriate methods for analyzing the data.

It is worth noting that most research studies, especially those that are ultimately published, usually contain multiple questions, including different types of questions. Whereas the definitive classification of a research question into one of these three types may be viewed as an academic exercise, comprehending the basic nature of the research question is an important part of understanding the research process.

In order to help the reader better understand the three types of research questions, we have included examples that have been adapted from published papers or theses and categorized according to the type of question being asked. It is noted that additional research questions may have been included in each study.

Descriptive Questions

Descriptive questions
Type of research question that seeks to describe phenomena or characteristics of a particular group of subjects.

As the name suggests, **descriptive questions** seek simply to describe phenomena or characteristics of a particular group of subjects being studied. Such questions describe what is. Data are typically gathered by asking questions of a group of individuals, observing their behavior, or measuring (testing) their performance on specified tasks. Descriptive questions are often the basis for survey research as well as qualitative research. An example of research centered around a descriptive question is illustrated by the Youth Risk Behavior Surveillance System (YRBSS) sponsored by the Centers for Disease Control and Prevention (CDC). The YRBSS consists of national, state, and large school district surveys of representative samples of high school students. Conducted every two years, these surveys monitor health risk behaviors among young people so that health and education agencies can more effectively target and improve programs. Consider the following examples:

What are the perceived barriers to leisure-time physical activity participation among Australian adults? (Cerin, Leslie, Sugiyama, and Owen 2010)

How do first year physical education teachers perceive the effectiveness of a mentoring program on their professional growth and teacher development? (Rikard and Banville 2010)

What is the extent of perceived ethnic/cultural violence among students in middle and high schools? (Hamdan and Martinez 2000)

What do physical education teachers think about the effect of block scheduling in secondary school physical education classes? (Bukowski and Stinson 2000)

Difference Questions

Difference questions seek to make comparisons between or within groups. They ask the question: Is there a difference? This type of question tends to be associated with experimental research, where at the simplest level a researcher is comparing an experimental group that has been exposed to some treatment to a control group that has not received the treatment. Similarly, comparisons that are made between pretest performance and posttest performance are also representative of research questions asking if there is a difference. Difference questions may also be the basis for nonexperimental research in which the researcher is interested in comparing one group to another on the basis of existing characteristics. For example, Faucette and colleagues (1995) used self-administered surveys to compare fourth grade boys' and girls' out-of-school physical activity levels and choices of activity. Examples of difference questions follow.

> **Difference questions** Type of research question that seeks to determine if there are differences between or within groups or conditions.

Do expert and novice dancers use similar strategies to learn appropriately challenging routines in domain-relevant conditions? (Poon and Rodgers 2000)

How does intrinsic motivation toward physical fitness testing differ according to award status and gender of upper elementary school children? (Domangue and Solmon 2010)

Does performing a forward lunge with a long step result in greater forces acting on the cruciate ligaments (ACL and PCL) than performing a forward lunge with a short step? (Escamilla et al. 2010)

Is there a difference in physical activity levels between adults with and without mental retardation? (Frey 2004)

Relationship Questions

Relationship questions investigate the degree to which two or more variables covary or are associated with each other. Rather than comparing groups, typically the researcher obtains measurements on two or more variables for a group of subjects

> **Relationship questions** Type of research question that seeks to investigate the relationship or association between two or more variables.

and then computes some index of association, often a correlation coefficient. The intent of such questions is simply to determine the extent to which the variables are related, not to establish cause-and-effect. The work by Welk and colleagues (2003) to investigate the relationship between various parental influences (e.g., role modeling, support behaviors, encouragement) and children's physical activity provides a good illustration of a relationship question. Several examples of relationship questions follow.

Is there an association between leisure-time physical activity and indicators of well-being and selected symptoms of medical conditions? (Brown, Mishra, Lee, and Bauman 2000)

What is the relationship between class size, lesson context, and students' engagement in physical activity during middle school physical education class? (McKenzie, Marshall, Sallis, and Conway 2000)

Is there an association between self-esteem and eating behaviors among collegiate female swimmers? (Fey 1998)

Is physical activity in childhood and adolescence a predictor of physical activity in young adulthood? (Telama, Yang, Laakso, and Viikari 1997)

Is there a relationship between middle school students' intrinsic motivation and their learning in school physical education? (Sun and Chen 2010)

DEFINING THE PROBLEM

Distilling
The process of narrowing an initial research question to a specific problem that is amenable to investigation.

Once the research question has been selected, the researcher must take the question and begin a process of **"distilling"** the question into a carefully defined problem that is amenable to investigation. This process normally commences with a thorough review of background literature in the problem area surrounding the research question. Such a literature review will go a long way in helping the researcher crystallize the research question, thus facilitating the development of a specific research problem. Before going much further, the researcher is now at a point to make a final determination as whether or not the problem should be studied. In making this decision, the researcher should consider three primary criteria.

1. **Does the problem interest you?**
   Arguably the most important criteria is your interest in the problem. It may be a splendid problem, but you should pass it by if you are not genuinely interested in it. You should realize that you will spend anywhere from approximately six months to well over a year working on the problem. People tend

to do a better job with a problem that was their own idea or something they created. Faculty advisors are sometimes reluctant to "give" a research topic to a graduate student for this reason. Even when a faculty advisor suggests a research topic, you would be advised to carefully consider the topic to insure that it interests you before proceeding with the research.

2. **Is the problem worthwhile?**

This criterion is often difficult to judge. Most individuals believe that the problem they are studying is important and worthwhile. Ultimately, a graduate student's thesis or dissertation committee will make a statement about the value of a problem when they approve the proposed research topic. The acceptance or rejection of a manuscript for publication in a professional journal is often based on how the reviewer or editor judges the worthiness of a research problem. Does the problem and its solution make a contribution to the body of knowledge within the field of study? Oftentimes the significance of a research problem can be established through either the theoretical or practical contribution that it will make to a field. Is the research problem timely? Is there a recognized demand for a solution to the problem? It is incumbent upon the researcher to answer these questions affirmatively and be able to justify and provide the rationale for these answers in the research proposal or report.

3. **Is the problem manageable?**

A researcher may have a deep interest in a particular problem, but he or she must determine if the problem is actually researchable. Moreover, it is important to select a problem that is not too large. Oftentimes a graduate student identifies a worthwhile problem in which he or she has an interest, but is unable to attack the problem in a meaningful fashion because the problem is too large and complex. Whereas it is important to contribute to building the road of knowledge within a particular area, this contribution may well take the form of a grain of sand as opposed to a large stone. This is particularly true for beginning researchers as they acquire an understanding of the research process. Does the researcher have sufficient training and expertise in the problem area to conduct the study? If not, can the expertise be acquired? Is a research problem feasible from the standpoint of time, expense, resources, and availability of data? All research studies involve certain expenses, whether they are for the purchase of electrodes, printing of questionnaires, postage, laboratory costs, travel, or the design of equipment. Who will pay these expenses? Sometimes an excellent research problem is conceived and developed only to find that the participants needed to produce the relevant data are unavailable. No subjects, no data, no study! Historical studies often require an extended period of time and can also be expensive and involve extensive travel as one seeks to obtain original materials and sources of information. Is the problem one that you can attack without prejudice? If the answer to this question is no, then it is better to pass the problem on to someone else. All researchers, beginners and veterans alike, need to be objective. Bias can creep into a study through the way participants are selected, instrumentation is developed, and procedures conducted. While it is desirable to have a strong conviction, letting this conviction mediate one's research efforts to the point of introducing bias in a study is out of place.

Purpose of the Study

Purpose statement
A specific statement expressing the researcher's intent or goal for conducting the study; normally indicates the variables or phenomenon of interest and information regarding the participants and setting of the study.

Once selected and appropriately delineated, the research problem becomes the focus of the research. The research problem is usually developed in the introductory section of a research report and is typically identified, clearly and succinctly, in a **purpose statement** that expresses the goals for the research study. Arguably, a purpose statement is the most important statement in a research proposal as well as the final thesis, dissertation, or published research paper. The purpose statement indicates the researcher's intent for conducting the research study. According to Locke, Spirduso, and Silverman (2007), a purpose statement expresses "why you want to do the study and what you intend to accomplish" (p. 9). Typically found as the last sentence or near the end introductory section, the structure and clarity of the purpose statement is extremely important. A well-written purpose statement should identify the key variables or phenomenon to be investigated and provide some information about the scope of study (i.e., research participants, setting, and treatment). Remember, the purpose statement tells what is to be done in the study. In addition, the language used in a purpose statement should suggest the basic type of research by indicating whether the study is descriptive, correlational, comparative, qualitative, or examining a cause-and-effect relationship. A purpose statement may take a variety of forms, but usually begins in a manner similar to one of the following:

1. "The purpose of this study was to . . ."
2. "The aim of this research was to . . ."
3. "This study was designed to . . ."
4. "The intent of this investigation was to . . ."

Note that when the final research report is written the purpose statement is worded in past tense since it is reporting of something that was previously done (i.e., "The purpose of this study *was* to . . ."). However, in the proposal stage of the research process, the purpose statement may be written in the present tense (i.e., "The purpose of this study is to . . ."). Since some advisors recommend that even the research proposal be written in past tense, students are advised to check with the chair of their thesis or dissertation committee to make certain they are using the preferred wording. Following are examples of purpose statements selected from published articles:

> The goal of this study was to determine whether Colorado on the Move could produce short-term increases in lifestyle physical activity. (Wyatt et al. 2004)
>
> The first purpose of this study was to report cardiovascular fitness levels, as measured using the 20-meter shuttle run test, for youths 8–18 years of age from a midwestern metropolitan area. Second, we make comparisons among midwestern youths' 20-meter shuttle run performance and their U.S. and international counterparts. (Beets and Pitetti 2004)
>
> The purpose of the present study was to examine the stability of physical self-perceptions across a short period of time (four days). (Raudsepp, Kais, and Hannus 2004)
>
> The purposes of this study were (a) to describe the prevalence of participation in moderate to vigorous physical activity and overweight and obesity and (b) to examine the associations between physical activity and weight status in students at a rural university. (Eisenmann, Bartee, and Damori 2004)

All types of research studies contain a researchable problem that serves as the focus of the purpose statement. However, the structure of a good purpose statement differs somewhat for quantitative and qualitative research. A purpose statement for a quantitative study tends to be specific and narrow, clearly identifying the major variables, whereas a purpose statement for a qualitative study may be somewhat broad in nature, identifying the central phenomenon or concept to be studied rather than specific variables. Consider the following examples:

A quantitative purpose statement:

> The purpose of this study was to investigate the relationship between young children's physical activity behavior and the attitude of their same-sex parent towards physical activity.

A qualitative purpose statement:

> The purpose of this qualitative study was to explore hazing rituals in interscholastic sports.

Note that both statements specify the major intent for conducting the research study. The quantitative statement is more specific, identifying children's physical activity and parental attitude as the key variables in this correlational study. On the other hand, the qualitative statement is more general, suggesting that the researcher wants to gain a deeper understanding of hazing rituals, the central phenomenon of interest. Also note that this statement identifies the study as a "qualitative" study.

Delimitations

Delimitations
Characteristics specified by the investigator that define the scope of the research study, in effect, "fencing it in."

In research circles, **delimitations** refer to the scope of the study. The delimitations of a study set the boundaries for the research, in effect, "fencing it in." For example, delimitations include characteristics of a study such as (1) type of research participant, (2) number of research participants, (3) measures to be collected, (4) instruments utilized in the study, (5) time and duration of the study, (6) setting, and (7) type of intervention or treatment. These are the parameters of a study that the researcher can control. Identifying the delimitations of a study is actually part of the process of defining (distilling) the problem. As the researcher narrows the question down to a researchable problem, many of the delimitations are established. Others are identified as the research plan and methodology are developed. In fact, an astute reader will be able to recognize important delimitations in a well-written purpose statement. For instance, consider the following purpose statement cited above:

> The purpose of this study was to report cardiovascular fitness levels, as measured using the 20-meter shuttle run test, for youths 8–18 years of age from a midwestern metropolitan area. (Beets and Pitetti 2004)

It is easy to see that this study was delimited to (1) cardiovascular fitness measured by a 20-meter shuttle run test, (2) youths 8–18 years old, and (3) youths living in a metropolitan area in the Midwest. Other delimitations are described in the "methods" section of the article.

Whereas most published papers do not contain a section entitled "delimitations," the format specified for many theses and dissertations include a specific subdivision of the manuscript for listing the delimitations of the study. In published papers, delimitations are usually embedded in the narrative contained within the "methods" section. The following example illustrates delimitations that were included in a thesis focusing on participation in Special Olympics:

1. Sixty-two adults with mild to moderate levels of mental retardation.
2. Individuals who reside in Northeast Iowa.
3. The experimental group consisted of athletes who participated in the Special Olympics Spring Games which took place in March 1998 in Northeast Iowa.
4. The control group consisted of an intact group of individuals residing at one of five group-living homes in Northeast Iowa.
5. The Rosenberg Self-Esteem Scale (as modified for purposes of clarity in regards to the particular group of subjects).
6. A two-week interval for pretest-posttest administration.

Limitations

In research terminology, **limitations** refer to weaknesses of the study. All studies have some weaknesses because compromises frequently have to be made in order to conform to the realities of a situation. Limitations are those things the researcher could not control, but that may have influenced the results of the study. The reader of a research report should always know at the outset those conditions of the study that could reflect negatively on the work in some way. Only those things that might affect the acceptability of the research findings should be reported. The researcher will, of course, try to eliminate extremely serious weaknesses before the study commenced. The process of carefully defining (distilling) the research problem necessarily involves identifying the major limitations associated with the research. Additional limitations may be identified as the researcher develops the research plan and then actually proceeds to implement it. Among the items that typically involve limitations to a study are the following:

- The research approach, design, method(s), and techniques
- Sampling problems
- Uncontrolled variables
- Faulty administration of tests or training programs
- Generalizability of the data
- Representativeness of research participants
- Compromises to internal and external validity
- Reliability and validity of research instruments

Whereas the number of limitations identified will vary depending upon the nature of the study, the research design, and the methodology utilized, it is generally recommended that the number of limitations be less than the number of delimitations presented. While it is important that the researcher recognize from the outset potential weaknesses of the study, an exceedingly long list of limitations raises serious questions about why so many facets of the research were not controlled, thus questioning the overall legitimacy of the research. In published papers, the author frequently will discuss the limitations of the research and the implications thereof within the "discussion" section of the manuscript. For instance, in the study of shuttle run performance cited earlier (Beets and Pitetti 2004), the authors note limitations in the "discussion" section pertaining to (1) sampling procedures, (2) unfamiliarity with test procedures, (3) the number of different people administering the tests, and (4) cultural differences. Sometimes, a separate section of the manuscript entitled "limitations" will present the weaknesses of the research. In a thesis or dissertation, it is common to see a specific subdivision of the manuscript called "limitations" in which the author

Limitations
Aspects of a research study that the investigator cannot control, that represent weaknesses to the study, and that may negatively affect the results.

will provide a listing of the weaknesses or perceived weaknesses of the study. This is illustrated by the following examples of limitations taken from the study regarding the Special Olympics:

1. Participants for the study were a convenience sample.
2. The participants' understanding of the research instrument's statements as they were intended.
3. Previous participation as a Special Olympics athlete.
4. Existence of research participants' involvement with organized recreation programs.
5. Participants' family setting may be a potential extraneous variable that could influence the findings.

Assumptions

Assumptions
Facts or conditions presumed to be true, yet not actually verified, that become underlying basics in the planning and implementation of the research study.

Assumptions are conditions that the researcher presumes to be true. They are conditions that are taken for granted. Assumptions are derived primarily from the literature, but may also come from the researcher's own knowledge of the problem area. In other words, what does the literature tell the researcher that can be assumed to be true for purposes of planning the study? The information gleaned from the literature during the process of defining (distilling) the problem frequently serves as the basis for much of the development of the research project, including the identification of assumptions that should be taken for granted. The literature provides information about a particular behavior, and sometimes contains factual evidence explaining the behavior. The researcher undertakes a study certain with the assumption that this information is correct. Assumptions are also made about the way the instrumentation, procedures, methods, and techniques will contribute to the study. The researcher may also assume that certain things that could not be controlled or documented may have happened in the study. In a study designed to investigate the effects of participation in Special Olympics on the self-esteem of adults with mental retardation, the following assumptions were made by the author:

1. The test instrument, as modified, was appropriate for the target population and was a valid and reliable measure of self-esteem.
2. The participants understood the directions as they were intended.
3. The participants completed the self-esteem inventory to the best of their ability.
4. The participants were a representative sample of adults with mental retardation who reside in the state of Iowa.
5. The interviewers were sufficiently trained and capable of utilizing the recommended survey procedures.

Additional examples of assumptions that are commonly made include the following:

- All research participants completed the questionnaire honestly and correctly.
- The research participants complied with the investigator's request to put forth maximal effort on all trials of the test.
- The instructors (or trainers) were capable of utilizing the prescribed teaching method.

Although published papers frequently do not explicitly state the underlying assumptions for a research study, a thesis or dissertation often contains a specific subdivision of the manuscript that includes a listing of assumptions that were made. This is illustrated above by the assumptions listed for the study on Special Olympics participation.

THE CONCEPT OF VARIABLES

The focus of the researcher's effort is always on the **variable.** A variable is a characteristic, trait, or attribute of a person or thing that can be classified or measured. Eye color, sex, and church preference are classifications. Skill, self-concept, strength, heart rate, and intelligence are variables that can be measured. The term *variable* indicates that a characteristic can have more than one value. There are two genders in the human race, male and female, and if both appear in a research project, then gender becomes a variable. When a characteristic does not vary, it is referred to as a *constant.* In a study of the manual dexterity of second-year nursing students, the characteristic, second-year, is a constant; it does not vary among the student nurses.

Variable
A characteristic, trait, or attribute of a person or thing that can take on more than one value and can be classified or measured.

Quantitative and Qualitative Variables

Variables can be *qualitative* or *categorical* if they are classified according to some characteristic, attribute, or property. People are categorized as to sex (male, female), eye color (blue, brown, green), church preference (Catholic, Protestant, Jewish), and political affiliation (Republican, Democrat, Independent). Qualitative variables are usually unmeasurable. Variables are called *quantitative* if they can be measured in a numerical sense. The heights of five starters on a basketball team may be 5'10", 6'2", 6'5", 6'8", and 7', respectively. Their ages range from 18 years, 6 months to 22 years, 3 months. There are two basic type of quantitative variables, *discrete* and *continuous*.

Discrete Variables. This type of variable is usually thought of as being a whole unit, one that cannot be fractionated or divided into smaller parts. Examples of discrete variables are football scores, and the number of correct answers on a test. Football scores are recorded in whole numbers (e.g., 3, 7, 10, 14) and cannot be divided into smaller parts like 7.5 or 11.75.

Continuous Variables. This type of variable can be divided into fractional amounts in large or small degrees. Strength and endurance scores, track and field times, height, weight, and girth measures are considered to be continuous variables. Time in a 100-meter dash is sometimes to the nearest tenth of a second, but in high-level competition it could be one one-hundredth of a second. The height of a person could be measured in feet and inches, in half-inches, or in quarter-inches, depending on the precision desired and the ability of the measuring instrument to measure height accurately.

Independent and Dependent Variables

Independent variable
The experimental or treatment variable in a study; it is the variable that is purposively manipulated or selected by the researcher in order to determine its effect on some observed phenomenon; it is antecedent to the dependent variable.

Dependent variable
The variable that is expected to change as a result of the independent variable; it is the variable that is observed or measured in a study.

In research, particularly experimental research, the terms **independent** and **dependent variables** are commonly used. Although sometimes confusing for beginning research students, recognizing the distinction between independent and dependent variables and being able to properly identify each in a research study is critically important in understanding the research process. The experimental approach involves observing what effect different amounts of one variable (independent) have on a second variable (dependent). The independent variable is referred to as the experimental treatment. It is the variable that is manipulated or purposively selected by the researcher in order to determine its effect on some observed phenomenon. The researcher controls what treatment will be selected and how much will be applied. The treatment, or independent, variable will not change during the research or as a result of the research. It is considered an antecedent or precursor to other variables. According to Ary, Jacobs, and Sorensen (2010), there are two types of independent variables, *active* and *attribute*. An active variable is one that is actually manipulated or selected by the researcher, such as method of training, form of reinforcement, or type of nutritional supplement. An attribute variable is one that cannot be actively manipulated or altered by the researcher since it represents a preexisting attribute or trait, such as gender, race, age, or grade level. Researchers are able to form comparison groups on the basis of such preexisting characteristics.

The dependent variable, on the other hand, is the one that is expected to change as a result of the treatment. It is the variable that is observed or measured in the research process. The dependent variable is not under the control of the researcher as it represents the response or outcome from the manipulation of the independent variable. It is the presumed consequence of the independent variable.

Said another way, the independent variable is expected to *cause* some *effect* on the dependent variable. The changed, or affected, variable is referred to as dependent because its value depends upon the value of the independent variable (Tuckman 1999). In many instances, the independent variable forms or defines comparison groups in research; the dependent variable generates data.

Following are some examples of independent and dependent variables:

Problem 1: A study is designed to investigate the effects of different brands of toothpaste (e.g., Colgate and Crest) on the prevention of dental cavities.
Independent variable: brand of toothpaste
Dependent variable: number of cavities

Problem 2: A researcher wants to compare a dosage of 1200 mg versus 2400 mg of a popular over-the-counter pain reliever on delayed onset muscle soreness (DOMS) following an intense exercise bout.
Independent variable: dosage level
Dependent variable: some measure of muscle soreness

Problem 3: An investigator seeks to study the effects of different types of incentives on participation in a weight-loss program.
Independent variable: type of incentive
Dependent variable: participation rates

Problem 4: A study is undertaken to investigate the effects of a movement education program on motor skill development among preschool children.
Independent variable: movement education program
Dependent variable: some measure of motor skill development

Some of the most common independent variables seen in kinesiology research are exercise, diet, medicines, drugs, motivation, programs, procedures, methods, techniques, gender, social class, attitude, and intelligence. Some of the most common dependent variables are performance, fitness, learning, attitude, knowledge, and behavior. It is also noted that variables may be used as an independent variable in one study and as a dependent variable in another study. Consider, for example, one experiment in which the investigator studies the effect of losing a game (independent) on motivation (dependent) among a group of athletes, while in another study the investigator studies the effect of motivation (independent) on physical performance (dependent). Motivation served as the dependent variable in one study and as the independent variable in the other. The purpose of the study determines whether a variable is considered independent or dependent.

While some research studies, as in the examples above, may have only one independent and one dependent variable, it is not uncommon for research studies to have more than one independent variable and/or more than one dependent variable. Consider the following examples:

Problem 5: A study is designed to investigate the effects of a new movement education unit taught in a second-grade physical education class on students' motor skill proficiency and leisure-time physical activity participation.
Independent variable: method of teaching (new movement education curriculum versus traditional unit)
Dependent variable: measure of motor skill proficiency (e.g., TGM-2) and accelerometer-based measure of physical activity

Problem 6: A researcher is interested in investigating the effects of a high-protein diet and two different modes of strength training on muscular strength development of college-age males.
Independent variable: type of diet and method of strength training
Dependent variable: muscular strength

Problem 7: An educational researcher seeks to determine the effects of block scheduling of classes on skill acquisition and attitude toward physical activity among junior high school students. Furthermore, the researcher is interested in determining if boys and girls respond to block scheduling differently.
Independent variable: type of scheduling (block versus traditional) and gender
Dependent variable: skill achievement and attitude toward physical activity

Extraneous Variables

Extraneous variable
Error-producing variable that could negatively affect the results of a research study if not adequately controlled.

While the independent variable is to serve as a stimulus to evoke a response from the dependent variable, there are usually other factors (variables) that could possibly cause the same response. In fact, it is quite likely that there are many possible variables that could have an effect on the dependent variable. To conclude that one type of physical fitness training is more effective than another, the researcher must be confident that other factors did not produce the same effect. Perhaps the most frequent and most serious mistake made by the beginning researcher is the failure to either control or account for the variables that could contribute error in an experiment. These error-producing variables are generally referred to as **extraneous variables.** Although some authors may also describe error-producing variables as intervening variables, modifying variables, or confounding variables, we prefer to use the term extraneous variable to refer to any factor that is a source of unwanted or error variance. The task of the researcher is to eliminate or somehow control the potential influence of extraneous variables. Methods of controlling extraneous variables are discussed below. The following examples illustrate the potential effect that extraneous variables could have on research findings.

A researcher studied the effect of motivation (independent) on the physical fitness test scores (dependent) of sixth-grade boys and girls. The two motivating conditions were team competition and level of aspiration (goal seeking). The subsequent finding that the group receiving level of aspiration was significantly better than the group receiving team competition was surprising because the literature contains much information proclaiming the superiority of team competition as a motivational vehicle. A detailed check into the composition of the groups participating under each condition revealed that they came from classes that were divided into high, average, and low academic achievement. The sixth graders who performed under the level of aspiration condition came from the high achievement category and possessed a mean intelligence quotient (IQ) of 132. The literature clearly indicates that, in general, the more intelligent an individual is, the easier it is to get that person "up," or motivated. So, IQ, a variable that was not included in the design of the study, served as an extraneous variable that slipped into the research situation, interacting with the dependent variable (fitness score) to make the condition (level of aspiration) look extremely potent and effective. The researcher presumed that IQ, while not a planned part of the study, was a substantive contributor to its results. This variable, like all extraneous variables, was not manipulated by the researcher.

There are many extraneous variables that can have a significant influence on the dependent variable and can invalidate research conclusions. Other such extraneous variables besides IQ, and depending on the specific type of experiment, are sex, socioeconomic level, teacher competence, personality, enthusiasm, physical health, emotional health, age, and the use of volunteers and intact groups as research participants. If a researcher conducted a study on the effect of three different methods of teaching outdoor education concepts on elementary students' appreciation and knowledge of the outdoors, with one instructor assigned to each method, instructor personality could play an important role in the ultimate results of the study. Extraneous variables are difficult, if not impossible, to control. A good design of a study can help to play down the effect of such variables. In the teacher personality example above, the outdoor education teachers could be screened for personality characteristics; the one with the desired personality would then be assigned to teach the outdoor education concepts under the three different methods. Teacher personality would be the same for all three groups of participants and so, in this case, the teacher personality variable would be controlled, or neutralized. However, it is assumed here that the teacher is equally effective in teaching with each method.

Control of Variables

It is critically important not only for the researcher but also for the consumer of the research literature to be able to identify the pertinent variables in a study. In designing a study, particularly an experimental study, the researcher should pay particular attention to controlling the influence of extraneous variables.

Many studies in kinesiology are conducted outside of the laboratory, using human research participants, and many variables surround the research situation which could alter the results in some substantive way. It becomes imperative that the researcher maintain as much control over these variables as possible so as to prevent or reduce their effect. At the same time it must be recognized that not every variable that could make a difference can be controlled. Following are some of the procedures that are frequently used in an attempt to control extraneous variables:

Random Selection of Research Participants.   When the laws of probability are permitted to operate in the selection of two or more experimental groups of participants, systematic bias is removed and the effect of extraneous variables is minimized. It is assumed that the groups are equal and that if any difference does exist, it is due to probability or chance factors (Best and Kahn 2005).

Equating or Matching by Some Criterion.   The participants are paired on some characteristic, such as age, sex, height, weight, ability, or the results of preliminary testing. After the pairing is completed, the members of each pair are assigned at random, one to the experimental group and the other to the control group. If a researcher wanted to use 15-, 16-, and 17-year-old boys and girls to study methods of developing flexibility, it might be desirable to match on age and gender so that the experimental and control groups would be comparable on those two variables at the beginning of the experiment. Each boy and girl in each age group would be randomly assigned to either the experimental or control group.

By matching participants it is also possible to reduce the variation among them because of chance differences in initial ability. It is a relatively simple matter to match on one or two characteristics. As the number of traits to match increases, so does the difficulty in obtaining accurate pairs.

Excluding the Variable.   A researcher may simply choose to not include a particular trait in the study. The intent is to eliminate the possible effects of a variable by holding the variable constant, thereby removing it from the study. This is sometimes referred to as *controlling for the variable*. For instance, if a researcher suspects that gender might influence the outcome of a study designed to investigate the effect of extrinsic motivation on weight loss, the researcher could control for gender by limiting the participants to only females. In this case, gender has been held constant by excluding males from the study. Similarly, research participants could be selected from only one age group or grade level, thus removing age and grade as variables.

Summary of Objectives

1. **Understand the various steps of the research process.**
   The research process involves several steps which vary
   according to the nature and purpose of the research being
   conducted. In general, the research process always involves
   identifying the research question, defining the problem,
   searching relevant literature, stating a hypothesis, designing
   and implementing a research plan, and analyzing and
   interpreting results.

2. **Recognize the different types of research questions.**
   Research questions are categorized by the type of information
   they are designed to investigate. Descriptive questions are
   used to obtain descriptive information; difference questions
   are used to make comparisons, and relationship questions
   seek to identify associations between variables.

3. **Understand those factors that must be considered when
   selecting a research question.** A good research question
   should not only focus on a problem of interest to the
   researcher; it should also address a worthwhile problem that
   holds some value for the discipline. It is also important that
   the problem be manageable, both in terms of the scope of
   the research and as it relates to the resources available to the
   researcher.

4. **Recognize the different types of variables.** The variable is
   always the focus of a research effort. Independent variables
   are carefully controlled or manipulated by the researcher,
   while dependent variables are those upon which measures
   are collected. Depending upon its nature, a variable could
   also be classified as either a qualitative or a quantitative
   variable.

3

Reviewing the Literature

OBJECTIVES

After selecting the research question, it is common for the novice researcher to want to jump right into developing the research plan and be eager to start the research project. While often challenging and time consuming, reviewing the literature is seen by many as being something that is tangential to the real purpose of the study. However, thoroughly reviewing the literature is an essential step in developing the research proposal, formulating hypotheses, and developing the research plan. This chapter discusses the purposes of reviewing the literature and recommends strategies for conducting a meaningful literature review.

After reading Chapter 3, you should be able to

1. Understand the importance of the literature review.
2. Recognize the various sources of literature.
3. Understand how to conduct a literature search.
4. Establish a system for taking notes and keeping track of sources and citations.

Reviewing the literature serves several purposes for the researcher. McMillan (2008) identifies seven specific purposes for reviewing the literature:

1. Refining the research problem
2. Establishing the conceptual or theoretical orientation
3. Developing the significance of the study
4. Identifying methodologies and procedures
5. Uncovering contradictory findings
6. Developing research hypotheses
7. Discovering new information

For many, particularly students with little experience in conducting research, reviewing the literature may stimulate interest in a particular problem area and lead to the selection of the research question. The knack of perusing the many journals and publications in a given area is a time-consuming, tedious task, even in today's world of the Internet and online searches. Time spent reading related literature is time well spent and will serve the investigator very well as the study proceeds. Knowledge of related research in your area of interest will go a long way in establishing your professional competence and enabling you to conduct meaningful research of your own.

THE IMPORTANCE OF REVIEWING THE LITERATURE

Once the general research question has been decided upon, the student should then begin a literature search in an attempt to obtain additional background information to assist in rounding out or fully defining the problem. Two basic kinds of literature should be consulted. **Conceptual literature** includes books and articles written by experts or authorities in a problem area. Through their writing they have passed on their ideas, opinions, and theories about what is good, bad, desirable, and undesirable in the problem area. Most of the time conceptual literature is not to be considered research literature as such, but the information disseminated frequently is based on research. A second type of literature is **related research.** This category includes previous studies in the problem area. Similar or related studies are reviewed to determine what is already known about the main issues inherent in the problem.

Conceptual literature
The conjectural, often abstract, literature that provides the theoretical underpinnings for a research study.

Related research literature
Scientific reports of previous research related to the problem area being studied.

In reality, the literature should be consulted throughout the research project. However, the majority of the review should be accomplished before the final plans for conducting the research have been completed. The first plunge into the literature will provide the novice researcher with a broader and deeper understanding of what facts are already known in the problem area. If a decision is made to actually investigate the problem, further review of the literature will provide helpful information on methods, techniques, instrumentation, and procedures for conducting the study.

As discussed in Chapter 2, the literature is a big help in providing the beginning researcher with an initial understanding of existing knowledge in the problem area. A thorough review of the literature should reveal links between your study and the existing body of knowledge related to the research question. Studies having no linkage to the existing knowledge base tend to produce isolated bits of information and seldom make significant contributions to the field (Ary, Jacobs, and Sorensen 2010). The information gained from the preliminary excursion into the literature helps to round out the problem. As the problem planning continues, the literature search becomes increasingly more pointed and specific. The review of literature provides an important link between existing knowledge and the problem being investigated. By showing how a research study compares to previous investigations, the research problem can be placed in the appropriate context. Related research becomes critical. Studies related to the proposed study are sought out in terms of problem, variable, and population similarity. The researcher will attempt to find out just how far inquiry into the problem has progressed. What is known and what is not known concerning the problem? Are there any gaps in the literature with respect to the relevant information surrounding the problem? These questions can be answered by a thorough literature search.

The researcher will also become knowledgeable about methodology and procedures for attacking the problem, as well as ideas on instrumentation and design. Conceptual and theoretical relationships among the key variables will be found. A major outcome of the literature search is that the researcher will develop a theoretical basis for the study and justification for its conduct. It has often been said that the more sound and thorough knowledge of the previous research, the better will be the planning of subsequent study in the problem area. As noted by Bookwalter and Bookwalter (1959) more than fifty years ago, "Knowledge of the literature in the field and critical insight into the research in the student's major field of interest is considered evidence of high scholarship."

It is recommended that the literature be searched by looking at the most current literature first, then working backward in time. This will familiarize the researcher with the newer methods, techniques, procedures, instrumentation, and data analysis designs that have been developed in the problem area. Chances are better that mistakes made in previous studies will have been corrected, old theories revised, new ones postulated, and more sophisticated designs developed. Based on our experience doing research and conducting literature reviews, we recommend beginning your literature search with the most recent 10 years. If you find too many sources, then limit the search to five years. One of the best sources of articles can be found in the reference list of a recent publication of a study closely related to your research problem. Again, background reading should be completed before final plans for conducting the study are made.

Searching the literature is hard and demanding work. It is absolutely essential that graduate students contemplating a research project for the first time build plenty of time for searching the literature into their schedules. The literature search can be a frustrating and not particularly romantic task. However, it can be exciting to increase the knowledge base on the topic to be researched. One of the more frustrating occurrences for the beginner is to discover that the proposed study, or closely related study, has already been done. In this situation the researcher must weigh the merits of replicating the previous study or of revising the proposed study to attack a different part of the overall problem.

SOURCES OF LITERATURE

Before we discuss the actual process of conducting a literature search, it is important that you have a basic understanding of the distinction between primary sources and secondary sources. Although there are many different types of literature, individual items in the literature can be classified into two broad categories: primary sources and secondary sources. Being able to identify sources as either primary or secondary is an important skill in conducting a literature search for research purposes. A *primary source* is an original article or report in which researchers report firsthand the results of their study, providing considerable detail regarding how the study was conducted. Primary sources are usually reported in scholarly journals. Whereas there are hundreds of scholarly journals publishing primary research reports applicable to the field of kinesiology, the quality of the journals varies greatly. It is also noted that most theses and dissertations represent primary sources, although these are often more difficult to obtain. A *secondary source* is one that summarizes, reviews, or discusses primary research, but is not a firsthand reporting of the research. Examples of secondary sources include textbooks, encyclopedias, scholarly books on a particular topic, and reviews. Although secondary sources often provide a useful overview of a particular topic and cite relevant research studies and primary sources, secondary sources generally do not contain the necessary detail and are not the same as having the researcher directly report the results of a research study. Primary sources are considered to be most valuable for the researcher and generally represent the majority of references cited in published research articles, theses, and dissertations. In fact, many college professors are known to require their students to use only primary sources in their literature review.

Both primary and secondary sources are important in the literature review process. Secondary sources generally provide an overview of a topic, often citing some of the key research studies that help shape the body of knowledge. These are often particularly useful to the novice researcher who is first delving into the scientific literature in order to get a general picture of the research that has been done on a topic. Two types of secondary sources may be particularly useful in providing an overview of an area: reviews and meta-analysis studies. Reviews of research frequently appear as individual articles appearing in scholarly journals or in dedicated review publications such as *Psychological Reviews* or *Exercise and Sport Science Reviews*. There are several excellent sources for reviews in the areas of kinesiology, education, psychology, physiology, and sociology. An example of a review published as an individual article in a scholarly journal is the article by Sherar and colleagues appearing in an issue of *Pediatric Exercise Science* (22[3], 2010), that discusses the research investigating the relationship between timing of biological maturity and physical activity. Reviews may also be published as a monograph or as a stand-alone publication. The *PCPFS Research Digest,* for example, a publication of the President's Council on Physical Fitness and Sports, frequently contains reviews of topics addressing physical activity, fitness, sports, and nutrition. Meta-analysis studies, on the other hand, involve a reanalysis of the results of a large number of published research studies on a topic. Meta-analysis studies are more than simply a comprehensive review of literature on a topic and are designed to quantitatively synthesize available research. The important point to note here is that meta-analysis studies, as is the case with review articles, normally include a lengthy list of references that relate to a specific topic. Moreover, most of these references represent primary research reports. Further discussion of meta-analysis is provided in Chapter 11 of this textbook.

Periodicals

Periodicals constitute a significant portion of the literary world. There are thousands and thousands of periodicals. But exactly what is a periodical? Quite simply, a periodical can be defined as a publication that is issued at regular intervals. Its regularity distinguishes it from other forms of publications such as books, monographs, and reviews. There are many types of periodicals which vary significantly in terms of purpose, audience, and content. In general, periodicals can be classified as either newspapers, popular press periodicals, trade periodicals, or scholarly periodicals. Newspapers consist of short articles and are nontechnical in nature. They tend to cover current events and issues and often provide firsthand reports or accounts of events. Popular press periodicals, or what we generally think of as simply "magazines," are publications that appeal to broad groups of readers. Articles in popular press periodicals tend to be shorter in length and do not usually contain highly specialized or technical language. Trade periodicals refer to magazines that are targeted at specific occupational groups and businesses. They contain shorter articles but tend to be aimed at those who share an occupation or business goal in common and offer insights into trends on particular aspects of the business or occupation. **Scholarly journals** are more highly specialized, contain a higher level of technical terms, and are usually intended for a more specific and limited segment of the population. Scholarly journals provide the firsthand reporting of research studies that serves to build the knowledge base in a field. Scholarly journals constitute the type of periodical most valuable for researchers. The various categories of periodicals as well as sample publications in each category are shown below:

Scholarly journals
A primary source of literature that provides the firsthand reporting of research studies that serves to building the knowledge base in a field.

Newspapers
- *Chicago Tribune*
- *New York Times*
- *Washington Post*
- *USA Today*
- *Des Moines Registrar*

Popular Press Magazines
- *Time*
- *National Geographic*
- *Sports Illustrated*

- *People*
- *Entertainment Weekly*

Trade/Professional Magazines
- *Advertising Age*
- *Psychology Today*
- *Beverage Industry*
- *American Spa*
- *The Progressive Farmer*

Scholarly Journals (in kinesiology)
- *Research Quarterly for Exercise and Sport*
- *Medicine & Science in Sport & Exercise*
- *Journal of Teaching in Physical Education*
- *Journal of Physical Activity and Health*
- *Pediatric Exercise Science*

Whereas all the previous publications are examples of periodicals, only scholarly journals constitute primary sources in which researchers report the results of their research studies. Scholarly journals represent the most importance source of information for literature reviews associated with scientific investigations. It is important to note, however, that just because an article is published in a scholarly journal does not automatically make it trustworthy and a significant contribution to the body of knowledge in the field. Moreover, just because a study is published does not mean it represents good research. As previously stated, journals vary greatly in terms of quality, making it important for consumers of research as well as aspiring researchers to recognize which journals in your field are considered to be high-quality publications.

Scholarly journals may be classified as either refereed or nonrefereed journals. Typically, the most prestigious scholarly journals in a field are **refereed or peer-reviewed journals,** meaning that the manuscripts undergo a careful evaluation by the editor and two or three reviewers who are respected experts in the field. A **nonrefereed journal** does not use external reviewers to evaluate submitted manuscripts, although the journal editor may examine the manuscript for its suitability for being published in the selected journal. In general, nonrefereed journals are considered to be of lessor quality.

Usually reviewers for scholarly journals are asked to make one of three recommendations regarding the disposition of the manuscript: (1) publish as submitted, (2) revise and resubmit, or (3) reject. Rarely is a manuscript accepted as submitted. If the manuscript is deemed publishable, yet needing changes of some type, the reviewers will likely offer specific suggestions for improving the quality of the

Refereed (peer-reviewed) journal
Type of scholarly journal in which the manuscripts undergo a careful evaluation by the editor and expert reviewers in the field.

Nonreferred journal
Type of scholarly journal in which the manuscripts are not evaluated by external reviewers, although they may be appraised by the journal editor.

manuscript and recommend that it be revised and resubmitted. To mitigate the possibility of reviewer bias, some journals use a blind review process in which the names of the authors of the manuscript are withheld from the reviewers. Depending upon the journal, many more manuscripts are submitted for publication than are actually accepted. The rejection rate of a scholarly journal, or what some consider as a selectivity index, is sometimes used as a general indicator of journal quality (i.e., the higher the rejection rate, the higher the quality).

Another method of evaluating the quality of a scholarly journal is based upon how frequently a journal's articles are cited by other scholars or researchers. An **impact factor** is a computed measure of the frequency with which the "average article" in a journal has been cited in a given period of time. To illustrate, an impact factor of 3.0 for a journal means that the "average article" published in this particular journal has been cited in 3.0 other articles within the defined time period, say the previous two years. Quite simply, the frequent citation of an article in other articles is an indication that the article is influential within its field. A product of Thomson Reuters (previously known as the Institute for Scientific Information [ISI]), the *Journal Citation Reports* (JCR) was first published in 1975 and now includes approximately 10,000 journals in science and social science. Although not all journals applicable to research in kinesiology are cited in JCR, considering a journal's *impact factor* provides a quantitative basis for judging the relative quality of scholarly journals. For additional information concerning kinesiology journals, you may wish to read the 2005 article by Cardinal and Thomas appearing in the *Research Quarterly for Exercise and Sport* (Vol. 76, S122–S134) or consult the listing of kinesiology journals and associated impact factors provided by the American Kinesiology Association at the following website: http://www.americankinesiology. org/journal-listing-and-impact-factors.

Impact factor
Computed index of the quality of a scholarly journal based upon the frequency with which a journal's articles are cited by other researchers.

SEARCHING THE LITERATURE

You must first be able to find research and related literature before you can interpret and use it. Searching the literature is a tedious and time-consuming task, yet it is critically important to the success of any research. Before starting the actual search process, the researcher should carefully define the research problem as specifically as possible. By doing so, the researcher has established an entry point into the literature surrounding the topic of interest. Even if you have only a general idea for a research topic, it is important to establish a starting point as you commence the literature review. Doing otherwise will result in a needless waste of time and effort. Depending upon the general research topic and the researcher's knowledge about the topic, consulting secondary sources such as textbooks or reviews is a logical first step in searching the literature. As your search proceeds and you become more knowledgeable about the literature, make note of terms that seem to define the content area. These terms should provide

---

TABLE 3.1 Steps in the Literature Review Process

1. Identify Topic
2. Review Secondary Sources and Known Primary Reports
3. Identify Key Terms
4. Select Database(s)
5. Conduct Search
6. Identify Relevant Publications (particularly primary sources)
7. Locate and Obtain Sources
8. Read and Document Selected Literature

---

you with a set of key words that will help you search the literature more efficiently as you move into the primary source literature. Although there is no guarantee of finding primary sources directly related to your research topic, following the sequence of steps shown in Table 3.1 will increase the likelihood of conducting a successful literature search and locating valuable articles and other related sources (see Table 3.1).

Conducting a Database Search

The advent of the computer has added great speed to the process of searching the literature. Searching electronic databases is certainly easier and faster than flipping through stacks of periodicals or looking through a mountain of print indexes, yet effective searching requires the student to have a basic understanding of databases and to master the skills necessary to perform successful searches. No one masters such intricate searching skills immediately; successful searching requires considerable experience in conducting searches. Students today want their literature search to yield a comprehensive list of relevant publications and, of course, with full text.

Many databases enable complex searches to be performed that would be much more difficult, if not impossible, using paper resources. These reference sources include indexes to journals and other publications (sometimes accompanied by the full text of the cited article), abstracts, statistical reference materials, and compilations of useful data. Learning to do a basic computer search for literature is a relatively simple matter. Select the key words, or descriptors, from the problem statement of the proposed research topic or from your initial reading of secondary sources. These key terms are important in that they will be used to search computerized databases to find associated literature. Once identified, these key words are entered into the search fields of the selected database software, which uses them to search for related information from the records maintained by the particular database. Results of the search produce a report with the titles and citation information of published articles, research reports, reviews, conference papers and proceedings, and other sources. Some computerized databases include a brief abstract describing the content of each reference, while a few provide full text access to articles. These reports are typically available almost immediately. The nature of searching electronic databases often yields many sources that are not relevant to the research problem, requiring the researcher to repeat the search using a different database as well as different key words. This highlights the importance of carefully selecting the key words and choosing the appropriate database.

Once you have identified the topic of interest and relevant key terms you must identify the database or databases that will be used for your literature search. A key part of a successful search strategy is choosing an appropriate database. Databases are generally classified as either *multidisciplinary*, such as Academic Search Premier, which is a general database containing records from many fields, or *specialized*, such as Medline, which emphasize a particular subject or discipline (see Table 3.2). There are numerous computerized databases. Among the many databases available, ERIC, PsycINFO, SPORT Discus, Academic Search Premier, Ingenta, and Medline, among others, are commonly used by kinesiology researchers. While it may be convenient to simply select a single database, rarely will one database be sufficient in providing the complete coverage of the topic under investigation.

Although a comprehensive listing of literature databases is beyond the scope of this textbook, we do want to mention one that may be particularly useful for finding research conducted by graduate students. The ProQuest Dissertations and Theses (PQDT) database includes abstracts of doctoral dissertations and master's theses dating back to 1861. Its hard copy form is Dissertation Abstracts. If you are not affiliated with a library that subscribes to PQDT, you can search for dissertations and theses through Dissertation Express (http://www.proquest.com/en-US/products/dissertations/disexpress.shtml), a service that lets you purchase unbound copies of PDFs of graduate works published by ProQuest.

TABLE 3.2 Selected Multidisciplinary and Specialized Databases

MULTIDISCIPLINARY	SPECIALIZED
Academic One File	ERIC
Academic Search Premier (EBSCO)	LexisNexis Academic
Ingenta	Medline
JSTOR	PsycINFO
Web of Science (ISI)	Science Direct
WilsonWeb	Sociological Abstracts
WorldCat	SPORT Discus

A literature search can be greatly facilitated by using a basic **Boolean search strategy** to probe electronic databases. Although not readily appreciated by novice researchers who may be more familiar with simply using Google on the Internet, using Boolean operators (AND, OR, and NOT) to narrow or broaden the scope of one's search increases the precision of searching today's computerized information systems. Using the Boolean operator AND serves to narrow the search by combining constructs so that references obtained must include all the specified constructs; using the Boolean operator OR serves to broaden the search by retrieving references that contain either of the constructs; and using the Boolean operator NOT narrows the search by excluding references that contain one or more of the constructs. Figure 3.1 illustrates the concept of Boolean operators using only two constructs.

No single search strategy fits all research queries. Although conducting a Boolean search using a combination of keywords is a powerful method of locating titles related to a particular topic, other techniques, such as using Library of Congress subject headings, may also prove to be helpful.

Because of its simplicity and ease of use, Google Scholar (scholar.google.com) has been extremely popular and deserves special mention. Google Scholar was released in 2004 as a free service provided by Google that enables users to search for academic articles and peer-reviewed literature. It's available on the open web and it's free to use, although it often guides you to full text articles that may not be free. But Google Scholar points the user to multiple versions of the same article, and as a result, may turn up a source that is freely available online. Google

Boolean search strategy
A strategy for searching electronic literature databases by using AND, OR, and NOT between search words.

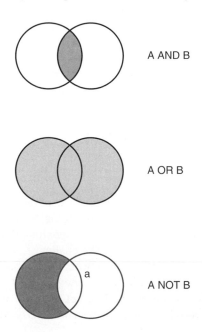

FIGURE 3.1
Venn Diagram Illustrating Boolean Searches.

Note: Shaded areas represent what a search retrieves from each logical statement.

Scholar is different from ordinary Google because it is limited to academic materials and it searches full text collections from multiple sources. Full text databases searched by Google Scholar include Ingenta, JSTOR, Project Muse, among others, as well as a variety of undisclosed academic publishers, professional societies, and universities. Google Scholar does not search all of the full text databases available, is less comprehensive, and does not allow for more advanced, sophisticated searches. Moreover, it is generally recognized that you will get more results by searching the databases directly. However, Google Scholar is a good place to start your search.

Once the database search is complete, you will obtain a listing of relevant references and, in most cases, a short summary or abstract of the article. Although full text access to articles may be possible with some database providers, generally the next step in the literature search process is to actually locate and obtain the pertinent articles or other sources. Keep in mind that your library may not have all the publications revealed in your literature search, although the material may be obtained through interlibrary loan or through a locator service available at many libraries. Be advised that additional costs may be involved. Once the publications have been obtained, now you are responsible for reading them. This may, in turn, lead you to additional sources.

Many computer reference sources are now available in most college and university libraries that subscribe to a variety of databases. The reference sources include indexes to journals and other publications, and may include the full text of the cited article, statistical reference materials, and compiled data. Most libraries utilize an online computerized information system that permits the researcher to gain immediate access to the needed literary citations. Graduate students typically learn to do a computer search in one of two ways: through a seminar-type course sponsored by the institution or their department; or with the help of a reference librarian highly skilled in using the various methods for retrieving information. We cannot overstate the importance of asking a reference librarian for assistance.

Searching the Internet

The Internet is a vast collection of interconnected computers throughout the world that provides access to a wealth of information. The resources available on the Internet are almost limitless. Today it is estimated that there are more than 2 billion web pages, accessible from computers located in libraries, classrooms, worksites, and even one's home. In fact, we are now seeing cellular phones and personal digital assistants (PDAs) with Internet access capability, thus making it possible to connect to the Internet almost anywhere. The challenge, however, is to find quality information. Special care must be taken when obtaining information from the Internet, because anyone can put up a website and post information. Thus, just because you locate information on the Internet does not mean that it is accurate and credible. It is important to carefully read Internet sources and evaluate their content on the basis of intent, bias, reputation of the author or publisher, and verifiable accuracy.

Internet Search Utilities. The easiest way of locating information on the Internet is to use some form of search utility that is available on the Web, namely subject directories, search engines, and metasearch engines. **Subject directories** are essentially Internet "yellow pages" in which you are able to peruse Internet sources according to subject area. Subjects are organized and located within a hierarchy of topical categories. Yahoo! is an example of a large and perhaps the most popular subject directory. WWW Virtual Library is another example of a subject directory. The primary advantage of subject directories is that the content has been reviewed and organized by a team of editors who have knowledge of specific disciplines, thus enhancing the relevance and quality of the resources assembled for a given topic. Yet, despite their organizational integrity, subject directories index a relatively small number of web pages compared to the number of pages examined by Internet search engines.

Subject directories
Internet "yellow pages" that enable the user to peruse World Wide Web sources according to subject areas.

Search engines are websites that enable you to search Internet databases for specific information, based upon entry of a key word or words. The search itself is performed in an automated fashion using a "spider" or "robot" that moves from website to website, capturing information from each site it visits in an attempt to find relevant matches to the key word provided. Google, Excite, Alta Vista, HotBot, and Northern Light are examples of Internet search engines. Search engines index millions of web pages and provide a quick, convenient way to search the Internet, although the relevance of the results is often less than desirable. Furthermore, the various search engines do not obtain consistent results since their databases may differ, thus suggesting that it is wise for the researcher to use several search engines.

Search engines
Websites that perform automated searches of Internet databases for specific information based upon specification of a key word or words.

A **metasearch engine** utilizes multiple search engines simultaneously to perform an Internet search of their databases. Within a short time, you get back results from several individual search engines, albeit only a portion of the results in any of the databases queried. Although no single metasearch engine includes all the search engines currently available, metasearch engines may be especially useful to researchers because of the inconsistent results obtained from each individual search engine. Dogpile, Copernic, Ixquick, and Metacrawler are examples of metasearch engines. Although the use of metasearch engines appears to hold much promise for the researcher, the user is somewhat limited in being able to specify search parameters, thus bringing to question the relevance of search results. In other words, the results obtained from a metasearch engine could easily yield large quantities of information, but only a relatively few sites are actually pertinent to the topic of interest.

Metasearch engine
Website that uses multiple search engines simultaneously to perform an Internet search.

With the ease of using a computer-based search of the Internet to locate information all over the world, it is both easy and tempting to cut and paste excerpts from documents. By so doing, one could easily forget to keep track of the source for the material, thus creating problems in the development of a reference list or, more seriously, increasing the chances of plagiarism occurring. It is important to

TABLE 3.3 Internet Search Utilities	
SUBJECT DIRECTORIES	
Academic Info	www.academicinfo.net
Britannica Internet Guide	www.britannica.com
Subject Guides A to Z	guides.lib.udel.edu/index.php
Wikipedia	www.wikipedia.org
Yahoo!	www.yahoo.com
SEARCH ENGINES	
Alta Vista	www.altavista.com
Excite	www.excite.com
Google	www.google.com
Lycos	www.lycos.com
Northern Light	www.northernlight.com
Yahoo Search	search.yahoo.com
METASEARCH ENGINES	
Chubba	www.chubba.com
Copernic	www.copernic.com
Dogpile	www.dogpile.com
Ixquick	www.ixquick.com
MetaCrawler	www.metacrawler.com

note the source of the material accessed over the Internet by maintaining an accurate citation for the material. In some cases it is necessary to record the actual URL and date accessed in the reference citation. Researchers should pay close attention to the reference format prescribed for electronic sources. The various style manuals (e.g., *APA, MLA,* or *Chicago*) contain detailed directions for citing sources obtained electronically.

Table 3.3 provides a listing of selected examples of each type of Internet search utility. Those interested in obtaining more information about Internet search capabilities, descriptions of the various directories, search engines, and metasearch engines, as well as strategies for successful Internet searching, may wish to consult the following websites:

- University of California Internet Resources (www.lib.berkeley.edu/TeachingLib/Guides/Internet)
- Search Engine Showdown (www.notess.com/search)
- Google Guide (googleguide.com)

Evaluating Information on the Web.   With the advent and development of the Internet, a massive amount of information is readily available by going online and clicking on a few websites. A variety of searchable electronic databases, as well as many full-text articles published in scholarly journals, are easily accessible, but so too is a lot of trash and questionable information. Anyone can develop a web page and post information for the whole world to see. So how does a researcher wade through this enormous quantity of material and locate quality information at credible Internet sites? A thorough discussion of this topic is beyond the scope of this textbook, but we believe the following questions represent a meaningful framework for evaluating information located on the Internet:

- **What is the source of the information?**
  Check the URL address. Check the domain of the website. Does it end with *edu* (education), *com* (commercial), *gov* (government), *org* (organization), or *net* (telecommunications)? Is the domain appropriate for the information sought? Is it someone's personal home page, often identified by a tilde (~) in the URL? If the source is an organization's website, then you should attempt to learn more about the organization.

- **Who is the author?**
  Is the author identified? Who wrote the document? Is the author someone that is well known or recognized within the field of study? Is there contact information for the author in order to request additional information? Is the author biased toward a particular viewpoint? Does the author have a "hidden agenda," such as promoting a product for sale?

- **Is the information current?**
  For some information, timeliness is important, and it is imperative to have current information. Does the document include a publication date or date of copyright? Is there an indication of when the information was gathered? If a date for the publication is not given, you may be able to check the website to determine the latest date the page was modified.

- **Are references provided?**
  In most scholarly work, you would expect a list of references documenting the sources of the information. Without proper documentation, the information presented on a website may not be any better than just one person's opinion on a topic.

- **Are links to other websites provided?**
  Many websites provide links to other sites on the Internet that provide related information on the topic. If provided, are the links to credible websites? Do the links actually work, and do they provide unbiased information on the topic?

In general, we advise you to use information obtained on the Internet very cautiously. Material published in professional journals and reputable textbooks is generally thought to be more credible and more trustworthy. The following websites at Johns Hopkins University and the University of California–Berkeley provide additional information pertaining to the evaluation of material available on the Internet:

www.library.jhu.edu/eresources.html

www.lib.berkeley.edu/TeachingLib/Guides/Internet/Evaluate.html

READING AND DOCUMENTING THE RESEARCH LITERATURE

After the literature search has been completed and promising sources identified, the sources have to be located. The majority of sources will probably be found in scholarly journals, although books, monographs, dissertations, reports, and Internet sites may also provide relevant information. The task of locating the desired references is generally dependent upon the type of publication. Most college and university libraries have computerized catalogs that list information about books, magazines, journals, newspapers, and other regularly published periodicals that these libraries hold. As previously discussed, locating information on the Internet usually requires the use of some form of search utility, including subject directories, search engines, and metasearch engines.

Once a source is located, the researcher studies it to evaluate its potential value to the proposed research. This is done by quickly reading the description of the source and by scanning the table of contents, index, and chapter summaries, or *abstract* if an article. Even though a title may seem to indicate that the content will be useful, frequently it is not. As the scanning process continues, a *working bibliography* is created that includes only those literature sources that are pertinent to the research problem being studied. Some sources identified during the literature search will be thrown out because they hold no promise of being helpful, while new ones may well be discovered that will be of use. The research focus may even change as the study develops. This, in turn, would render changes in the working bibliography. During this critical review of the literature, note taking is kept very brief, since the primary purpose is to judge the appropriateness of the various sources for the research problem.

When it has been determined which sources will be valuable to the proposed study, each one must be read in depth, while at the same time thinking about, reflecting upon, and analyzing what is being said. Particular attention should be given to the problem, hypotheses, procedures, findings, and discussion or implications. While doing **critical reading,** it is essential that the researcher take notes. This has been referred to as developing an annotated bibliography. Even today, with the widespread availability of computers and other electronic equipment, the use of index cards for note taking remains a time honored method for abstracting

Critical reading
The process of reading a large amount of literature while thinking about, reflecting upon, and critically analyzing what is being said.

an article or report. Each card will contain source notes pertaining to the items that have a close relationship to the proposed research. Bibliographic management tools or online applications such as EndNote, ProCite, or RefWorks generally include a notes or abstract field within the database that may be used to record pertinent information from the article or report. Whatever the method, it is important to accurately note all the bibliographic information for each source. Typically, this information includes the author's last name and initials; title of the journal article, book, report, or review; volume or issue number, year, and month of the journal; publisher of the book; date of publication; edition; page numbers of the article or book reference; library call number; and the Internet address (URL) of an online source.

Notes should be taken only from the sources most pertinent to the current problem of interest. In transcribing notes from the source to cards or bibliographic management systems, use extreme care to ensure accuracy. If any of the information will be quoted directly when it appears in the research paper, use quotation marks to identify those items. Record page numbers accurately.

After the notes have been taken from all relevant and pertinent sources, the researcher should gain insight into agreements, differences, relationships, and trends in the literature. When two or more sources do not agree, both sides of the issue should be noted. Beginning researchers sometimes have the mistaken idea that they should seek out only those hypotheses, findings, and conclusions with which they agree.

While notes gathered from reading scholarly journals usually will be the most profitable, notes from speeches, lectures, class discussions, interviews, letters, and even television programs can sometimes provide useful information to a literature review. The point is that no stone should be left unturned during the literature search. It is recognized that with the easy access to copy machines, many graduate students will be tempted to duplicate book chapters and journal articles and highlight appropriate information. With the increasing availability of full-text articles, temptation exists to simply print out relevant information. This is a common way of "taking notes" today. Moreover, it is possible to use an article reproduction or delivery service such as IngentaConnect (www.ingenta.com), among others, to obtain photocopies or PDFs on a fee basis for articles not otherwise available. It is recommended, however, that photocopying be limited to only the key articles or reports; otherwise the expense becomes too great and the task of handling hundreds of sheets of paper becomes onerous. The technique of actually taking notes, rather than merely photocopying every article, will also help researchers focus on the key elements of the report being read and will enhance their understanding of the given topic. Being able to identify the key elements and important findings in published research reports reflects one's ability to critically review the literature and is a mark of the scholarly expertise of the researcher.

Summary of Objectives

1. **Understand the importance of the literature review.**
   Reviewing relevant literature is a crucial step in the research process. Reading related studies and journal articles helps the researcher to better grasp the depth of research already done on a given subject and to better understand the methodology and procedures that have already been applied to it.

2. **Recognize the various sources of literature.** Primary sources, secondary sources—literature exists in many different forms. Periodicals include newspapers, popular magazines, trade publications, and scholarly journals. Moreover, literature is readily available on the Internet and can often be downloaded to computers or handheld devices. Being able to recognize the different forms of literature and choosing literature appropriate for scientific endeavors is an important skill required for any researcher.

3. **Understand how to conduct a literature search.** A firm understanding of how to conduct a computerized search of appropriate literature databases can be extremely helpful in conducting research. With the vast amount of information available today, researchers must be able to efficiently and effectively search appropriate literature sources. Researchers may also use search engines, subject directories, and metasearch engines to obtain information from the Internet.

4. **Establish a system for taking notes and keeping track of sources and citations.** Reading and taking notes is the crux of the process of literature review. Researchers at every level must understand the importance of taking copious notes and know how to carefully reference all material culled from other sources. Keeping track of citations is an important part of this process.

4

Reading and Evaluating Research Reports

OBJECTIVES

A published research report is often the culmination of the research process. The ability to read, understand, and critically evaluate research reports is an important expectation of the professional consumer of the research literature. Although the content will differ, developing a familiarity with the general format of a research report is a first step in becoming an informed consumer. The astute reader should be able to judge the content of the various sections and discern the overall quality of the report and the underlying research.

After reading Chapter 4, you should be able to

1. Explain the purpose of research reports.
2. Understand the various sections of a research report and the information required within each section.
3. Critique and evaluate a research report.

As previously discussed, each of us is a consumer of research information in one way or another. As our knowledge has advanced, the world in which we live has changed dramatically. Our growth as a society is directly related to the knowledge we have acquired through scientific research. Consider the changes that have occurred as a result of the invention of the computer and the exponential growth in computing technologies. We are inundated with product research in our everyday lives—whenever we read the newspaper, listen to the radio, watch television, or browse the Internet. As professionals, our programs and practices are shaped by the results of research in kinesiology. Whether you are a physical education teacher, a school nurse, an exercise specialist, a youth sport coach, or the director of a corporate wellness program, you have an obligation to those you serve to provide appropriate programs and services in an effectual manner. Keeping abreast of the contemporary knowledge in your field is essential. Therefore, as a research consumer, you will undoubtedly have cause to read and evaluate research reports.

    A quintessential characteristic of the scientific method is the public disclosure of the findings and the knowledge acquired. Therefore, the culmination of the research process is the disclosure, in one form or another, of the findings of the research study. Frequently, this means a written research report published in a professional journal. A research report is really

TABLE 4.1 Typical Contents within a Research Report

- Preliminary Information
  - Title
  - Author and organizational affiliation
  - Acknowledgments (if any)
  - Abstract
- Introduction
  - Background information and literature review
  - Rationale for study
  - Purpose statement
  - Hypotheses or research questions
- Methods
  - Participants
  - Instrumentation
  - Procedures
  - Statistical analysis
- Results
  - Presentation of data
- Discussion
  - Conclusions
  - Recommendations
- References
- Appendix (if appropriate)

nothing more than a report summarizing the researchers' activities and the results of the study. Although there may be some variation in terminology as well as in the arrangement of the different sections, almost all published research reports follow a similar format. In general, research reports typically include the following main sections: introduction, methods, results, discussion, and references. The outline shown in Table 4.1 illustrates a typical format used in published research reports. In the remainder of this chapter, you will learn more about the content of research reports and you will acquire information to help you evaluate such reports.

PRELIMINARY INFORMATION

Preliminary items
Introductory material in a published research report may include title, author, institution, acknowledgments, and abstract.

The **preliminary items** usually include the title, author and organizational affiliation, acknowledgments (if applicable), and abstract.

The title of the research article should be clear and concise, yet accurately reflect the content of the research study. A title should generally be less than 15 words in length, should identify the key variables, and should provide some information about the scope of the study. Since indexing and Internet searching are tied to the key words of an article, authors should carefully select words for the title.

The authors' names usually appear beneath the article title and, typically, are ordered in accordance with the relative contributions made to the research study. The institutional or organizational affiliation of each author usually appears in a footnote or in a special box located on the first page of the article. In some journals, the highest degree earned, special titles (for example, FACSM, designating Fellow, American College of Sports Medicine), and the current position of each author are also presented. Moreover, the mailing address or e-mail address of the primary author is usually provided in order to facilitate communication by readers who may have questions or want article reprints.

Authors often acknowledge individuals who have contributed in some way to the research or to the writing of the report. The acknowledgments may include persons who have assisted with the design of the study, with data collection, and/ or with statistical analysis, or someone who has reviewed the manuscript. In addition, specific acknowledgment should be made of any sponsoring agency or funding source. **Acknowledgments** usually appear in an author's note that is located either at the beginning or end of the article, depending upon the journal. See Example 4.1.

Journal **abstracts,** typically 150 to 200 words long, depending upon the journal, are usually located at the beginning of the article, immediately following the title and authors' names. Quite frequently, abstracts are set in a special type (i.e., italics) or indented to distinguish them from the main article. An abstract is a brief summary of the research study and should include a succinct description of the problem, information about the participants and methods used to investigate the problem, a concise summation of the findings, and conclusions drawn from the study. According to Huck (2000, 2), "the sole purpose of the abstract is to provide readers with an overview of the material they will encounter in the remaining portions of the article." Inasmuch as an abstract should provide an overview of a research study, it is inappropriate for an abstract to simply state "The results are provided," or "The conclusions and recommendations are presented." Example 4.2 illustrates a variety of published abstracts. It should be noted that not all journals require abstracts. Additional information about abstracts is presented in Chapter 17.

Acknowledgments
Preliminary item in a research report in which the author lists the contributions of others who have assisted with the research.

Abstract
Preliminary item in a research report that provides a brief summary of the research study.

Acknowledgments

Support for the RENO Diet Heart Study has been provided by grant #HL34589 from the National Heart, Lung, and Blood Institute of the National Institutes of Health. The authors are grateful to Michaela Kiernen for technical assistance, to Linda Bartoshuk, PhD, for guidance and insight, and to Catherine Sananes Katz, PhD, for critical review of the manuscript.

EXAMPLE 4.1
Acknowledgments

From Katz, D. L., Brunner, R. L., St. Jeor, S. T., Scott, B., Jekel, J. F., and Brownell, K. D. (1998). Dietary fat consumption in a cohort of American adults, 1985–1991: Covariates, secular trends, and compliance with guidelines. *American Journal of Health Promotion,* 12(6), 382–390.

EXAMPLE 4.2

Abstracts

1: From Wen, L. M., van der Ploeg, H. P., Kite, J., Cashmore, A., and Rissel, C. (2010). A validation study of assessing physical activity and sedentary behavior in children aged 3 to 5 years. *Pediatric Exercise Science,* 22(3), 408–420.

2: From Etnier, J. L. and Landers, D. M. (1998). Motor performance and motor learning as a function of age and fitness. *Research Quarterly for Exercise and Sport,* 69(2), 139–146.

Abstract [1]

Assessing young children's physical activity and sedentary behavior can be challenging and costly. This study aimed to assess the validity of a brief survey about activity preferences as a proxy of physical activity and of a 7-day activity diary, both completed by the parents and using accelerometers as a reference measure. Thirty-four parents and their children (aged 3–5 years) who attended childcare centers in Sydney (Australia) were recruited for the study. Parents were asked to complete a 9-item brief survey about activity preferences of their child and a 7-day diary recording the child's physical activity and sedentary behaviors. Both measures were compared with accelerometer data collected from the child over the same period as the diary survey. The findings suggest that parent-completed diaries have acceptable correlation coefficients with accelerometer measures and could be considered in future research assessing physical activity and sedentary behavior of children aged 3–5 years.

Abstract [2]

Past studies have shown that electroencephalographic alpha activity increases as people learn to perform a novel motor task. Additionally, it has been suggested that motor performance and learning decline as people age beyond 60 years, and it has been hypothesized that physical fitness may attenuate this decline through its impact on the cerebral environment. This study was designed to replicate past research by assessing changes in alpha activity as a function of learning and to extend past research by examining differences in motor performance, motor learning, and alpha activity as a function of age and fitness. VO_2max was assessed in 41 older (ages 60–80 years) and 42 younger (ages 20–30 years) participants. Participants were randomly assigned to experimental or control conditions, which differed in the amount of practice received. Participants performed trials on the mirror star trace on both an acquisition and a retention day. Results indicated that younger participants performed better and had greater learning than older participants. Fitness was not found to impact either performance or learning. Participants in the experimental group improved more than those in the control group and maintained this difference at retention, which suggests that learning occurred. Associated with these improvements in performance capabilities was an increase in alpha power.

INTRODUCTION

The **introduction section** normally appears immediately following the abstract and often is presented in published form without the use of a heading preceding the content. The introductory section of an article generally contains two primary elements: (a) background information and (b) a statement describing the purpose of the study. Some articles may also include the researcher's hypotheses. A well-written introduction section will not only enable the reader to clearly understand the problem being investigated but also provide critical background literature that helps the reader understand why the author conducted the study.

Typically, the background portion of the introduction acquaints the reader with the problem and establishes the foundation and rationale for conducting the study. The length of this portion of the introduction varies substantially depending upon the nature of the problem being investigated and the amount of related literature. It may be as short as only a single paragraph, but more likely it will be several paragraphs in length. Because of space limitations in most journals, the **background information** does not represent a comprehensive review of literature of the topic being studied, but it should include references to the most important and timely literature. In explaining the underlying basis for their study, authors will often point to gaps in the existing literature, contradictory results or unexpected findings from previous research, and the likely practical benefits to be derived from their study. It is important that the authors make the connection between their study and similar research or published materials.

The author(s) will usually state the specific **purpose statement** near the end of the introduction section, although it could be positioned anywhere in the introduction. It is usually pretty easy to locate the purpose statement, as researchers often use wording such as

- "The purpose of this study was to . . . "
- "This study was designed to . . . "
- "This investigation sought to . . . "
- "The present study explored . . . "

The statement of purpose is often only one sentence long, although it could be a couple of sentences, or even a short paragraph. A well-written purpose statement will enable the reader to identify the key variables in the study as well as understand something about the scope of the study. Examples of purpose statements from published articles are shown in Example 4.3. Although it is becoming less common, authors will occasionally state their research hypotheses in a paragraph immediately following the purpose statement. It is rare today for authors of published articles to state the hypothesis in the null form, preferring instead to specify the research hypothesis, or the predicted outcome of the study. In lieu of stating

Introduction section
The introductory portion of a research report that provides background information and develops the rationale for conducting the study.

Background information
Important literature on the topic being investigated that is cited in the introductory section of a research report, thus establishing the foundation for the study.

Purpose statement
A specific statement expressing the researcher's intent or goal for conducting the study.

EXAMPLE 4.3
Purpose Statements
1: From Thomas, D. Q., Bowdoin, B. A., Brown, D. D., and McCaw, S. T. (1998). Nasal strips and mouthpieces do not affect power output during anaerobic exercise. *Research Quarterly for Exercise and Sport,* 69(2), 201–204.
2: From Agbuga, B., Xiang, P., and McBride, R. (2010). Achievement goals and their relations to children's disruptive behaviors in an after-school physical activity program. *Journal of Teaching in Physical Education,* 29(3), 278–294.
3: From O'Neill, D. E. T., Thayer, R. E., Taylor, A. W., Dzialoznski, T. M., and Noble, E. G. (2000). Effects of short-term resistance training on muscle strength and morphology in the elderly. *Journal of Aging and Physical Activity,* 8(4), 312–324.
4: From Eisenmann, J. C., Sarzynski, M. A., Tucker, J., and Heelan, K. A. (2010). Maternal prepregnancy overweight and offspring fatness and blood pressure: Role of physical activity. *Pediatric Exercise Science,* 22(3), 369–378.

Purpose Statement [1]

Therefore, the purpose of this study was to determine the effect of utilizing nasal strips or athletic mouthpieces or both on anaerobic exercise performance.

Purpose Statement [2]

In sum, this study used the trichotomous model to examine achievement goals and their relations to disruptive behaviors among elementary school students in an after-school physical activity program. Specifically, the following research questions were addressed: (a) What achievement goals do students endorse in their after-school physical activity classes? (b) To what extent do students demonstrate disruptive behaviors in their after-school physical activity classes? And (c) What are the relationships between children's achievement goals and disruptive behaviors?

Purpose Statement [3]

The aim of the present study was to examine muscles of elderly participants after an 8-week resistance-training regimen, using information provided by biopsy sampling to assess the extent of change in selected muscle-fiber characteristics.

Purpose Statement [4]

The primary purpose of this study was to examine the combined influence of maternal prepregnancy weight status and offspring physical activity on offspring fatness and BP.

---

hypotheses, sometimes authors may provide a listing of research questions that the study proposes to answer. Regardless of the specific format and organization, after reading an introduction section the reader should have a clear understanding of what is being studied and why it is being studied.

Methods section
Section of a research report that describes the research participants, instrumentation, and procedures for data collection.

METHODS

The next major part of most published research articles is the **methods section,** generally identifiable by a section heading titled, *Methods, Methodology, Procedures,* or something similar. Here the author provides a description of the research participants, research instruments, and procedures for the administration of treatments as well as for data collection. Sometimes the author will also provide information about the data analysis. It is fairly common for each of these parts to be presented as a specific subsection, complete with a subheading, within the methods section of a published research report. The methods section tends to be highly structured and should contain detailed statements explaining the methodology used to conduct the study. Ideally, the entire methods section should be written in such a way that would enable an interested and qualified reader to replicate the study using the same methodology.

Research Participants

Typically, the first part of the methods section is used to describe the **research participants** (subjects). This should include information about the target population, the number of participants, and how they were selected. In addition, pertinent characteristics of the participants, such as age, gender, grade level, socioeconomic level, ethnicity, and any other characteristics that may have a bearing on the problem being studied should be described. If appropriate to the study, the author should also describe how participants were assigned to comparison groups or treatment groups. It is important that the author carefully describe how the research participants were obtained, including a description of the population, thus enabling the reader to make a judgment about the generalizability of the results. Were they volunteers? Were they randomly selected? What selection criteria were established? What sampling technique was used? Chapter 7 provides a full description of various sampling techniques and the process of selecting research participants. When sampling procedures are not well defined, it is wise to believe that a convenience sample was used. See Example 4.4 for examples of excerpts from published articles describing research participants.

Research participants
People participating in a research study; portion of the methods section of a research report used to present information about the people being studied.

Instrumentation

This subsection of a journal article should contain a description of data collection instruments, materials, and any equipment or apparatus used in the study. Given the diverse nature of kinesiology research, **instrumentation** may vary substantially. For some researchers, instrumentation is largely a paper-and-pencil variety and may include tests, checklists, scales, inventories, questionnaires, interview schedules, or observation reports. Other researchers, however, utilize specialized equipment for data collection, such as skinfold calipers, timing devices, strength gauges, metabolic measurement systems, cinematographic equipment, and heart monitors, among others. Furthermore, some researchers utilize standardized performance tests, such as sport skills tests or physical fitness tests as their means of collecting data.

    Whereas space limitations within the journal may prohibit the actual reproduction of a written instrument in the article itself, authors should provide a complete

Instrumentation
Portion of the methods section of a research report describing the measuring instrument or equipment, such as a questionnaire, test, or inventory, used to collect data from the research participants.

EXAMPLE 4.4
Methods: Research
Participants

1: From Weiss, M. R.,
McCullagh, P., Smith, A. L.,
and Berlant, A. R. (1998).
Observational learning and the
fearful child: Influence of peer
models on swimming skill
performance and psychological
responses. *Research Quarterly
for Exercise and Sport,* 69(4),
380–394.
2: From Papaioannou, A. (1998).
Students' perceptions of the
physical education class
environment for boys and girls
and the perceived motivational
climate. *Research Quarterly
for Exercise and Sport,* 69(3),
267–275.

Participants [1]

Children were recruited from community school or nonschool youth programs. Program instructors and parents were asked to identify children who had minimal swimming experience, were fearful of the water, and had low self-confidence. In all, 24 children (18 boys and 6 girls) met these criteria. Their average age was 6.2 years ($SD = .90$), 62.5% ($n = 15$) had taken formal swimming lessons, and they averaged 9.5 ($SD = 11.4$; range = 0 to 40) weeks of swimming lesson experience. Children were matched to group by age and lesson experience, and then groups were randomly assigned to one of three model type conditions: control, peer mastery, and peer coping. All parents provided informed consent prior to study procedures, and children signed an assent form on the first day of the study prior to any swimming skill or questionnaire assessments.

Participants [2]

The 310 adolescents participating in this study were enrolled in six junior high schools ($n = 77$ boys, $n = 64$ girls; M age = 13.5 years, $SD = 1.5$) and six senior high schools ($n = 76$ boys, $n = 93$ girls; M age = 16.5 years, $SD = 1.5$). All physical education classes were coeducational and taught by 12 physical education teachers, 3 male and 3 female teachers in junior high schools and 3 male and 3 female teachers in senior high schools. These schools were randomly selected from the total number of schools in Thessaloniki, Greece, a town with 1 million residents.

description of the instrument, including pertinent psychometric properties (i.e., validity and reliability), if available. Similarly, equipment or research apparatus should be thoroughly described, including evidence of its technical properties. Sometimes illustrations or photographs of testing equipment may be used to supplement the written description.

Researchers utilizing published instruments or commercially available equipment often cite manufacturer's specifications or the work of other researchers as the basis of asserting the validity and reliability of the chosen instrument. If the measuring instrument is new and specifically designed for the study described in the article, the authors would be expected to go to greater lengths describing the development of the instrument as well as pertinent validity and reliability evidence. The main concern for the author(s) is to establish that the instrumentation used in the study was appropriate for the particular research problem and that it enabled the researchers to collect accurate and credible information. Example 4.5 provides illustrations of instrumentation sections in published articles.

Instrumentation [1]

Intrinsic motivation was assessed using a sport-oriented version of the Intrinsic Motivation Inventory (IMI; McAuley, Duncan, & Tammen, 1989). An original version of the IMI was used by R. Ryan and his colleagues (e.g., Plant & Ryan, 1985; R. Ryan, Mims, & Koestner, 1983) as a multidimensional measure of subjects' intrinsic motivation for a specific achievement activity. McAuley et al.'s sport-oriented version of the IMI contains 16 items that assess four components of intrinsic motivation, including interest-enjoyment, perceived competence, effort-importance, and tension-pressure. McAuley et al. reported acceptable psychometric properties for the four subscales.

A fifth subscale was included in the current study questionnaire based on suggestions by McAuley et al. (1989). This additional subscale, labeled *perceived choice,* included four items to assess the degree to which athletes believe they are participating in their sport by personal choice. The four items include the following: (a) "I participate in this sport because I want to", (b) "I would quit this sport if I could", (c) "Working hard in this sport is something I choose to do", and (d) "When my eligibility is up I will quit this sport."

Each item on the IMI is followed by a 7-point Likert-type scale, with response choices ranging from *strongly disagree* to *strongly agree.* Subjects are asked to indicate their agreement or disagreement with each statement by circling the appropriate response.

Instrumentation [2]

Based on a comprehensive review of the literature, a 12-item instrument was developed to assess subjects' perceived self-efficacy in performing life-saving skills and the impact of training on subjects' willingness to act during an emergency and in the presence of noted barriers. The instrument consisted of four demographic items (age, gender, race, and education level) and five background items (level of previous training, first aid requirement for college major or job, reasons for taking the first aid course, field of study, and previous experience in giving first aid and CPR). The instrument also contained questions based on Bandura's self-efficacy model. Efficacy expectations, outcome expectations, and outcome values subscales consisted of three items each. The remaining questions contained three items examining subjects'

EXAMPLE 4.5
Methods: Instrumentation
1: From Amorose, A. J. and Horn, T. S. (2000). Intrinsic motivation: Relationships with collegiate athletes' gender, scholarship status, and perceptions of their coaches' behavior. *Journal of Sport and Exercise Psychology,* 22(1), 63–84.
2: From Kandakai, T. L. and King, K. A. (1999). Perceived self-efficacy in performing lifesaving skills: An assessment of the American Red Cross's responding to emergencies course. *Journal of Health Education,* 30(4), 235–241.

(Continued)

EXAMPLE 4.5
Concluded

willingness to perform lifesaving skills in the presence of specified barriers.

To establish face validity, items in the survey instrument were constructed based on a comprehensive review of the literature. Content validity was established by distributing the instrument to three national experts in survey research and one national expert on the self-efficacy model. Experts were defined as individuals who were recognized authorities on survey research or the self-efficacy model and who had recently published articles on these topics. Recommendations offered by experts were taken under consideration and appropriate revisions were made to the survey instrument. Stability reliability was assessed utilizing a sample of 25 male and female undergraduate college students who were given the instrument twice, 5 days apart.

Procedures

Procedures
Portion of the methods section of a research report that includes a description of data collection procedures, experimental treatments, and how they were administered; a step-by-step description of how the study was conducted.

The **procedures** portion of the methods section includes a description of data collection procedures as well as experimental treatments and how they were administered. Basically this is a description, step by step, of how the researcher conducted the study. Where was the study performed? What did the research participants do? What did the researcher do? Who collected the data? How long did it take? What safeguards were provided? The procedures should be presented with sufficient detail and clarity that another researcher would be able to follow the steps described and replicate the study. You might consider this to be the "recipe" for conducting the study.

For experimental studies, this section should also include a description of the research design, clearly identifying the independent and dependent variables, and describing the experimental treatments. It is important that the research design be appropriate to the solution of the research problem and be relatively free of threats to the validity of the study. See Chapter 8 for a more thorough discussion of internal and external validity. All studies will include a description of the data collection procedures. These procedures should be appropriate to the research participants and should correctly use the selected measuring instruments. Although not seen in all published research articles, sometimes a description of the **data analysis** procedures will be included here. This approach is typical in theses and dissertations. Otherwise, the data analysis procedures are described in the results section. Examples of procedures sections are shown in Example 4.6.

Data analysis
The methods of manipulating and analyzing the collected data to reveal relevant information.

Data Collection [1]

Each participant completed a continuous graded treadmill test using the Bruce protocol (Bruce, Kusumi, & Hosmer, 1973) to determine both HRmax and VO_2max. The treadmill tests were performed under the supervision of specifically trained, qualified medical personnel throughout the day over a collection period of approximately 6 months. During each maximal exercise test, oxygen consumption was measured continuously by open-circuit spirometry using a Beckman metabolic Cart (Beckman Instruments, Schiller Park, IL). A participant's heart rate response was determined electrocardiographically from the V_5 position. For that purpose, electrocardiogram chart paper recordings were obtained during the last 30 s of each completed exercise stage and continuously once a participant signaled that he or she was approaching exhaustion. Individual HRmax was defined as the highest heart rate achieved (15-s R-R interval count), which usually occurred during the last minute of exercise.

Data Collection [2]

On a separate day, subjects returned to the laboratory 3 h after eating. Subjects did not ingest caffeine overnight or before the test. Subjects again warmed up at $14 \text{ km} \cdot \text{h}^{-1}$ for 5 min. Subjects then completed two submaximal workloads, one at $16.1 \text{ km} \cdot \text{h}^{-1}$ and the other at current 10-km race pace, with all subjects utilizing the same calibrated treadmill (Powerjog EG30, Birmingham, England). Each workload was undertaken for 6 min separated by a rest period of 5 min. VO_2, V_E, RER, and HR were measured continuously and results averaged over 15-s intervals. Mean values of the last 60 s were designated as steady state values for data analysis. A venous blood sample was obtained exactly 1 min after exercise for each workload for determination of plasma ammonia and plasma lactate concentrations. Samples were immediately centrifuged at 4°C at 3000 rpm and plasma was obtained. Plasma ammonia was assayed spectrophotometrically in duplicate within 2 h (NH_3 kit, Boehringer Mannheim), and plasma was stored for later spectrophotometric analysis of lactate in duplicate (bioMerieux lactate PAP, Boehringer Mannheim).

EXAMPLE 4.6
Methods: Procedures

1: From Engels, H. J., Zhu, W., and Moffatt, R. J. (1998). An empirical evaluation of the prediction of maximal heart rate. *Research Quarterly for Exercise and Sport,* 69(1), 94–98.

2: From Weston, A. R., Mbambo, Z., and Myburgh, K. H. (2000). Running economy of African and Caucasian distance runners. *Medicine and Science in Sports and Exercise,* 32(6), 1130–1134.

RESULTS

The **results section** of a published article is where the researcher reports the results of the data collection efforts as well as the outcomes of the various statistical treatments that were applied to the data. If the data analysis procedures were not previously discussed under the methods section, that information would be presented here. For many readers of research reports, the results section is the most difficult part to read and understand because of all the statistical information and numerical data. As a consequence, many readers simply skip over the results section. Yet in order to become an astute consumer of the research literature, you will need to develop some level of competence in reading and understanding results sections. Chapters 13 and 14 describe common descriptive and inferential statistical techniques frequently seen in the research literature. For a more in-depth explanation of the various statistical techniques, readers are referred to basic statistics textbooks such as Harris (1998) or Gravetter and Wallnau (2008).

The nature of the research problem will determine, to a large extent, the type of statistical technique that is used. We previously saw that research questions generally fall into three categories: descriptive, relationship, and difference. Statistical techniques can also be grouped into these same three categories. Therefore, if the reader of a research article can identify the type of questions(s) being asked, this is a first step in understanding what general category of statistics is required to answer the question. It is important to note that a single research study will usually contain more than one research question; therefore, it is likely that several different statistical techniques will be used within a single study. Consequently, the results section will likely include the outcomes of several statistical techniques.

Results sections should not contain a discussion, explanation, or interpretation of the results (Tuckman 1999). This information will follow in the discussion section. Demographic information about the research participants, if not previously presented in the methods section, is usually presented first, followed by the more substantive findings related to the research questions. Results sections are often organized around each hypothesis or each research question of the study. Most articles, regardless of the type of research, will generally report basic descriptive statistics, such as means, standard deviations, frequencies, and percentages for the key variables. Studies asking relationship questions as well as those asking difference questions will also report correlational statistics and inferential statistics, as appropriate. The use of tables and figures to complement the information reported in the text of published articles is commonplace. Tables and figures should always follow their contextual reference.

While it is impossible to indicate exactly what information should be presented in a results section, some general guidelines may be helpful. Ultimately, the nature of the research problem being studied and the statistical procedures utilized will go a long way in determining the precise content in the results section. In accordance with the recommendations of Tuckman (1999), we suggest that the following elements, if appropriate for the study, should be included in a results section:

1. A brief restatement of each hypothesis
2. An indication of the descriptive statistics used (e.g., means, standard deviations)
3. An indication of the inferential statistics used (e.g., t-test, ANOVA, correlations)
4. Specification of the significance level used for hypothesis testing
5. A brief statement identifying the statistical assumptions examined
6. The anticipated effect size and power of the statistical test used
7. The results of the statistical tests (including t-values, F-ratios, probability levels, and degrees of freedom, if appropriate)
8. The magnitude of the effect obtained
9. An indication as to whether the null hypothesis was accepted or rejected

In qualitative studies, researchers often have notes from interviews or field observations that must be organized and synthesized. Qualitative researchers generally do not have numerical data to report or analyze. Consequently, the results section of a qualitative study takes on a different appearance, one that is largely a narrative presentation of the findings, often supported by the words of the participants, including direct quotations. More information about qualitative research is found in chapter 10 of this textbook.

Example 4.7 presents examples of results sections from various published reports. Note that each example represents only a portion of the complete section in the published article. Several examples also refer to tables or figures that have not been reproduced here.

DISCUSSION

The **discussion section** of a journal article contains a nontechnical explanation of the results. Basically, the discussion section is where the author presents the outcomes of the study. Here, the author provides his or her interpretation of the findings, culminating with a conclusion that provides an answer to the research problem. Note that some authors may include in the paper a separate section

Discussion section Section of a research report containing a nontechnical explanation or interpretation of the results, culminating with the researcher's conclusions.

EXAMPLE 4.7
Results

1: From Prohaska, T. R., Peters, K., and Warren, J. S. (2000). Sources of attrition in a church-based exercise program for older African-Americans. *American Journal of Health Promotion,* 14(6), 380–385.

2: From Amorose, A. J. and Horn, T. S. (2000). Intrinsic motivation: Relationships with collegiate athletes' gender, scholarship status, and perceptions of their coaches' behavior. *Journal of Sport and Exercise Psychology,* 22(1), 63–84.

3: From Spencer, L. (1999). College freshmen smokers versus nonsmokers: Academic, social and emotional expectations and attitudes toward college. *Journal of Health Education,* 30(5), 274–281.

4: From Etnier, J. L. and Landers, D. M. (1988). Motor performance and motor learning as a function of age and fitness. *Research Quarterly for Exercise and Sport,* 69(2), 139–146.

Results [1]

A total of 53 (43%) older adults had dropped out of the exercise program within 4 months. There were no demographic differences found between those who dropped out of the exercise program and those who remained, except for education level. Education level differed significantly between the two groups; a greater proportion of the attrition group reported less than a 12th-grade education ($x^2 = 7.33$, $p < .05$).

Health differences were found between the exercise attrition group and those who completed the program (Table 2). Compared with those who continued in the exercise program, the attrition group reported poorer self-ratings of health ($x^2 = 6.0$, $p < .05$), a greater frequency of not having enough energy to do the things they need to do ($x^2 = 6.57$, $p < .05$), and that they climbed fewer flights of stairs per day. If the PAR-Q scale had been used as an eligibility screening tool, a greater proportion of attrition group individuals would have been considered ineligible for the program, as more of them reported having one or more problems on the revised PAR-Q scale indicating greater health risk ($x^2 = 3.58$, $p = .058$).

Results [2]

Intrinsic Motivation, Gender, and Scholarship Status. To test whether athletes' intrinsic motivation would vary as a function of their gender, scholarship status, and perceived percentage of athletes on scholarship, a 2 × 3 × 2 (gender by scholarship status by scholarship percentage) MANOVA was conducted. The dependent variables for this analysis were the five subscale scores from the IMI (interest-enjoyment, perceived competence, effort-importance, perceived choice, and tension-pressure). The independent variables were gender (male, female), scholarship status (full, partial, none) and perceived scholarship percentage (low: ≤ 70%, high: ≥ 75%). The descriptive statistics for each group are presented in Table 3.

Due to the nonorthogonal nature of the research design, the significance of the main and interaction effects was tested in hierarchical fashion (Finn, 1974; Tabachnick & Fidell, 1996). This procedure revealed a nonsignificant three-way (gender by scholarship status by scholarship percentage) interaction effect. In addition, the Scholarship Status × Scholarship Percentage interaction, the Gender × Scholarship Status

(Continued)

EXAMPLE 4.7
Continued

interaction, and the Gender $\times$ Scholarship Percentage interaction were all nonsignificant. The scholarship percentage main effect was also nonsignificant. However, both the scholarship status main effect, Wilks's lambda $= .94$, $F(10, 740) = 2.37$, $p < .01$, and the gender main effect, Wilks's lambda $= .97$, $F(5, 370) = 2.39$, $p < .04$, were significant.

Results [3]

The Freshman Survey with tobacco-related questions was completed by 544 first-semester freshmen. Both genders were fairly equally represented, with 305 (56%) females and 232 (43%) males completing the survey (7 students did not indicate gender). Unfortunately, the survey instrument did not include a question about race or ethnicity; however, other sources provided this information about the entire freshman class ($n = 1142$). Eighty-three percent ($n = 943$) of the class was white, 7% ($n = 83$) was African-American, 6% ($n = 69$) was Hispanic, 3% ($n = 29$) was Asian, one was Native American, and 1% ($n = 17$) did not indicate ethnicity.

Sixty-six percent of respondents ($n = 360$) reported that they have never been smokers. Twenty-seven percent ($n = 148$) reported smoking either regularly (more than 1 day per week) or occasionally (1 day per week or less). Specifically, regular smokers were more prevalent ($n = 91$) than occasional smokers ($n = 57$). Among all smokers, 86 (58%) were female, 56 (38%) were male, and 6 (4%) did not indicate gender. Only 7% of respondents ($n = 36$) reported being former smokers. Among current smokers, the average age of smoking initiation was 16 years, with a range of 8–18 years. Former smokers began smoking at age 14 and smoked for 2 years before quitting, on average.

Results [4]

Demographic data are presented in Table 1 as a function of Age Group, Fitness Group, and Treatment Group. Results showed no significant difference in years of education since high school as a function of Age Group, Fitness Group, or Treatment Group ($p > .05$). There was a significant main effect for Fitness Group on weight, $F(1,79) = 11.03$, $p < .001$, such that fit participants ($M = 76.03$ kg, $SD = 9.12$) weighed significantly less than unfit participants ($M = 83.86$ kg, $SD = 11.80$). There was also a significant main effect for Age Group on self-reported

(Continued)

EXAMPLE 4.7
Concluded

physical activity level, $F(1, 79) = 13.91$, $p < .001$, such that the scores for the older participants ($M = 11.63$, $SD = 7.51$) were significantly higher than those for the younger ones ($M = 7.09$, $SD = 1.32$). For VO_2 max, there was a significant main effect for Age Group, $F(1, 79) = 146.14$, $p < .001$, such that younger participants ($M = 43.05$ ml/kg/min, $SD = 9.15$) were significantly more fit than older participants ($M = 28.30$ ml/kg/min, $SD = 9.82$). Examination of the time interval between acquisition and retention trials indicated that there was not a significant difference as a function of Age Group, Fitness Group, Treatment Group, or the interactions of these variables, $F(1, 75) = 0.00 - 2.65$, $p > .05$. Importantly, for the older participants, there was no significant difference in years since retirement as a function of Fitness Group, Treatment Group, or their interaction ($p > .05$).

Conclusions
A closing portion of a research report in which the author provides an answer to the research problem.

labeled **Conclusions.** The discussion section is often the least structured of the research report, enabling the author to take considerable latitude in the writing. However, if the study was set up to test hypotheses, the discussion section should include a report on the results of each hypothesis test. Tuckman (1999) suggests that the discussion section of a research report serves six major functions:

- **To summarize the findings**—a rather straightforward function is to provide a summary of the major findings in the form of conclusions, thus providing the reader with an overall picture of the results.

- **To interpret the study's findings**—the author's explanation or interpretation of what the results mean. (Note: We would propose that this may be the most important function of the discussion section.)

- **To integrate the findings**—an attempt to synthesize the various findings, both expected and unexpected, to achieve meaningful conclusions and generalizations.

- **To theorize**—occasionally, a study generates a number of interrelated findings that might serve as the basis for theory development, either as support for existing theory or for the establishment of original theory.

Recommendations
Portion of a research report, often included in the discussion section, in which the researcher presents suggestions for professional practice and/ or further research based upon the findings of the current research study.

- **To recommend or apply**—since results from research frequently have implications for enhancing or altering professional practices, the discussion section provides the venue for making such **recommendations.**

- **To suggest extensions**—inevitably, the results of a research study give rise to more questions; the discussion section of a report often includes recommendations for future research.

While each of these functions may not be served in the discussion section of every published research report, it is important to realize the breadth of possible content. It is common for the discussion section to begin with a brief restatement of the purpose of the study, followed by a general statement summarizing the results. This is usually followed with a more detailed discussion of the specific findings. The discussion section generally does not contain the statistical notation and numerical information found in reporting the results, but usually consists of a narrative discussion in which the author summarizes and explains what the results mean, often attempting to explain why the results turned out as they did. In explaining the results, the author attempts to connect the results of the study with appropriate theory, professional practice, and the related literature. The author should be careful to avoid reaching conclusions that are not supported by the results of the study. Moreover, the author should present only implications and recommendations that are based on the results of the study, not on what the author had hoped to be true. Sometimes the author cautions the reader about possible misinterpretations, pointing out the limitations associated with the research. A common error made by researchers as well as by consumers of the research literature is to overgeneralize the results, that is, attempt to apply the findings and resultant conclusions to settings or populations that are not warranted by the study. Generalizability of research findings is discussed in more detail in Chapter 8 under the topic "external validity." Example 4.8 provides excerpts taken from discussion sections in published reports. Please note that each excerpt is only a portion of a complete section.

Discussion [1]

This study supports the literature that shows males are more likely to be current users of smokeless tobacco over females[1,6,9,24,25] and smokeless tobacco use increases with age.[3,6,8] However, the ethnic diversity of use found is very different from what is reported in the literature. This study found that Hispanics were more likely to be current users (11.4%) than Whites (4.2%), Blacks (2.1%), or Others (6.8%). Studies have reported Hispanics have a higher prevalence of smoking and using smokeless tobacco than Black or "other" ethnic groups,[6,8,25–27] but none of those studies reported higher use in Hispanics than in Whites. Since North Carolina is a tobacco-producing state, perhaps patterns of use are different compared to national samples. This fact makes interpretation of these results difficult and underscores the need for further research on smokeless tobacco use in ethnic minority groups.

(Continued)

EXAMPLE 4.8
Discussions
1: From Lewis, P. C., Harrell, J. S., Deng, S., and Bradley, C. (1999). Smokeless tobacco use in adolescents: The cardiovascular health in children study. *Journal of School Health,* 69(8), 320–325.
2: From Behlendorf, B., MacRae, P. G., and Vos Strache, C. (1999). Children's perceptions of physical activity for adults: Competence and appropriateness. *Journal of Aging and Physical Activity,* 7(4), 354–373.
3: From Cheatham, C. C., Mahon, A. D., Brown, J. D., and Bolster, D. R. (2000). Cardiovascular responses during prolonged exercise at ventilatory threshold. *Medicine and Science in Sports and Exercise,* 32(3), 1080–1087.

EXAMPLE 4.8
Concluded

Discussion [2]

Competence

As hypothesized, age was the most significant factor in determining the perceived competence of the adults involved in the three physical activities. The main effect for age accounted for 61% of the variance, whereas type of physical activity accounted for 8% and gender accounted for 0%. The results indicate that the older adults were perceived as less competent than the middle-aged adults, who were viewed as less competent than the young adults. These findings support those of Ostrow et al. (1987), who reported that preschoolers' perceptions of motor skill proficiency decreased as the age of the referent person increased from 20 to 40 to 60 to 80 years. Similarly, Kite and Johnson (1988) found in their meta-analysis that measures of competence in older adults were more negatively rated than in young adults. They cautioned that it is unlikely that older people are evaluated more negatively than young people on all dimensions. For example, the elderly might be seen as less competent or physically attractive than young people but might not be seen as less kind, friendly, or satisfied (Deaux & Lewis, 1984). A multidimensional approach that includes physical, cognitive, social, and affective aspects of older adults might be more informative and lead to greater insights in understanding age effects on perceived competence.

Discussion [3]

In conclusion, the results of this study indicate that the cardiovascular responses to prolonged exercise are similar in boys and men. Specifically, the magnitude of cardiovascular drift is similar between boys and men, although there is a tendency for the increase in HR and decrease in SV to be somewhat higher in adults. In addition, the cardiovascular responses during prolonged exercise at VT are similar to previous studies examining prolonged exercise in children and adults relative to VO_{2max}. Therefore, it seems that the cardiovascular responses to prolonged constant-load exercise are somewhat independent of whether the intensity is below or above VT, and thus individual differences in VT may not be a concern during prolonged constant-load exercise, although whether this idea applies to exercise at equal intensities above VT is unclear and worthy of future research.

REFERENCES AND APPENDIX

Following the text of the published article will be a list of **references.** This list includes all books, journal articles, or other sources that were cited by the author. The format of the reference list will vary according to the publication guidelines of the specific journal. Regardless of the style manual specified, every item in the reference list should have been cited in the text of the paper and every source cited in the paper should be included in the reference list. The reference list is an excellent place to obtain information about articles, books, or other sources that pertain to the topic under investigation.

Readers are advised to carefully note the references cited, taking into consideration such factors as the date of publication and the nature of the journal or publication source. For instance, an article in which most of the references are 25–30 years old should be viewed cautiously. While there may be legitimate reasons for a preponderance of old references, an astute reader of the research literature should at least ask the question, "Why?" In addition, a lengthy reference list does not necessarily mean a quality article. Locke, Spirduso, and Silverman (2007) point out that the use of nonselective references may be an indication of poor scholarship and may reflect the inability of the author to differentiate between the trivial and the important in research.

Some published articles may also include a notes section or appendix at the end of the article. A notes section is a likely place to locate acknowledgments and may be positioned either at the beginning of the article or at the end, depending upon the requirements of the journal. Although less likely to be seen in published articles because of space limitations, appendixes may be used to include copies of questionnaires, inventories, tabular information, special materials, or even illustrations of testing equipment.

References
Lists of all books, journal articles, or other sources cited by the author in a research report.

CRITIQUING A RESEARCH ARTICLE

The mere fact that a research study has been completed or even published does not necessarily mean that the study was good or that it was reported correctly (Gay, Mills, and Airasian, 2008). The astute reader and wise consumer of the research literature should be able to critically read research reports and make an informed judgment about the quality of the research and the resultant report. While some published articles undergo a rigorous review process by experts in the field before they are published, others may be published with little or no critical review. Ultimately, it is up to you, the reader, to judge the quality of the study. You should be able to read a research report and make an informed judgment about the adequacy of the research study as well as written report. Therefore, the information that follows is designed to assist you in making this informed judgment.

Criteria

Criteria for critiquing an article
Basic standards or guidelines for evaluating a research report or proposal.

The **criteria for critiquing an article** are the same criteria a researcher could apply to a manuscript being developed. Many research methods books present a framework for evaluating research, including a list of criteria for evaluating an article or other research publication. These lists differ to some degree but are generally similar. The majority of the criteria on these lists usually apply to any article or research publication, particularly ones based on experimental research. Due to the variety of research conducted, no article or research publication should be expected to fulfill all the criteria on any list.

The authors of this book have developed an unreferenced list of criteria for evaluating research in kinesiology. It is organized similar to the outline described earlier in the chapter: (1) introductory section, including the review of related literature, (2) methods, (3) results, (4) discussion, (5) references, and (6) appendix. A *series of questions for evaluating a research paper,* similar in organization to those previously presented, appears in Example 4.9.

EXAMPLE 4.9
Checklist for Evaluating a Research Paper

Questions to Ask when Evaluating a Research Report

Because of the wide diversity of types of research projects, as well as the multitude of approaches that may very well be taken with any single problem, it is not possible to present either an outline or a checklist that would be appropriate for all cases. Nevertheless, the researcher as well as an astute reader should be able to answer the questions listed below. Obviously, if a question does not apply, it should be disregarded. Those that do apply should merit positive answers by the investigator or the reader.

1. Introductory Section

Does the title succinctly reflect the focus of the research?

Have unnecessary words been avoided?

Is the title too long or too short?

Do the introductory paragraphs capture the interest of the reader?

Is the background information sufficient to justify the study?

Has an adequate rationale for the study been developed?

Has a theoretical foundation for the study been established?

Has the problem been delimited in such a fashion that it can be pursued realistically?

Is the purpose of the study clear?

(Continued)

EXAMPLE 4.9
Continued

Are the key variables identified?

Does the purpose statement provide information about the scope of the study?

Are specific hypotheses or questions to be answered stated?

Has an important problem been selected, the study of which will make a worthwhile contribution to the field?

2. Review of Related Literature

Is the literature relevant to the topic?

Is the review of literature comprehensive in nature?

Were references drawn from recent literature?

Is a wide variety of sources represented?

Is the literature review based mostly on primary sources?

Is the review well organized?

Has the literature been critically reviewed?

Are references cited accurately in accordance with the appropriate editorial style?

3. Methods Section

Is the research design appropriate to the problem?

Will the design permit testing the stated hypotheses or answering the research questions?

Is the population of interest clearly identified?

Were the sampling procedures clearly specified?

Is the sample size appropriate for the problem and the research approach selected?

Is the sample representative of the population of interest?

Have provisions for obtaining informed consent of the participants been explained?

Are the research instruments and their use adequately described?

Is a rationale provided for the selection of the various instruments?

Were the reliability and validity of the research instruments reported?

(Continued)

EXAMPLE 4.9
Concluded

Are the instruments appropriate for the participants in the study?

If an instrument was developed specifically for the study, are instrument development and validation procedures described?

Are the procedures described in sufficient detail so that the study could be replicated by another researcher?

Were critical extraneous variables either held constant or randomized among participants of all groups?

Were the appropriate statistical procedures selected?

Was the significance level for the hypothesis testing specified in advance?

4. Results Section

Are the data clearly presented?

Are the results for all hypotheses tests presented?

Are figures, tables, and other charts well organized and appropriately used?

5. Discussion Section

Have the statistics been appropriately interpreted?

Are the conclusions consistent with the obtained results?

Are the conclusions justified by the data reported and free from personal bias?

Are the conclusions appropriately discussed in light of previous research and related literature?

Are plausible explanations provided for the findings?

Are generalizations limited to the stated population of interest?

Are the limitations of the study acknowledged?

Does the author present reasonable implications based upon the results of the study?

Are recommendations given for future research?

6. References

Are complete references presented for all sources cited in the research report?

Are references cited accurately in accordance with the appropriate editorial style?

7. Appendix

Are sample questionnaires, forms, letters, and so forth used in the study included in the appendix?

Evaluating the Research Report

Articles in journals associated with well-qualified manuscript reviewers will have few if any faults, since any faults in the manuscript either caused it to be rejected or were corrected before it was published. Also, keep in mind that all researchers and manuscript reviewers have their own ideas concerning how research should be conducted and what are the most important evaluation criteria. Readers of an article often see certain things they think could be improved, but these may just be opinions. It is always easier to criticize the research of others than to conduct the research yourself.

Earlier in this chapter, the parts of a research report were discussed, starting with the title and ending with the references. These parts were discussed from the standpoint of reading and understanding the article. Keep in mind that many articles are written assuming the reader has had at least one graduate-level course in the general area of the research. Further, there are certain terms unique to research writing. Thus, do not be too discouraged if you do not understand all research articles.

If the title of the article does not interest you, it is doubtful you will read further. If you do read the abstract, look for the statement of the purpose for the research study, the research participants and methods used in the study, and the major findings and conclusions.

In the introduction and review of related literature section, look for why the research was needed, a review of articles bearing on the conduct of the study, and a statement of purpose for the study. After reading the procedures and methods section, you should have a good understanding of the type and number of research participants involved as well as the procedures and methods used in the study. Further, you should feel that the study was well conducted. If you do not feel the study was well conducted, there may be no reason to read further.

Most readers of a research article falling within their area of expertise can understand the information up to the results section. The results section may be difficult to understand if your statistical knowledge is limited or if quite advanced statistical techniques are used. To the best of your ability, determine if the appropriate statistical techniques were correctly applied and, more importantly, whether the results have been accurately stated. The discussion and conclusions section is based on the results of the study. If you do not fully understand the results section, you may have to accept some of the discussions and conclusions not knowing whether they are totally correct; worse yet, you may not understand them. Even if you do not fully understand the results of discussion and conclusions sections, you may find some comfort in the fact that the reviewers of the manuscript found their presentation acceptable. However, the danger remains that, due to lack of knowledge, you may misinterpret the information set forth in these two sections.

The reference section may be of particular interest to you if you want to evaluate the quality of the books and journals cited in the literature review. Also, the references may be valuable to your own research study.

Summary of Objectives

1. **Explain the purpose of research reports.** The research report is the culmination of the research process, a summary of the researchers' activities and the results of the study.

2. **Understand the various sections of a research report and the information required within each section.** A research report generally consists of several sections. Preliminary items include title, author, organizational affiliation, acknowledgments, and abstract. Background information and purpose statement are included in the introduction. Methods, results, discussion and references are provided in subsequent sections.

3. **Critique and evaluate a research report.** Critiquing and evaluating a research report involve thoroughly examining each section for format, presentation, and content.

Developing the Research Plan 5

The process of developing a research project involves many interrelated elements. We have previously discussed various types of research and approaches to scientific inquiry. We have addressed the nature of research problems and the importance of reviewing the related literature. Now, it is important to consider the details of a research plan, which include the research approach, methodological steps, instruments to be used, and how the instruments will be administered to capture the data needed on the selected variables under study.

After reading Chapter 5, you should be able to

1. Describe four basic research approaches.
2. Understand the role of hypotheses and hypothesis testing in the research process.
3. Explain the three methods of collecting data, and know the various techniques available for each.
4. State the criteria for selecting an appropriate research instrument.

Once the research question has been identified and the investigator has distilled or narrowed the question into a researchable problem that is amenable to investigation, the next stage of the research process is designing the plan of attack. You might think of this as preparing "the recipe for conducting the study." By following the "recipe," the investigator will gather information or data that will eventually lead to the question being answered. The plan of attack prescribes an orderly, systematic procedure for collecting the desired information. Although the specific procedure one follows will vary considerably depending upon the nature of the research problem and the approach taken, all types of research studies will include an explicit plan for conducting the research.

SELECTING THE RESEARCH APPROACH

In Chapter 1 we discussed various systems for classifying research and provided a description of the types of research that are most prevalent in kinesiology. As previously stated, the general purpose of research is to increase our understanding and the body of knowledge within a given field, yet there are substantial differences in the approach one may take in pursuit of this end. Regardless of the approach taken, however, all research involves elements of observation, description, and the analysis of what happens under certain circumstances (Best and Kahn 2005). Once a definitive problem has been identified and a thorough search of the literature has been accomplished, it is incumbent upon the researcher to decide on the best approach to take in systematically collecting the data, or information, needed to solve the research problem. According to Drew, Hardman, and Hosp (2008), the approach selected will depend on several factors: the nature of the research problem, the setting in which the research is to be conducted, the disciplinary perspective of the researcher, and the background of the researcher.

There is not a single way of conducting research. Many different approaches and procedures have been developed; the researcher must choose from these. We have found that the system proposed by Best and Kahn (2005) helps students, as well as veteran researchers, better understand the general approaches that may be taken in research. Best and Kahn suggest that practically all studies fall under one, or a combination, of the following **research approaches:**

Research approaches
General procedures that a researcher may take in investigating the problem of interest; may include historical, descriptive, qualitative, or experimental methods.

- *Historical*—describes *what was* in order to discover generalizations that help to understand the past and the present.
- *Descriptive*—uses quantitative methods to describe *what is* in order to gain an understanding of conditions that currently exist and the relationship between existing variables that are not manipulated.
- *Qualitative*—uses a variety of methods to explore existing phenomenon in a natural environment that generally yield nonquantitative information in order to describe *what is*.
- *Experimental*—describes *what will be* when certain variables of interest are controlled or manipulated in order to seek causal relationships between variables.

In general, the nature of the research problem will go a long way in determining what approach is best suited as the method of attack for obtaining the required knowledge. For example, if one wants to trace the evolution of youth sport programs in the United States in order to better understand the basis for today's programs, an historical approach is needed. Research whose purpose is to investigate the effect of teaching method on sport skill development is seeking to establish a cause-and-effect relationship and thus would use an experimental approach. Such an approach would enable the researcher to deliberately manipulate the independent variable (teaching method in this example) while controlling all other variables and then observe the subsequent effect on the dependent variable (sport skill development). A descriptive approach utilizing survey methodology is called for when a researcher is interested in ascertaining the attitudes of physical education teachers toward the use of technology in the classroom. Similarly, a correlational study in which an investigator seeks to determine the relationship between television-viewing behavior and physical fitness level of adolescent females utilizes a descriptive approach. In this situation there is no manipulation of the variables, only descriptions of the variables and their relationships as they naturally occur. A qualitative approach would best enable a researcher to investigate the nature of hazing and induction rituals practiced by a local high school sports team. The researcher would likely engage in extensive interviews with members of the local sports team to ascertain the perspective of those doing the hazing as well as that of those being hazed. As the previous examples illustrate, the very nature of the research problem coupled with the intent of the researcher will generally reveal the preferred approach to be taken. Each of the four research approaches presented here is discussed more thoroughly in subsequent chapters in the textbook.

HYPOTHESES

Statements of **hypothesis** are important to almost all research projects. Most researchers proceed in their studies with the idea that a certain outcome will result. This idea is then stated as a "tentative explanation of the relationship between two or more variables" (Best and Kahn 2005). The predicted outcome is referred to as a **research hypothesis.** It has been hypothesized that extensive use of anabolic steroids by athletes leads to the deterioration of certain body parts and to disease. Many research studies have been done on the relationship between steroid use and serious illness, and the results have generally supported the hypothesis: *There is a relationship.*

In general, research hypotheses possess these characteristics:

1. They are based on theory or previous research findings.
2. They state a relationship between at least two variables.
3. They are simple and clear statements with no vague terms clouding the relationships.
4. They are testable; that is, the stated variables can be measured, and theoretical or previous research knowledge exists to permit a clear and testable hypothesis.
5. They have the capability of being refuted; the prediction can be evaluated in terms of "yes, it occurred" or "no, it did not occur."
6. They are related to available techniques of design, procedure, and statistical analysis.

Research hypotheses can be stated in a **directional** or a **nondirectional** manner. If, based on previous research, the researcher believes that a particular relationship or

Hypothesis
A tentative explanation or prediction of the eventual outcome of a research problem.

Research hypothesis
A tentative explanation or prediction of the eventual outcome of a research problem; normally this is the outcome expected by the investigator.

Directional hypothesis
Type of research hypothesis that is posited when the researcher has reason to believe that a particular relationship or difference exists.

Nondirectional hypothesis
Type of research hypothesis that is posited when the researcher has no reason to believe that a difference or relationship exists in any direction.

difference exists between groups of research participants, he or she will state the hypothesis directionally, or in the direction of the expected result.

> *Directional hypothesis:* Children with a high IQ are more easily motivated than children with a low IQ.

The researcher is predicting that there is a difference between children in how easily they are motivated and that this difference favors or is in the direction of those with high IQs. A nondirectional hypothesis is stated when the researcher has no reason to believe that a difference or relationship exists in any direction.

> *Nondirectional hypothesis:* There is a difference between the motivational level of children with a high IQ and those children with a low IQ.

In this case the researcher expects a difference but does not indicate the direction it will take. The topic of the directional versus the nondirectional hypothesis has implications regarding the statistical analysis and will be discussed further in a later chapter.

The number of research hypotheses in a given study will depend upon the number of research questions being asked and the number of variables being investigated. The more variables, the greater the number of relationships; hence, the greater the number of hypotheses. This point is related to the scope of the study, which increases as the number of hypotheses increases. All research hypotheses are stated (1) in the present tense and (2) before collecting data on the variables.

Null (statistical) hypothesis
Hypothesis used for statistical testing purposes that proposes that there is no difference between comparison groups or no relationship between variables; hypothesis stating that the independent variable has "no effect" on the dependent variable.

The research hypothesis is not tested directly by the data. Rather, the research hypothesis is transformed into a **null (statistical) hypothesis,** symbolized by H_o, that is tested by the data. The null hypothesis states that there is no difference between the groups being studied or no relationship between the variables of interest. For example:

> *Research hypothesis:* Preschool children exposed to a classroom-based physical activity intervention program will demonstrate higher levels of physical fitness than children who have not been exposed to this program.
>
> *Null or statistical hypothesis:* There is no difference in the physical fitness of preschool children who have participated in a classroom-based physical activity intervention program and children who have not participated in the program.

The statistical procedures used for analyzing research data can test only hypotheses stated in the form of a null hypothesis. Moreover, hypotheses are neither proved nor disproved. Hypothesis testing involves determining the likelihood (probability) that the outcome observed is due to chance occurrence. If the data support the null hypothesis, it will be accepted (technically, we should say that we fail to reject the null hypothesis); if the data refute the null hypothesis, it will be rejected. Usually, the research and null hypotheses are stated in opposite terms. The research hypothesis is a positive statement of expected outcome, while the null hypothesis simply states that no difference or no relationship will be found.

> *Research hypothesis:* Young children who have completed a nutrition education program will have a lower total caloric intake and a lower body mass index (BMI) than those children who have not received the nutrition education program.

> *Null hypothesis:* There is no difference in the total caloric intake and body mass index (BMI) among young children who have participated in a nutrition education program and those who have not received nutrition education.

If on the basis of an appropriate statistical test the researcher fails to reject the null hypothesis, he or she concludes that the nutrition education program is not effective in reducing caloric intake or body mass index. On the other hand, if the statistical test shows a significant difference between those children receiving the nutrition education program and those not exposed to the program, the null hypothesis should be rejected. The researcher then concludes that the program was effective in reducing caloric intake and body mass index. In this case the research hypothesis is accepted.

In most instances, a researcher goes into a study hoping to find a difference or hoping to find a relationship between variables. In some situations, however, a researcher may go into an investigation expecting no difference. If this occurs, then the research hypothesis is stated the same way as the null hypothesis. In this case, whatever action is taken on the statistical hypothesis, as dictated by the data, will also be taken on the research hypothesis.

Stating hypotheses helps to make a researcher's thought process about the research situation more concrete. If a prediction of a specific outcome is made, this forces more thorough consideration of which research techniques, methods, test instruments, and data-collecting procedures should be employed. Hypotheses also help set up the way the data will be analyzed and how the final report will be organized and written.

Inasmuch as hypotheses are founded upon the research problem, they serve to guide the researcher in the selection of the approach and methods to be used to attack the problem. Hypotheses serve to focus the design of the study on the methods that are needed to collect the data that are required to test the null hypotheses. Once the research topic has been reduced to a specific and manageable problem and the type of approach needed to study it has been determined, the researcher then states the hypotheses or, more specifically, the predicted outcome(s) of the study.

All experimental studies and those descriptive investigations in which comparisons are made will have hypotheses. Readers of those studies deserve to know what the researcher expected would be revealed by the experiment or the descriptive comparison. Hypotheses are also appropriate for causal-comparative research and correlational research. Simple descriptive and historical studies generally would not have hypotheses, although occasionally the researcher, by virtue of his or her experience or based on the literature, would want to make a prediction of the outcome and thus would include hypotheses. As a general rule, qualitative researchers do not state hypotheses *a priori,* but may formulate hypotheses based upon the results of their studies. A hypothesis is warranted whenever a reasonable expectation of outcome is anticipated. Usually the hypothesis will indicate an expected relationship between the variables (e.g., characteristics, traits, attributes) being investigated. The researcher may have several objectives for a research project, and a hypothesis should be stated for each one. The usual intent of a research study is to predict a series of outcomes based on the objectives of the research problem. Once the research data have been collected, the hypotheses are tested to determine whether they are true or false.

What happens if the research hypotheses are not supported by the results of the study? A frequent misconception is that the research was faulty and is of no value. Perfectly well-conducted research can reveal data that do not support what was expected. In such a situation, the researcher should review the assumptions that served as the basis for the hypotheses, the theoretical relationships involved, and the design of the study. On the other hand, the truth may be that the research hypotheses should have been rejected. There really may be no relationship between the variables of interest or no difference between the comparison groups. A finding of no significant difference between comparison groups or of no significant relationship may be just as important as a finding in which the null hypothesis is rejected.

DATA-COLLECTING METHODS AND TECHNIQUES

Observation techniques Methods for collecting information in which the participants are observed by the researcher, either directly or indirectly, and relevant data recorded.

Measurement techniques Methods for collecting information in which participants are directly tested or measured on the characteristics of interest; may include physical measures, cognitive measures, and affective measures.

Questioning techniques Methods for collecting information in which the participants are asked to respond to questions posed by the researcher; may include self-report questionnaires, personal or group interviews, or telephone interviews.

The research process includes three different methods of procuring information, or data. They are **observation, measurement,** and **questioning.** The researcher may watch individuals perform and record relevant data about them; he/she may test research participants or apply a device to them to measure certain qualities; or he/she may ask research participants questions to obtain information that cannot be obtained in any other way. Each of these methods of gathering data, along with numerous examples of each, is discussed more completely in the sections that follow. It is important to realize that there are a variety of techniques that may be used to carry out each of these methods. Furthermore, depending on the scope and objectives of the study, a single research project may incorporate several methods and techniques.

Observation Techniques

Direct Observation.   Under the direct technique, research participants are cognizant of being observed and they usually know why they are being observed. Often in direct observation the researcher will observe and record ongoing behavior as it naturally occurs. This is referred to as *naturalistic* observation. For example, researchers have used naturalistic observations to study behaviors of girls and boys in regular school physical education classes. In other situations the researcher could observe behavior in settings or situations that have been specifically created for purposes of the research. Such a technique is generally called *contrived* observation. For example, in a study to investigate the response to cheating in sports competition, the researcher engaged a confederate (an accomplice) to purposively cheat during the game or match in order to observe the reaction of his or her opponent. In both the descriptive and qualitative approach, the research participants can be observed in a contrived research setting or in a natural, real-world environment. In the historical approach, direct observation is accomplished retroactively by viewing museum artifacts, antiques, photographs, and printed material.

Sometimes the researcher's presence might cause a change in the research participants that would inhibit them from reacting in a natural way, thus resulting in invalid data. The phenomenon in which research participants do not behave naturally when being observed is referred to as *reactivity*. In some cases where reactivity is a concern, it is important to the study that research participants be directly observed, but unaware they are being watched. For example, elementary school children, knowing they were going to be observed performing a series of motor skill activities, might get nervous and feel intimidated, or become hyperactive in their behavior and not perform to their true ability. In this case, direct observation could be accomplished through the use of a one-way mirror, so the youngsters would not know they were being watched. Videotaping research participants' overt behavior is often used with observational research. Sometimes this may accompany the direct observation by the researcher and in other situations the video camera could just be running discreetly. Such an approach using disguised observation, however, raises ethical concerns as this may be considered an invasion of privacy.

Some types of research in biomechanics are based on analyzing visual records of human movement, often involving sports performance. High-speed cinematography using a specialized camera records the movement and the resulting film or tape is subsequently analyzed using specialized computer software. This technique is often used to investigate the performance of elite athletes. Although based upon the direct observation and recording of human movement, the nature of the methodology is quite different from the other observational methods described.

Participant Observation.   In the technique of **participant observation,** the researcher or observer participates in the same activities as the people being observed.

Participant observation
An observational technique in which the researcher or observer participates in the setting and in the same activities as the people being observed.

This represents one type of naturalistic observation and is a technique often used in qualitative research. For example, a researcher is studying the attitude and behavior of teenage campers and participates in a two-week camp experience, engaging in all activities, attending meetings, and so forth. The young campers know that the researcher is an outside person who wants to learn as much as possible about teenage camper attitude and behavior. Sometimes the researcher's participation in the research setting may unwittingly affect participants in one way or another. Also, to the extent that the researcher becomes immersed in the lives of the people being observed, he or she may lose the ability to observe and record the behavior of others objectively. In certain instances it may be appropriate that the researcher's identity is unknown to the research participants, but again ethical concerns must be considered.

Measurement Techniques

Almost anything can measured one way or another (e.g., attitudes, knowledge, opinions, movement patterns, sport skills, and physiological characteristics). As Wood (2006, 3) states, ". . . we are measured 'from womb to tomb' in the sense that measures are taken on humans prior to birth (e.g., sonograms) and throughout one's life (e.g. measures of physical growth and development, intellectual capacity, academic ability, job performance, attitudes, opinions, and so on). Then at the very end of life, we are measured for the box!" Some of these qualities can be measured directly, whereas others, mostly affective behaviors, are measured indirectly. Measurement techniques in research involve testing or assessing the research participants in some way to gather the information or data required by the research question. Research in kinesiology often involves movement and the measurement of various outcomes associated with the movement. In fact, the overt nature of movement makes it somewhat easier to measure than affective behaviors or psychological traits which must rely on indirect methods to capture the construct of interest. Physical measures, cognitive measures, and affective measures are presented here. Although these three categories of measures by no means exhaust the possibilities, they are ones commonly seen in kinesiology research.

Physical Measures.   The very nature of the activity inherent in the field of kinesiology provides countless opportunities for physical measures. Some variables, such as height or the distance jumped, can be measured directly and the measurement procedure is usually quite straightforward. Physical education and the various areas of exercise science have produced a large variety of tests, equipment, and techniques to measure physiological characteristics, motor behavior, sport skills, anthropometric attributes, and biomechanical variables. Depending upon the problem being investigated, researchers in kinesiology may utilize equipment valued at thousands and thousands of dollars to obtain measures of body composition, e.g., units for Dual X-ray absorptiometry (DEXA) or whole body air plethysmography (Bod Pod); muscular strength, e.g., electronic isokinetic dynamometers; cardiorespiratory endurance, e.g., metabolic measurement systems; force production, e.g., force platforms; and countless other aspects of human movement. We also see researchers use less-expensive field techniques (e.g., skinfold measurements, pull-up test, 1-mile run/walk test, or medicine ball throw) to obtain measures on these same characteristics of human movement plus many others. Each measurement technique has its own advantages and disadvantages. For research purposes, arguably the most important consideration is the validity of the measure. Without having confidence in the information or data collected, conclusions based on these data will inevitably be questioned. Validity concerns aside, the choice of which measure to use in a research project often comes down to costs, the accessibility to the needed equipment, and practicality of use. The measures available from which to choose will be highly dependent upon the area of specialization (e.g., exercise physiology, athletic training, pedagogy) and the setting for the research. A thorough and comprehensive description of the various physical measures used in kinesiology research is beyond the scope this textbook.

Cognitive Measures.   Whereas assessing knowledge is an integral component of most educational programs, the collection of cognitive measures in kinesiological research is less common. Yet, research studies in kinesiology have sought to measure knowledge about physical activity, health, fitness, and sports, among other things. Many nutrition education interventions or health-related fitness programs include knowledge objectives. A recent study by one of the authors designed to improve dietary practices and physical activity behaviors among elementary school children included a knowledge component related to reading food labels. In another example, Morrow and colleagues (2004) used a telephone interview to assess the knowledge of adult Americans regarding their understanding of current physical activity recommendations. The development of cognitive measures for research purposes largely follows the same principles that guide the development of knowledge tests for education purposes. Item difficulty, the ability to discriminate, and the efficiency of responses are relevant characteristics for cognitive measures. You may want to consult a measurement textbook, such as Baumgartner, Jackson, Mahar, and Rowe (2007), for a more thorough discussion of constructing knowledge tests.

Affective Measures.   Affective characteristics such as opinion, attitude, personality, motivation, self-efficacy, mood, anxiety, and frustration are generally more difficult to measure accurately than are physical or cognitive variables. However, recent years have seen a tremendous growth in research in kinesiology in which the outcome variables of interest are affective in nature. Sport and exercise psychologists are interested in identifying personality characteristics that predispose an individual to participate in various sports, or they wish to identify what psycho-social factors affect a child's physical activity behavior, or they seek to better understand "burn-out" in sports. Physical education teachers and pedagogy professionals may be interested in assessing the attitudes of children toward school physical education or perhaps the children's level of self-esteem. In each of these situations, the construct of interest involves an affective measure. Instruments developed to measure these variables have typically been paper-and-pencil self-report scales. In fact, hundreds of instruments have been developed that purport to measure these affective factors. Since the willingness of the research participant to provide accurate and truthful information is key to the usefulness of such self-report instruments, validity and reliability consideration are paramount. Researchers will typically try to select an instrument that has previously been published and validated rather than construct a new one. Unfortunately, not all of the available instruments have been scientifically developed and may lack acceptable reliability and validity. Therefore, it is incumbent on the researcher to critically examine and carefully check the suitability of available instruments and then to choose wisely the most appropriate instrument for one's research study.

You might see the terms *inventory, scale,* and *questionnaire* used to describe affective measures. Researchers in the social and behavioral sciences, including kinesiology, do not use a consistent terminology to distinguish between the various measures. Typically, an inventory is an instrument on which the research participant is presented with a list of statements and asked to mark yes-no, true-false, or agree-disagree. Scales are devices used by researchers to attempt to quantify responses to various concepts and variables. A scale is actually an instrument with gradations or levels that is used to assign a numerical value to an individual's response to a concept, subject, or characteristic of interest. **Scaling techniques** measure the degree to which the research participant values or exhibits the desired construct. Some affective measures, however, are dichotomous in nature, in which the respondent simply indicates whether a particular feeling, belief, or characteristic is present or not. Generally, however, scales yield either ordinal or interval data. Scales can be used to obtain data on almost any topic, object, or subject. Attitudes, opinions, values, perceptions, and even behaviors are frequently measured by some scaling device. Moreover, evaluation and assessment are often accomplished through the use of various scaling techniques. An excellent review of measures and measurement issues of the major constructs in sport and exercise psychology is provided in *Advances in Sport and Exercise Psychology Measurement* (Duda 1998). In addition, the *Directory of Psychological Tests in the Sport and Exercise Sciences* (Ostrow 2002) summarizes information on 314 psychological scales, questionnaires, and inventories specific to sport and exercise settings. Following are descriptions of some of the more common types of affective measures used in kinesiology research.

Likert Scale. One of the most widely used and versatile type of scales, a **Likert scale** is designed to measure the degree to which an individual exhibits a particular

Scaling techniques
Methods for measuring the degree to which a research participant values or exhibits a concept or characteristic of interest; uses a graded response format that assigns values to the strength or intensity of one's responses.

Likert scale
A type of scaling technique by which respondents are presented with a series of statements and asked to indicate the degree to which they agree or disagree.

attitude, belief, characteristic of interest, or opinion about something along a continuum of responses. Developed in the 1930s by Rensis Likert, Likert scales are called summated-rating scales because a person's score on the scale is computed by summing the numerical value assigned to the various responses provided by the research participant. Usually a Likert scale asks respondents to indicate whether they agree or disagree with a statement. A 5-point Likert scale is most common, but variations also include scales having 4, 6, 7, and even 9 points. For a 5-point Likert scale, the continuum of responses runs from strongly agree (SA), to agree (A), undecided (U), disagree (D), and strongly disagree (SD). Researchers have debated about whether to include a neutral point or category (e.g., "don't know," "undecided," or "no opinion") on the scale, thereby forcing the respondent to "get off the fence." If a neutral category is included, then the scale will consist of an even number of points on the scale. An example of an item from a Likert scale is shown below.

I feel that I have some really good friends among my teammates.

strongly agree   agree   undecided   disagree   strongly disagree

Although there is some debate among authorities, Likert scales are generally developed on the basis that the response categories are equally spaced. That is, the distance between agree and strongly agree is treated as a one-point distance that is equivalent to the distance between successive categories and any other one-point difference on the scale (Gravetter and Forzano 2009; Nunnally 1978). This equal spacing between response points on the scale permits the data to be treated as interval-level scores, thus enabling the responses to be treated statistically. If the intervals on a Likert scale are not presumed to be equal, but rather ordinal in nature, a sum of the responses is not legitimate and the scale would need to be analyzed item by item.

Semantic Differential Scale.   Sometimes called a bipolar adjective scale, this is a technique that has been shown to be quite versatile and useful for measuring attitudes, opinions, or other affective attributes. On a **semantic differential scale,** participants are asked to make judgments about a concept or object based on the use of a list of bipolar adjectives (e.g., happy–sad, bad–good, strong–weak). There are nearly always at least eight different pairs of adjectives, and quite often there are a dozen or more. Respondents then place an "x" or checkmark at one of the spaces along the scale between the contrasting adjectives to indicate their feeling or attitude toward the concept being presented. Typically seven spaces (or points) between the bipolar adjectives are presented, although this number could vary up or down slightly. The responses are then assigned a numerical value based on the number

Semantic differential scale
A type of scaling technique in which respondents are asked to make judgments about a concept of interest using a continuum consisting of bipolar adjectives.

of spaces along the scale (e.g., from 1 to 7, with a value of 7 representing the most positive response). An example of items from a semantic differential scale designed to measure one's feelings toward "athletes" is shown below.

Good	___ ___ ___ ___ ___ ___ ___	Bad
Weak	___ ___ ___ ___ ___ ___ ___	Strong
Pleasant	___ ___ ___ ___ ___ ___ ___	Unpleasant

The numerical values assigned may be considered as interval-level scores and thus the data may be treated statistically. A participant receives a total score for the scale by adding the responses (numerical value) from each item. In order to minimize a response set (that is, a tendency to answer a large number of items in the same way, such as choosing the extreme right end for each item) the adjective pairs making up the scale are listed in both directions. That is, on some pairs the leftmost adjective represents the positive or more favorable response, and on other pairs the rightmost adjective represents the positive or more favorable response. Research has shown that when developed correctly, semantic differential scales assess three dimensions of the participant's feelings toward the concept: evaluation (fair–unfair), potency (strong–weak), and activity (active–passive) (Osgood, Suci, and Tannenbaum 1957). For more information about this technique, readers are referred to Neutens and Rubinson (2002) and Nunnally (1978).

Rating Scale. Whereas both Likert scales and semantic differential scales could be considered as a special type of rating scale, we are using the term *rating scale* more generically to refer to a wide range of instruments whose format is designed to capture one's impression or behavior related to a particular concept or item. A typical rating scale asks respondents to choose one response category from several options provided on a predetermined scale. These scales can be numerical, verbal, or graphic in appearance. A *numerical rating scale* is used when items are to be judged on a single dimension, such as importance, using a simple linear scale with equal intervals between scale points.

How important to you is daily physical education for elementary age children?

Extremely Unimportant   1   2   3   4   5   6   Extremely Important

The RPE Scale (Ratings of Perceived Exertion Scale) created by Borg (1962) is a type of numerical rating scale used by exercise physiologists to measure participants' perceived effort or physical exertion.

Similar to a Likert scale in format, one of the more common rating scales is called a *verbal frequency scale*, but rather than measuring the degree of agreement with a concept, the scale seeks to determine *how often* an action has been taken. The following example illustrates an item from a verbal frequency scale used to assess parental influence on children's physical activity behavior.

How often do you exercise with your child?

always	often	sometimes	rarely	never

At times, a researcher may want to assess the relativity among items, such as choices among products, services, ideas, etc. A *forced ranking scale* requires the respondent to rank-order a limited set of options according to preference or importance. An example of a forced ranking scale is shown below.

Please rank the carriers listed below in order of your preference for cell phone service. Place a 1 next to the carrier you prefer most, a 2 by your second choice, and so forth.

_____ AT & T

_____ Verizon

_____ Sprint

_____ T-Mobile

Alreck and Settle (2004) provide additional examples of rating scales and discuss the characteristics of the many types of scales currently available.

Structured-Alternative Scale.   Although not a specific type of scale, per se, this technique involves a unique question and response format designed to reduce the tendency to provide a socially desirable response. Originally created by Harter (1982) for her Perceived Competence Scale for Children, the format has been adapted for a number of scales used by sport and exercise psychologists to measure various psycho-social attributes. The Physical Self-Perception Profile (PSPP) developed by Fox and Corbin (1989) to assess perceptions of self-competence in the physical domain is one such example. Brustad's (1993) Children's Attraction to Physical Activity Scale (CAPA) also uses a structured-alternative format to assess affect reactions to physical activity participation. These instruments use a 4-point structured-alternative format in which the respondent must first decide which of two opposing statements best describes them, and then choose whether the statement is *kind of true* or *really true* for them. A scale score can be computed by adding the responses, some of which have been reverse scored, for all items on the scale and dividing by the number of items to give a score that can range from 1 to 4. The following illustrates an item based on a structured-alternative response format.

REALLY TRUE FOR ME	SORT OF TRUE FOR ME				SORT OF TRUE FOR ME	REALLY TRUE FOR ME
☐	☐	Some teens try hard to stay in good shape	**BUT**	Other teens don't try to stay in good shape	☐	☐

Questioning Techniques

Questioning techniques include a variety of methods in which the research participant is merely asked to respond to questions presented by the investigator or a research assistant. These techniques frequently take the form of self-report questionnaires or some type of personal interview. Survey research is used extensively in the social and behavioral sciences and is the predominant form of questioning technique in kinesiology research. It would be difficult to find an adult who has not participated in some type of survey, and this method is becoming more commonplace in research involving children and adolescents. With survey research, a researcher is not required to observe one's behavior or introduce a measurement technique, but simply asks questions to research participants about their attitudes, opinions, or behaviors. Today, there are five popular methods of collecting survey data: personal interviewing, telephone interviewing, mailed surveys, Internet or online surveys, and administered surveys. The selection of the data collection method depends on the researcher's access to the population of interest, the type of information sought, time requirements, costs, and resources available. Readers are referred to books such as Alreck and Settle (2004) and Dillman (2008), among others, for a comprehensive discussion of survey research techniques. More information is also presented in Chapter 9 of this book. Regardless of the method of data collection, one of the keys to the success of survey research is the development of meaningful questions.

Structured Questionnaire.   Also called the *closed-ended questionnaire,* the **structured questionnaire** instrument includes questions that can be answered with yes-no or true-false responses, or by selecting an answer from a list of suggested (multiple-choice) responses. The short, quick response format takes less time and effort from the research participants and tends to be fairly objective. The analysis of the data from this type of instrument is relatively simple.

Structured questionnaire
Type of measurement instrument that includes questions along with prescribed response alernatives from which the respondents must choose, such as yes-no or multiple-choice items; also called a *closed-ended questionnaire*.

The following example illustrates a closed-ended question in which the respondent selects only one of the possible alternatives provided:

Which of the following professional basketball players do you think is the greatest of all time? (Check only one.)

_____ Kobe Bryant

_____ Bill Russell

_____ Michael Jordan

_____ Lebron James

_____ Oscar Robinson

The following example from a survey of coaches shows a multiple-response question in which the respondent can select one or more of the alternatives:

Please indicate the method you use to keep up-to-date on current coaching practices. Check all that apply.

_____ media (newspaper, TV, radio, etc.)

_____ professional conferences or clinics

_____ coaching journals or newsletters

_____ talking with other coaches

_____ Internet

Unstructured Questionnaire.   Also called the *open-ended* or *essay question-naire,* the **unstructured questionnaire** allows research participants to respond to a question in their own words. A primary advantage of an open-ended question is that it allows the respondent the greatest flexibility in choosing how to answer. While this format tends to produce answers of greater depth, it takes considerable time on the part of the respondent. It requires a highly motivated person to wade through several open-ended questions. This type of questionnaire is frequently used in exploratory situations, those in which the researcher is trying to gain information that may or may not exist in any particular manner, shape, or form. The unstructured item is not always easily tabulated, analyzed, and interpreted. The following examples from a study to investigate faculty opinions of intercollegiate athletic programs illustrate the use of open-ended questions:

> What do you think about the practice of funding intercollegiate athletic programs from general academic funds?

> In your view, what are the primary benefits of an intercollegiate athletic program?

Structured Interview.   In large measure, the structured interview technique is an oral questionnaire. The researcher poses the questions, along with the expected

**Unstructured
questionnaire**
Type of measurement instrument that includes questions for which the response alternatives are not listed and respondents will answer freely in their own words; also called an *open-ended questionnaire*.

answers, much the same as the structured questionnaire. The questions are asked in order and no repetition is permitted. Questions other than those listed are not permitted. The questions and expected answers are written down in what is called an *interview guide* or *schedule.* Distinct advantages of this technique are that (1) less bias prevails because whatever is in the guide is asked without alteration, and (2) the interviewer may not need to know a lot about the research topic being studied. Public opinion pollsters frequently use this technique by employing high school or college students as interviewers. They are screened for good interpersonal skills (essential to this technique) and then are sent out to do the interviewing without a lot of information concerning the variables and dynamics involved. Social marketing strategies frequently employ this technique through telephone interviews, asking product preference questions of the unsuspecting household member. While all of us are familiar with the annoying telemarketing calls that seem to always come at the wrong time, structured telephone interviews represent a common technique that provides valuable information for many purposes.

Unstructured Interview.

This technique utilizes no set format of questions and expected answers. The open-ended question format applies in that the person being interviewed is supposed to answer in his or her own words and provide all relevant information in as long or brief a period of time as is necessary. The interviewer may have a guide with possible questions, but is not tied to it. Usually the interviewer will be knowledgeable of the problem area being studied and will select questions accordingly. There usually is no set order for the questions and they can be repeated to ensure complete understanding on the part of the interviewee. No question implies a particular response. One major advantage of this technique is that follow-up or clarifying questions can be asked to preclude misconceptions on the part of both the interviewer and interviewee. Good interpersonal skills on the part of the interviewers are important, but perhaps even more so is the amount of knowledge they have concerning the research topic to which the questions are tied. Limited knowledge about the research topic provides a dull, boring, and weak data collection interview. The more informed interviewers are, the better decisions or judgments they will make as the interview process unfolds.

Focus Group Interview.

Focus group interview
An interviewing technique where a group of participants are interviewed together.

A relatively new technique to kinesiology research, focus group interviews have become a popular qualitative research technique for gathering information in some disciplines. The results of **focus group interviews** have made significant contributions to product-marketing research as well as program evaluations in public health. Greenbaum (1998) indicates that there are three major types of focus groups: full groups, minigroups, and telephone groups. Full focus groups, the most common of the three, typically involve 8 to 12 individuals who discuss a particular topic or issue under the guidance of a group facilitator or moderator. The moderator poses questions to the group, leads the group discussion to insure that it stays on track, and attempts to stimulate discussion from all participants. Often, focus group interviews are video or audio recorded in order to minimize the need for the moderator to record the views expressed. Alternatively, a research assistant could be utilized to record pertinent information during the conduct of the focus group. It is noted that focus groups are qualitative in nature and generally do not represent scientifically drawn samples, thus there are substantial limitations in being able to generalize the results to larger populations. Further discussion of focus group interviews is presented in Chapter 10.

Delphi Technique.   This technique is unique as a questioning method and is used to get consensus from a defined group of individuals on a specific issue. Individuals respond to the questions to produce the collective input of the group. Then each one reviews his or her position based upon group trends and revises that position as warranted. Ultimately, a group consensus is obtained. The **Delphi technique** has not been extensively used in kinesiology, but has wide application potential for some topics in the field. In brief, the Delphi technique is accomplished through the following procedures (Neutens and Rubinson 2002):

Delphi technique
A method of data collection using questioning techniques to obtain a consensus from a defined group of individuals on a specific issue.

1. Identify group members whose consensus opinions are sought.
2. Use initial questionnaire to solicit concerns, goals, and problems for which consensus is sought (e.g., knowledge competencies needed for a particular field of study, such as adapted physical education teachers, health educators, outdoor educators, and exercise specialists).
3. Arrange initial results in a second questionnaire. Each member ranks these items in terms of importance.
4. Present a third questionnaire containing an initial trend toward consensus on each item along with each member's initial response. Again each item is rated.
5. Administer a fourth questionnaire. It contains the data obtained from the third questionnaire and each member's most recent ranking. A consensus trend appears as the items are ranked for the third and final time.
6. Present the data from the fourth questionnaire, representing the final group consensus.

Getting Honest Answers

Although the use of various questioning techniques for acquiring data is very popular in social, behavioral, and educational research, including kinesiology, the method is not without its critics. A foremost concern for all self-report techniques is obtaining accurate and truthful responses from the research participants. For various reasons, respondents may be reluctant to answer the questions or to answer completely and truthfully. This is particularly true when being questioned about sensitive issues. People may be embarrassed or afraid to give truthful answers; they may underreport attitudes or behaviors they wish to hide or they may overstate positive behaviors or generally accepted beliefs, something called *social desirability bias*. Another concern often cited with survey research relates to sampling errors of one type or another. For instance, there may be a bias of some type that differentiates between those people who return a mailed or Internet survey and those who do not return the survey. For example, a survey designed to collect information about one's exercise behaviors is more likely to be returned by those individuals who exercise regularly or have positive feelings towards exercise and physical activity. The individuals who return the surveys are not likely to be representative of the entire group that receives them. This is called a *nonresponse bias*. Interview techniques are not immune to unintentional errors or bias contributing to the problem of getting honest responses. A unique challenge associated with interviewing is to avoid *interviewer bias*, the tendency of actions by the interviewer to influence how a respondent answers questions. Survey researchers try to minimize these and other sources of error or bias through careful planning and implementation of the data collection technique.

SELECTING THE APPROPRIATE METHOD AND INSTRUMENT

The selection of the data-gathering method(s) and associated instrument is always based on the type of data needed to solve the research problem, and many underlying factors must be considered. The researcher will examine the needs of the research in terms of (1) the suitability of the specific technique and instrument, (2) the demands of the research participants, (3) the cost in terms of energy, money, and time that will be required, and (4) personal ability to handle the selected methods and techniques, including data analysis procedures. Each of the various methods of data collection has its own advantages and disadvantages. The problem of the research implies a certain kind of data obtained by the selected research approach. The approach will incorporate one of the methods that will be carried out by the use of specific instruments or techniques. Moreover, once the researcher has decided on the general method of data collection (e.g., observation, measurement, questioning, or a combination of methods), the process of selecting the specific instrument from the hundreds or even thousands that are available or perhaps developing a new instrument is often a major undertaking.

Data-Collecting Instruments

Data-collecting instruments
The tools or procedures used by the researcher to collect relevant data pertaining to the research problem.

A **data-collecting instrument** is any paper-and-pencil test or measure, mechanical or electronic equipment measure, or physical performance test used to collect information (data) on the variable under study. The choice of the instrument to be used in the data collection process involves deciding whether it will be one that has already been developed and will be used as it is, one that already exists but will be revised, or one that will be new and needs to be developed. This decision will be based on the needs of the research and what instruments are available.

Whenever data are to be collected, the researcher must keep in mind that, at a minimum, there are three characteristics or attributes data must have to be worth using in a research study. These characteristics are **objectivity,** which is the degree to which multiple scorers agree on the values of collected measures/scores (also called "rater reliability"); **reliability,** which is the degree to which a measure is consistent; and **validity,** which is the degree to which interpretations of test scores or measures derived from a measuring instrument lead to correct conclusions.

Selecting the Research Instrument

Selecting a research instrument for any project is usually the result of a thorough search of the literature. The researcher who wants to study the effect of improved physical fitness on the self-concept of adolescents will probably find that several tests measuring self-concept are available. The Piers-Harris Children's Self-Concept Scale, originally developed over thirty years ago, has been widely used by kinesiology researchers to measure the self-concept of adolescents and would represent one such instrument. If you were interested in measuring self-esteem rather than self-concept, the Rosenberg Self-Esteem Scale would be a research instrument that should be considered.

Once it is determined that such an instrument exists, the next step is to assess its acceptability. Whether the instrument is *reliable* (measures consistently), whether it is *objective* (free of tester bias), and whether it is *valid* (truthfulness, measures what it is supposed to measure) are important characteristics in this part of the process. Quite frequently an instrument will be selected on the basis of its reliability and validity as reported by the researchers who have used it in earlier studies. If measures of reliability and validity are not provided, various statistical techniques can be applied to determine the reliability and validity of the instrument. Further information about these important attributes and how they are determined are discussed in Chapter 15. Sometimes, researchers must make their own determination of the reliability and validity of the instrument they plan to use. Part of determining validity is analyzing whether or not the instrument is *appropriate.* Can the research participants meet the demands of the instrument, or is it too hard or too easy for them? The vocabulary of an instrument may be appropriate for one age group and not for another. The same can be true for certain physical performance tests. If the instrument is not appropriate, it will not produce valid data. Without reliability and validity, the data are of no use in answering the research question.

Objectivity
The degree to which multiple scorers agree on the values of collected measures or scores; also called *rater reliability*.

Reliability
Degree to which a measure is consistent.

Validity
The degree to which interpretations of test scores or measures derived from a measuring instrument lead to correct conclusions.

In selecting an instrument, a researcher will also consider other criteria. How easy the test is to administer, how much it costs in time and money, and how easy it is to score are other factors the researcher must consider. Ideally, the researcher selects the most reliable and valid instrument. In reality, however, if that test is difficult, time-consuming, costly, and very demanding of the research participant, the researcher may instead select a test that is a little less reliable and valid, but is easier to handle, has a shorter administrative time span, is less costly, and is less demanding of the research participants.

Revising the Instrument

Quite often a researcher locates an instrument that is not quite acceptable for the intended research situation, in which case the instrument must be revised. Permission should be obtained before revising a published paper-and-pencil instrument originally developed by someone else. Permission is sometimes needed to revise a physical performance instrument. As a matter of professional courtesy, a researcher should request permission from the original author/developer to modify a proprietary instrument. When a standardized, copyrighted instrument is used or revised, permission from the instrument's publisher is required.

Changes in an original instrument may take many forms, but are usually done to better fit a particular group of research participants. Self-concept has been studied with different age groups, sexes, and races, and various kinds of disabled populations. Obviously, one instrument designed to measure self-concept cannot be used with all subject groups. The same can be said concerning the study of countless numbers of variables of a research interest. Collins, in her 1989 study of body figure perceptions and preferences among male and female preadolescent children, used a pictorial instrument modified from the original instrument developed in 1983 that used adult male and female participants (Stunkard, Sorenson, and Schulsinger 1983). Basically, the major change was that Collins revised the Stunkard adult figure drawings to reflect the figures of children. She also used seven figures for each gender, while Stunkard used nine figures. Revising an instrument may change its reliability and validity, and new measures may need to be determined for the revised instrument if changes are major enough. Note: Reliability and validity of an instrument are often specific to the age and gender of the research participants.

Instrument Development

It is difficult and time-consuming to develop an instrument and this procedure is avoided by both veteran and beginning researchers whenever possible. The task is undertaken only when it becomes obvious that no paper-and-pencil, electronic or mechanical, or physical performance test or instrument exists to generate the needed research data.

The starting point for instrument development is, once again, the literature. All of the dynamics in the prospective research problem must be thoroughly understood, and what instruments are available to use as models must be known before the instrument development process begins. Suppose a researcher is interested in determining the motivation of high school students for participating or not participating in athletics. The dynamics involved in this phenomenon are many and are comprised of intellectual, sociological, psychological, and physiological components. A complete review of the literature must include related research and conceptual articles reflecting each of those components and what instruments others have used. The knowledge accrued from such a review will provide the basis for determining the content of the instrument. That is, what type of questions and/or statements will contribute most in the attempt to measure the motivation students have, or do not have, for athletic involvement during high school?

The usual next step is to select the questions or statements and produce a tentative instrument. In writing these research items, the researcher is careful to see that each item will provide a reasonable estimate of each relevant component of the athletic motivation problem. If, for example, one of the components related to athletic participation is the student's perception of whether or not athletic participation will enhance the chances of being successful in life, then the researcher's task is to develop questions or statements that will provide an estimate of this component. If the students perceive that athletic participation will enhance their self-concept and status among their peers, the instrument should contain items that will provide a measurable estimate of these components.

Once the tentative instrument has been developed, it should be submitted to a jury of experts or committee of authorities. The researcher invites selected individuals, who are considered to have expertise in the problem area, to review the content of the instrument. These can be people who have taught, researched, or written in the problem area. The task of the jury members is to review the research questions or statements and revise them as needed. Which items should be rewritten? Should any of the items be deleted? Should items be added? Which items are most significant to the essence of the problem? Which are relatively insignificant? Needless to say, the work of the jury suggests careful attention to the elimination of instrument flaws. Submitting the proposed instrument to a jury of experts is an excellent way to increase the content validity of the proposed measurement instrument. In most instances the instrument is submitted to the jury only once, but it may be necessary to repeat the procedure two or more times.

The next step in the instrument development process is the pilot study or preliminary investigation. The intended instrument is administered to selected research participants from the same population who will make up the actual research sample, but who are *not* included in the actual sample of research participants. The pilot study serves as a trial run of the instrument to see if it is in further need of revision. The objectives of a pilot study are (1) to determine whether or not research participants are likely to understand the content items in the instrument, (2) to determine whether the instrument will provide the needed data, (3) to familiarize the researcher and any assistants with instrument administration procedures, (4) to obtain a set of data for trying out the proposed data treatment techniques, and (5) to first determine the reliability and then the validity of the instrument.

The researcher will further revise the instrument if the pilot study shows change to be necessary. A pilot study may not always be needed, but is a valuable research tool. The knowledge that the instrument is sufficient and will yield reliable and valid data, that the planned instrument administration procedure is appropriate, and that the planned attack on the research problem is the proper approach are the typical payoffs for conducting a pilot study. The actual research study may not be completely without problems, but the prospects of severe trouble occurring are diminished by having performed a test run. With a successful pilot study, the researcher can claim a finalized instrument.

This discussion of instrument development happens to be for a paper-and-pencil instrument. However, the same basic steps occur in the process of developing any instrument. These steps are:

- Survey the literature.
- Develop a tentative instrument.
- Reflect upon and revise the instrument.
- Obtain opinions of experts concerning the instrument.
- Revise the instrument as needed.
- Conduct a pilot study.
- Revise the instrument as needed.
- Use the instrument.

Summary of Objectives

1. **Describe four basic research approaches.** The research problem can be attacked using a variety of approaches, including historical, descriptive (quantitative), qualitative, and experimental. The nature of the research problem coupled with the intent of the researcher will generally point to a preferred research approach.

2. **Understand the role of hypotheses and hypothesis testing in the research process.** Formulating hypotheses provides direction in the research approach and guides the researcher

in designing data collection methods and techniques that will elicit the information needed to complete the study.

3. **Explain the three methods of collecting data, and know the various techniques available for each.** The research process includes three methods for procuring information. The observation method uses techniques such as direct, indirect, and participant observation. Measurement uses scales, inventories, physical and cognitive measures, and other techniques to assess and evaluate. Questioning is another common method of data collection, and can make use of a variety of techniques including questionnaires and interviews.

4. **State the criteria for selecting an appropriate research instrument.** A research instrument must be reliable, objective, and valid. In addition to these criteria, the researcher must also consider an instrument's availability, cost, and ease of use. Developing a research instrument involves several steps, including reviewing existing literature, creating a tentative instrument, and a series of reviews, revisions, and tests.

6

Ethical Concerns in Research

OBJECTIVES

The public acceptance of the scientific method as a source of knowledge is founded, at least in part, on the integrity associated with the process. While it is impossible to legislate ethics, the scientific community has sought to develop ethical standards that provide direction for conducting research. The effectiveness of such standards is ultimately dependent upon the adherence and practices of individual researchers. Since most research in kinesiology involves the use of human research participants in one way or another, it is important for researchers to consider the ethical principles and regulations that guide their research activities.

After reading Chapter 6, you should be able to

1. Discuss various instances of ethical misconduct in research involving humans.
2. Identify ethical codes and federal regulations that serve to guide research in the United States.
3. Understand the importance of informed consent in research involving human participants.
4. Understand the role and function of Institutional Review Boards in approving research activities.
5. Explain ethical considerations involved in the disclosure of research results.

As researchers work to contribute to the knowledge of a profession, they engage in a variety of activities that are critical to making the scientific method an effective and credible source of information in the search for truth. While the scientific method, with its orderly, systematic nature and built-in series of checks, has evolved to become highly respected as a source of knowledge, the integrity of this very system is founded upon the professional conduct of the researcher. Dishonest, fraudulent, or unethical researchers can circumvent the scientific method. While the quest for knowledge is important to a profession, and the application of such knowledge is important to professional practices and to society as a whole, we must also concern ourselves with the ethics of the researcher and the rights and well-being of the research participants.

THE BASIS OF ETHICS IN RESEARCH

History has taught us that without moral principles, protective measures, and a system of ethical standards that oblige researchers to follow certain rules, scientific misconduct and dishonesty will occur. It is noted, however, that the mere existence of ethical standards does not guarantee ethical behavior by researchers. Ultimately, it is the responsibility of individual researchers to conduct themselves in a way that promotes integrity and honesty throughout the scientific method. The following examples illustrate scientific inquiry gone askew.

Nazi Germany Experimentation during World War II

Perhaps the most grievous examples of unethical behavior in research were the "medical experiments" of Nazi scientists during World War II (**Nazi experimentation**). The charges brought against twenty-three German physicians in the Nuremberg War Crime Trials (the "Doctors' Trial") for their "medical experiments" upon prisoners, concentration camp inmates, and other living human subjects without the consent of these people shocked the world and exposed the dark side of humanity. The trials documented charges that, in the course of these "medical experiments," the doctors subjected thousands of people to cruelties, tortures, and other inhuman acts. Most of the people were murdered. Experiments included, but were not limited to, the following:

> *Freezing Experiments.* These experiments were designed to determine how long it would take to lower the temperature of the human body to the point of death and also to determine how best to re-warm a frozen victim. Prisoners were outfitted in aviator uniforms or stripped naked and either placed in an icy tank of water or strapped to a stretcher and placed outside in freezing temperatures. Methods for re-warming a frozen body included placing the victim under extremely hot sunlamps, immersing the victim in a hot bath and slowly increasing the temperature, or internal irrigation whereby hot water was forced into the stomach, bladder, and intestines. The investigators claimed that they hoped to determine the most effective means of treating persons who had been frozen.

> *Malaria Experiments.* Prisoners and concentration camp inmates were purposively exposed to mosquitoes that were known to carry the malaria virus, or were given direct injections of the virus, in order to investigate the effect of various antimalarial compounds. After having contracted malaria, the subjects were treated with various drugs to test their relative efficacy. Testimony revealed that victims not dying of malaria often suffered substantial and debilitating side effects from the various

Nazi experimentation
Medical experiments conducted by German scientists during World War II, that subjected unwilling participants to extreme cruelty and inhuman treatment.

compounds being tested. The alleged intent of these experiments was to determine effective immunization and treatment for malaria.

High-Altitude Experiments. Supposedly to investigate the limits of human endurance and existence at extremely high altitudes, Nazi physicians placed concentration camp inmates in a low-pressure chamber capable of reproducing atmospheric conditions and pressures prevailing at extremely high altitudes. As the simulated altitude was progressively increased, victims experienced excruciating pain, spasmodic convulsions, grave injury, and, frequently, death—due to an enormous amount of air embolism that developed in the brain, coronary vessels, and other internal organs.

Nuremberg Code
Basic principles of ethical conduct that govern research involving human participants that were developed as a result of Nuremburg trials of German scientists.

The international outrage over the atrocities revealed at the Nuremberg War Crime Trials led to the development of the **Nuremberg Code,** a set of basic principles to govern the ethical conduct of research involving human participants. Although the code focused on biomedical experiments, since its publication in 1947 it has been widely recognized as the starting point for systematic protection of human participants in all areas of research. A detailed account of the Nuremberg war crimes trial of Nazi doctors and the horrific experiments in the name of science is discussed in the book *Doctors from Hell* (Spitz 2005).

Tuskegee Syphilis Study

Even as the Nuremberg War Crime Trials were being conducted, the United States Public Health Service supported a research project that constituted an example of unethical behavior, and blatant misconduct—in the name of science. In 1932, the United States Public Health Service initiated a study in Macon County, Alabama, to investigate the long-term effects of untreated syphilis. At the time, Macon County was poor, semi-illiterate, and reportedly had the highest syphilis rate in the country, 36 percent, compared to less than 1 percent for the nation as a whole. While funding to support a treatment program was "not available," researchers believed that the high rate of syphilis in Macon County warranted further investigation. Moreover, there was speculation among some medical personnel that African Americans responded differently to the disease than did other racial groups. So the decision was made to conduct a prospective study and follow the long-term effects, all the way until death, of untreated syphilis among African Americans living in Macon County. It is also noted that at the time the study commenced, no cure for syphilis was available.

Various inducements, such as free physical examinations, free treatment for minor health problems, food, transportation to and from the clinic, and a burial stipend of $50, were used to recruit 399 males with syphilis and another 200-plus controls without syphilis to be a part of the study. (The burial stipend was needed in order to obtain permission to perform autopsies upon the death of the research participants.) Recruitment was easy. Most of the study participants had little money and almost no access to medical care. In some instances, this represented the first opportunity ever to receive a medical examination. The participants, however, were never told the real nature of the study and were not afforded the opportunity to provide informed consent. In fact, many were never told they had syphilis, and others thought they were being treated for "bad blood," a term that presumably was a synonym for syphilis. In reality, however, they were either not treated or provided only aspirin and an iron supplement to relieve some of the symptoms.

The periodic examinations for monitoring the course of the disease continued year after year. Moreover, treatment for syphilis was withheld, even after the discovery and widespread use of penicillin to treat syphilis in the 1940s. In order to preserve the integrity of the "experiment" and prevent treatment of those infected individuals by other doctors, the Public Health Service solicited and obtained agreements from local health departments as well as from the U.S. Army (for those individuals who were drafted) to not treat those participants in the study who were detected to have syphilis. The study continued for forty years. In 1972, an article in the *Washington Star* by Jean Heller exposed the story about the **Tuskegee Syphilis Study** and led to its termination. Following a series of congressional hearings on the matter, in 1974 the government agreed to an out-of-court settlement of approximately $10 million, paying each living participant $37,500 and the heirs of each deceased participant $15,000 altogether. In 1997, President Bill Clinton, speaking on behalf of the U.S. government, formally apologized for the syphilis study. James Jones's classic book, *Bad Blood: The Tuskegee Syphilis Experiment* (1993), provides an authentic account of how a government agency deliberately deceived and betrayed a highly vulnerable population in the name of science. Another excellent source of information about the infamous study by the U.S. Public Health Service is *Tuskegee's Truths: Rethinking the Tuskegee Syphilis Study* (Reverby 2000).

History contains other examples of experiments in which researchers have perpetrated unthinkable acts on unsuspecting research participants. The human radiation experiments conducted in the United States from the end of World War II to the mid-1970s represents one such example. Those interested in reading more about instances of scientific misconduct may wish to consult sources such as *Human Experimentation: When Research Is Evil* (McCuen 1998) or *In the Name of Science: A History of Secret Programs, Medical Research, and Human Experimentation* (Goliszek 2003).

Tuskegee Syphilis Study
U.S. Public Health Service research study conducted in mid-1900s that is infamous for the maltreatment of the participants.

REGULATION OF RESEARCH AND PROTECTION OF RESEARCH PARTICIPANTS

Ethics is concerned with human behavior from a perspective of right or wrong. According to Drowatzky (1996), "ethical statements are developed to prescribe behavior as directives that tell us what we ought to do in the situations we encounter."

Ethics
Moral principles that define one's values in terms of acceptable behaviors.

Ethical statements essentially define our values in terms of acceptable behaviors, telling us what we ought to do. It is important to note that ethics applies to our daily life, just as it does to research activities. But ethics may vary from one person to another, from one group to another, and from one culture to another. How, then, can we define normative ethics that apply to all individuals in all situations? Proponents of **situational ethics** argue that no general rules can be applied to all situations, that each action is unique and must be evaluated on its own merits, or lack thereof. In other words, "it depends." Others, however, believe that fundamental ethical principles can be formulated and that behavioral norms constitute the basis for such an ethical system (Drowatzky 1996).

Situational ethics
Ethical paradigm that proposes that no general rules can be applied to all situations and that ethics are situational specific.

The philosophical debate notwithstanding, governments and organizations have generally embraced a normative approach to ethics. While it is recognized that no ethical standards or codes will totally prevent scientific misconduct, it is also recognized that without ethical standards to serve as guiding principles for appropriate behaviors, responsible conduct in research may be jeopardized and scientific knowledge devalued. Developed in 1947, the Nuremberg Code (see Box 6.1) represents the first attempt to develop ethical standards for the conduct of research

BOX 6.1
The Nuremberg Code

(Trials of War Criminals before the Nuremberg Military Tribunals under Control Council Law No. 10, 1949.)

The Nuremberg Code

1. The voluntary consent of the human subject is absolutely essential. This means that the person involved should have legal capacity to give consent; should be so situated as to be able to exercise free power of choice, without the intervention of any element of force, fraud, deceit, duress, over-reaching, or other ulterior form of constraint or coercion; and should have sufficient knowledge and comprehension of the elements of the subject matter involved, as to enable him to make an understanding and enlightened decision. This latter element requires that, before the acceptance of an affirmative decision by the experimental subject, there should be made known to him the nature, duration, and purpose of the experiment; the method and means by which it is to be conducted; all inconveniences and hazards reasonably to be expected; and the effects upon his health or person, which may possibly come from his participation in the experiment.

Box 6.1
Concluded

The duty and responsibility for ascertaining the quality of the consent rests upon each individual who initiates, directs or engages in the experiment. It is a personal duty and responsibility which may not be delegated to another with impunity.

2. The experiment should be such as to yield fruitful results for the good of society, unprocurable by other methods or means of study, and not random and unnecessary in nature.

3. The experiment should be so designed and based on the results of animal experimentation and a knowledge of the natural history of the disease or other problem under study, that the anticipated results will justify the performance of the experiment.

4. The experiment should be so conducted as to avoid all unnecessary physical and mental suffering and injury.

5. No experiment should be conducted, where there is an *a priori* reason to believe that death or disabling injury will occur; except, perhaps, in those experiments where the experimental physicians also serve as subjects.

6. The degree of risk to be taken should never exceed that determined by the humanitarian importance of the problem to be solved by the experiment.

7. Proper preparations should be made and adequate facilities provided to protect the experimental subject against even remote possibilities of injury, disability, or death.

8. The experiment should be conducted only by scientifically qualified persons. The highest degree of skill and care should be required through all stages of the experiment of those who conduct or engage in the experiment.

9. During the course of the experiment, the human subject should be at liberty to bring the experiment to an end, if he has reached the physical or mental state, where continuation of the experiment seemed to him to be impossible.

10. During the course of the experiment, the scientist in charge must be prepared to terminate the experiment at any stage, if he has probable cause to believe, in the exercise of the good faith, superior skill and careful judgement required of him, that a continuation of the experiment is likely to result in injury, disability, or death to the experimental subject.

involving human participants and has become the prototype for other ethical guidelines developed since.

The World Medical Association (WMA) subsequently codified ethical guidelines for medical research involving human subjects in its *Declaration of Helsinki: Recommendations Guiding Medical Doctors in Biomedical Research Involving Human Subjects* (1964). The **Helsinki Declaration,** as it has come to be known, has since been revised slightly and reaffirmed by the World Medical Assembly of the WMA on multiple occasions, most recently in 2008. Readers should consult the website of the WMA for a complete description of the international code of medical ethics: (www.wma.net/en/30publications/10policies/b3/index.html).

A variety of regulations protecting human research participants have been established in the United States. The **scientific misconduct** associated with the Tuskegee Syphilis Study, government-sponsored human radiation experiments between 1944 and 1974, and other incidents of nonconsensual experiments on human participants led Congress in 1974 to pass the National Research Act, establishing the National Commission for the Protection of Human Subjects of Biomedical and Behavioral Research. The commission was charged with formulating ethical principles and guidelines for conducting research activities with human participants. The resultant **Belmont Report** (1979) serves as the fundamental document for current federal regulations for the protection of human participants in biomedical and behavioral research in the United States. Three basic ethical principles were set forth in the report:

1. **Respect for persons.** Proclaiming respect for individuals as autonomous agents capable of self-determination, and special protection to persons of diminished autonomy.
2. **Beneficence.** Obligating researchers to protect persons from harm, and to maximize possible benefits and minimize possible harms.
3. **Justice.** Requiring that the benefits and burdens of the research be fairly distributed, thus impacting upon the selection of research participants.

The complete Belmont Report is available on the web at the following address: www.hhs.gov/ohrp/humansubjects/guidance/belmont.htm

In response to the commission's recommendations, the Department of Health, Education, and Welfare (now the Department of Health and Human Services, DHHS) and the Food and Drug Administration (FDA) enacted in 1981 major revisions to their existing policies concerning research involving human participants. These basic government regulations have since been revised, most recently in 2009, and currently serve as the federal rules and regulations that govern research involving human participants in the United States. The DHHS regulations, those most applicable to kinesiology researchers, are codified in federal law as Title 45, Part 46 of the

---

Helsinki Declaration
Ethical guidelines defined by the World Medical Association for medical research involving human participants.

Scientific misconduct
The fabrication, falsification, plagiarism, or other practices that seriously deviate from those commonly accepted by the scientific community for proposing, conducting, or reporting research.

Belmont Report
The fundamental document that provides current federal regulations for the protection of human participants in research in the United States.

Respect for persons
Ethical principle proclaiming respect for individuals involved as participants in research studies.

Beneficence
Ethical principle obligating researchers to protect persons from harm and to maximize possible benefits and minimize possible harms.

Justice
Ethical principle requiring that the benefits and burdens of research be fairly distributed, thus impacting upon the selection of research participants.

Code of Federal Regulations (**45 C.F.R. 46**) July 14, 2009. These regulations are sometimes called the **"Common Rule."** Subpart A constitutes the Federal Policy for the Protection of Human Subjects. The policies established therein are applicable (with certain exceptions specified) to all research activities involving human research participants conducted, supported, or otherwise regulated by any federal department or agency (45 C.F.R. 46, 2009). Moreover, the code requires that all research protocols involving human research participants be reviewed by an **Institutional Review Board** (IRB) to ensure compliance with the requirements set forth in this policy. For further information you may wish to consult with your local Institutional Review Board or read the entire federal code at the following website: www.hhs.gov/ohrp/humansubjects/guidance/45cfr46.htm.

In 2000, the DHHS established the Office of Human Research Protections (OHRP) to assume responsibility for the development, coordination, and monitoring of policies relative to the protection of human research participants. This office maintains oversight of compliance polices and provides educational guidance materials on the protection of human research participants. The OHRP website provides a wealth of information concerning ethical standards and the protection of human participants: www.hhs.gov/ohrp.

In addition to the ethical standards and regulations promulgated by the federal government, many professional associations have developed ethical codes of conduct to guide the research activities of their members. The American Psychological Association (APA), for instance, issued its first code of ethics in 1953 and has subsequently revised the code several times, most recently in 2010 (American Psychological Association 2010). Other associations publishing ethical standards or research guidelines that may be of interest to kinesiology researchers include, among others: American College of Sports Medicine (ACSM), American Educational Research Association (AERA), American Sociological Association (ASA), and the Research Consortium of the American Alliance for Health, Physical Education, Recreation and Dance (AAHPERD). Whereas the ethical standards of professional associations typically relate to all practices pertinent to its members, some standards relate specifically to research practices. The following websites provide online access to the code of ethics for the respective associations:

American Psychological Association (APA)

www.apa.org/ethics/code/index.aspx

American Educational Research Association (AERA)

www.aera.net/AboutAERA/default.aspx?menu_id=90&id=717

American Sociological Association (ASA)

www.asanet.org/members/ecoderev.html

AAHPERD Research Consortium

www.aahperd.org/rc/about/codeofethics.cfm

---

45 C.F.R. 46
Specific federal law, referred to as the **Common Rule,** that establishes regulations governing research involving human participants in the United States.

Common Rule
The general name for federal law 45 C.F.R. 46 that establishes regulations governing research involving human participants in the United States.

Institutional Review Board (IRB)
Local committee established by an institution whose purpose is to ensure the protection of human participants involved in research activities.

INFORMED CONSENT

Informed consent
Explicit statement informing potential research participants of the purposes, procedures, risks, and benefits of a research project; provides an acknowledgment that participation is done so voluntarily.

The first provision of the Nuremberg Code and arguably the most important pillar underlying ethical standards governing research involving human participants states that "the voluntary consent of the human subject is absolutely essential." Inherent to this principle are four important elements: (1) research participants are made fully aware of the nature and purpose of the research project, (2) consent is voluntarily given, (3) the person involved has the legal capacity to give consent, and (4) the responsibility for obtaining consent rests with the researcher. Thus, **informed consent** is often seen as the key aspect of obtaining approval for conducting research involving human participants. A sample informed consent form is shown in Example 6.1.

EXAMPLE 6.1
Sample Informed Consent Template

Name of Institution

Informed Consent

(Sample for Adult Participants—Use 2nd Person Language Except for Agreement Statement)

Project Title: (as it appears on the IRB application)

Name of Investigator(s): _____

Invitation to Participate: You must provide a formal invitation to take part in the research project. For example: "You are invited to participate in a research project conducted through NAME OF UNIVERSITY. The University requires that you give your signed agreement to participate in this project. The following information is provided to help you make an informed decision about whether or not to participate."

Nature and Purpose: State clearly and accurately what the study is designed to discover or establish.

Explanation of Procedures: Describe all procedures to be followed, including their purpose(s), duration, frequency, use of any audio or video recording, what will happen to the data/information at the end of the study. Include enough detail that the participant has a reasonable idea of what he/she will be doing and what they will be asked about. State any anticipated circumstances where the participant's participation may end without regard to the participant's consent.

Discomfort and Risks: Describe any physical, psychological, social, legal, and/or economic risk(s) or cost(s) resulting from the project. If there are

---

EXAMPLE 6.1
Continued

no more than minimal risks—discomfort, burden, inconvenience—this should be so stated. This may be stated in one of several ways: Risks to participation are minimal. Risks to participation are similar to those experienced in day-to-day life. There are no foreseeable risks to participation.

Benefits and Compensation: Describe any direct benefit(s) that may result from the study. Benefits would include improved physical or mental health (e.g., from treatment), improved skills, etc. Compensation is distinct from benefits and would include cash, gifts, or academic credit provided for the person's time or travel expenses. If the individual participant will receive no direct benefit, this should be stated. If applicable, describe how voluntary or involuntary withdrawal or termination affects benefits. Note that compensation should be equivalent across participant groups and cannot be used to coerce participation. That is, if compensation for time is provided, then a portion of the compensation must be provided (pro-rated) even if the person terminates their involvement prior to completing the study.

Confidentiality: State the way the participant's confidentiality will be maintained: persons or organizations to whom information from the study will be furnished, nature of the information furnished, purpose of the disclosure. For example: "Information obtained during this study which could identify you will be kept confidential. The summarized findings with no identifying information may be published in an academic journal or presented at a scholarly conference."

Right to Refuse or Withdraw: Provide information about the voluntary nature of participation and the ability of the participant to stop at any time without penalty. For example: "Your participation is completely voluntary. You are free to withdraw from participation at any time or to choose not to participate at all, and by doing so, you will not be penalized or lose benefits to which you are otherwise entitled."

Questions: Participants should be able to seek additional information about the project. For example: "If you have questions about the study or desire information in the future regarding your participation or the study generally, you can contact (investigator) at (xxx) xxx-xxxx or (if appropriate) the project investigator's faculty advisor _____ in the Department of _____, (xxx) xxx-xxxx. You can also contact the office of the IRB Administrator, NAME OF UNIVERSITY, at (xxx) xxx-xxxx, for answers to questions about rights of research participants and the participant review process."

(Continued)

EXAMPLE 6.1
Concluded

Agreement: Include the following statement

> I am fully aware of the nature and extent of my participation in this project as stated above and the possible risks arising from it. I hereby agree to participate in this project. I acknowledge that I have received a copy of this consent statement. I am 18 years of age or older.

_____   _____

(Signature of participant)   (Date)

_____

(Printed name of participant)

_____   _____

(Signature of investigator)   (Date)

_____   _____

(Signature of instructor/advisor)   (Date)

In the United States, the Department of Health and Human Services articulates the requirements for informed consent in 45 C.F.R. Subpart A, Section 46.116 (2009). As set forth in these regulations, the basic elements of informed consent should include:

1. a statement that the study involves research, an explanation of the purposes of the research and the expected duration of the subject's participation, a description of the procedures to be followed, and identification of any procedures which are experimental;
2. a description of any reasonably foreseeable risks or discomforts to the subject;
3. a description of any benefits to the subject or to others which may reasonably be expected from the research;
4. a disclosure of appropriate alternative procedures or courses of treatment, if any, that might be advantageous to the subject;
5. a statement describing the extent, if any, to which confidentiality of records identifying the subject will be maintained;
6. for research involving more than minimal risk, an explanation as to whether any compensation is available, and whether any medical treatments are

available, if injury occurs and, if so, what these consist of, or where further information may be obtained;

7. an explanation of whom to contact for answers to pertinent questions about the research and research subjects' rights, and whom to contact in the event of a research-related injury to the subject; and

8. a statement that participation is voluntary, refusal to participate will involve no penalty or loss of benefits to which the subject is otherwise entitled, and the subject may discontinue participation at any time without penalty or loss of benefits to which the subject is otherwise entitled.

Furthermore, when appropriate, one or more of the following elements of information shall also be provided to each subject:

1. a statement that the particular treatment or procedure may involve risks to the subject (or to the embryo or fetus, if the subject is or may become pregnant) which are currently unforeseeable;

2. anticipated circumstances under which the subject's participation may be terminated by the investigator without regard to the subject's consent;

3. any additional costs to the subject that may result from participation in the research;

4. the consequences of a subject's decision to withdraw from the research, and procedures for orderly termination of participation by the subject;

5. A statement that significant new findings developed during the course of the research which may relate to the subject's willingness to continue participation will be provided to the subject; and

6. the approximate number of subjects involved in the study.

Many institutions provide sample consent documents or templates that may be adapted for a variety of research studies. An example of such a template appears in Example 6.1. In addition, for research involving vulnerable groups such as children, prisoners, or pregnant women, federal guidelines prescribe additional protections. Since a considerable amount of kinesiology research involves the participation of children, it is important to note that regulations require written parental permission before the minor child can participate in a research project. Moreover, if the prospective research participants are children, the regulations require the **assent** of the child or minor and the permission of the parent(s). There are certain situations, however, when parental permission may be inappropriate. One of the more challenging issues facing researchers interested in investigating children in

Assent
Statement of consent or agreement made by a child regarding his or her involvement in a research project.

public schools is obtaining parental permission. Sending permission forms home with children is notoriously unreliable, often resulting in a low response rate, which may make it impossible to obtain scientifically valid results. "Passive consent" has been permitted in school-based research in some situations in response to the difficulties of obtaining written permission from parents. The passive consent process involves notifying parents that a research study is about to take place and giving them the opportunity to state that they do not want their children to participate, thus opting-out of the research. However, passive consent is *not* recognized in the federal regulations and passive consent is *not* equivalent to informed consent. The provisions of the Common Rule (45 C.F.R. 46) specify that parental or guardian permission for children to participate in research must be secured in advance of their participation in the research or waived in accordance with the criteria specified in the regulations. Thus, passive consent is, in effect, a waiver of parental permission and must be approved by an IRB according to the same criteria used for waiving informed consent. Researchers using children as research participants are encouraged to review the federal regulations for the protection of human subjects, 45 C.F.R. Subpart D (www.hhs.gov/ohrp/humansubjects/guidance/45cfr46.htm) as well as local IRB policy concerning the acquisition of informed consent. An example of a minor assent document is shown in Example 6.2.

EXAMPLE 6.2
Sample Minor
Assent Form

Minor Assent Form

Survey Phase

Project Title: <u>Physical Activity Behaviors of Children and Adolescents</u>

Name of Principal Investigator: <u>I. M. A. Researcher</u>

I, _____, have been told that one of my parents/guardians has given permission for me to participate in a research project about my exercise behavior. This will require me to complete a survey that asks questions about my exercise habits and my interests in physical activity. There are no right or wrong answers on the survey.

I understand that my participation is voluntary. I have been told that I can stop participating in the project at any time. If I choose to stop or decide that I don't want to participate in the project at all, nothing bad will happen to me. I have been told that my grade in school will not be affected in any way.

_____   _____

(Name)   (Date)

Although the federal requirements concerning informed consent are relatively straightforward, questions often arise about how much information the participant needs to know before consent can be given. Researchers often cite the Hawthorne effect or placebo effect in pointing out that participants in experimental studies may act differently if they are fully informed of the study, thus necessitating the use of deception in the research design. This deception might take the form of misleading the research participant or withholding information about the true nature of the study. Furthermore, it is recognized that some qualitative studies involving participant observation may not be possible if full disclosure is made *a priori.* As a result of legitimate dilemmas such as these, IRBs have been given the right to waive or alter requirements for informed consent if (and only if) it is clear that (1) the goals of the research cannot be accomplished if full disclosure is made; (2) the undisclosed risks are minimal; (3) the rights and welfare of the research participants are not adversely affected; and (4) when appropriate, participants will be debriefed and provided the research results (Belmont Report 1979). Nevertheless, there is continuing debate among scholars regarding the appropriateness of deceptive procedures in research methodology. It is also noted that federal regulations permit IRBs to waive the requirement to obtain a signed consent form in certain circumstances, a process referred to as waiver of documentation of consent. This is often the case in survey research in which the research presents no more than minimal risk of harm to the participants, the principal risk would be from a breach of confidentiality, and the only record linking the participant and the research would be the consent document.

Prospective participants in a research study must be able to comprehend the information they are provided with respect to the study. The presentation of information should be adapted to the participant's capacity to understand it and researchers should strive to write informed consent forms that are understandable to the prospective research participants. This involves avoiding the use of technical jargon as much as possible and writing at the reading level of the desired participants. Cardinal, Martin, and Sachs (1996) recommend that if the researcher is uncertain of the reading level of the target audience, informed consent forms should be written at or below the eighth-grade reading level. For further information on this topic, see Cardinal (2000), Ogloff and Otto (1991), and LoVerde, Prochazka, and Byyny (1989). Readability statistics, such as the Flesch-Kincaid Scale, are often included as options on major word-processing programs and may be useful to researchers for checking the reading level of informed consent documents.

Inasmuch as informed consent is the cornerstone of ethical principles regarding the participation of humans in research, professional associations such as the American Psychological Association (APA) and the American Education Research Association (AERA), among others, as well as leading journals in the kinesiology field, such as *Medicine and Science in Sports and Exercise* and *Research Quarterly for Exercise and Sport,* have developed policy statements regarding informed consent and the use of human research participants. Moreover, authors of research-based manuscripts in these and other professional journals are typically required to include some statement about the acquisition of informed consent from research participants.

For further information about informed consent, researchers are advised to consult materials published by the Office of Human Research Protections (OHRP) of the Department of Health and Human Services as well as their local IRB. The OHRP website contains considerable policy information about the protection of human research participants, in addition to useful guidelines designed to assist the researcher.

Policy and guidance information:
www.hhs.gov/ohrp/policy/index.html

Informed consent checklist:
www/hhs.ohrp/policy/consentckls.html

Human subjects regulations decision charts:
www.hhs.gov/ohrp/policy/checklists/decisioncharts.html

PRIVACY AND CONFIDENTIALITY

One of the major ethical concerns associated with conducting research involving human participants pertains to the issues of privacy and confidentiality. Yet there is considerable debate over the precise definitions of these two terms. Some experts argue that the terms can be used interchangeably, while others argue that they are completely distinct. While further debate about the definitions of privacy and confidentiality is beyond the scope of this book, it does seem clear that the terms are closely related. The definitions that follow are consistent with federal guidelines concerning research involving human participants. **Privacy** refers to the capacity of individuals to control when and under what conditions others will have access to their behaviors, beliefs, and values. That is, it is simply the control we have over information about ourselves. **Confidentiality** refers to the ability to link information or data to a person's identity. The expectation is that information that an individual has disclosed will not be divulged to others without permission. Confidentiality, then, pertains to how the personal information that is disclosed may be used.

Virtually any research endeavor in which the investigator seeks to obtain information about human participants brings forward the issues of privacy and confidentiality. Normally, these issues are addressed through informed consent, in which the prospective research participant, by indicating his or her consent to participate in the study, is providing authorization for the researcher to have access to certain specified personal information. Privacy issues do arise, however, in situations in which a researcher seeks to obtain information from student records, medical records, or client files. It is noted that the Family Educational Rights and Privacy Act (FERPA) describes the process researchers must use and requires parental permission for access to records of, or identifiable information about,

Privacy
The capacity of individuals to control when and under what conditions others will have access to their behaviors, beliefs, and values.

Confidentiality
The ability to link information or data collected during a research study to a person's identity.

children in public schools. Schools may disclose, without parental permission, "directory information" such as a student's name, address, telephone number, dates of attendance, etc. For more information and guidance, search the term FERPA at the Department of Education's website (www.ed.gov). The Health Insurance and Portability and Accountability Act (HIPAA), commonly referred to as the Privacy Rule, provides extensive regulations regarding the privacy and disclosure of individually identifiable health information (called protected health information or PHI) that is contained in medical records. Researchers proposing to use medical records as a source of data are encouraged to review HIPAA requirements (www.hhs.gov/ocr/privacy/hippa/understanding/index.html). The use of covert observation or participant observation, however, presents even more serious concerns regarding privacy. While it is not possible to specify precisely the methods a researcher might take to reduce problems associated with privacy in such cases, it is incumbent upon the researcher to take all reasonable and appropriate action to honor a person's right to privacy. Researchers would be well advised to consult with their local IRB in situations where privacy may be an issue.

Additionally, the informed consent form should indicate how the researcher will go about protecting the confidentiality of the participants. In most cases, the researcher is interested in group data and will aggregate individual scores or information. Confidentiality is a major factor in determining whether certain types of research projects involving education tests, surveys, interviews, or the observation of public behavior may be considered exempt from federal policy governing research.

According to federal policy (45 C.F.R. 46), researchers are responsible for insuring confidentiality of personal information obtained from human research participants unless express permission to the contrary is granted by the research participant. Procedures that the researcher might take to insure the confidentiality of his or her research participants include:

- Obtain anonymous information (best example being survey research in which responses are obtained with no identifying information).
- Code data in such a manner that identifying information is eliminated.
- Substitute surrogate names or information that could identify the participants.
- Do not release or report individual data.
- Limit access to data that could reveal a participant's identity. (For example, only the principal investigator would have access to the data.)
- Report the data only in aggregate form.
- Use computerized methods for encrypting and storing data.

Where research involves collecting data about sensitive issues (such as illegal behaviors, alcohol or drug use, or sexual behaviors), it is essential that researchers are able to provide assurances of confidentiality to the participants. In fact, in certain instances researchers are able to obtain a "certificate of confidentiality" that protects the identities of research participants or research data even against subpoena by law enforcement agencies. In general, the more sensitive the data being collected, the more attentive the researcher needs to be in protecting confidentiality.

RESEARCH INVOLVING ANIMALS

Although the general nature of kinesiology research precludes the frequent use of animals in research endeavors, it is not uncommon to see in some professional journals in our field the results of learning studies or biomedical studies utilizing animals. Animal research has long been a part of biomedical research and has produced significant benefits for humans. Questions have arisen, however, about the way animals are selected and treated as research participants.

Governmental agencies and professional associations have issued ethical guidelines and regulations for the utilization and care of animals in testing and research. While various guidelines for the proper care and use of animals in research have existed for many years, the *U.S. Government Principles for the Utilization and Care of Vertebrate Animals Used in Testing, Research, and Training* (Interagency Research Animal Committee 1985) is a primary directive in the United States. In general, the guidelines relate to the transportation, care, and use of vertebrate animals in ways that are judged to be scientifically, technically, and humanely appropriate. Similar regulations are included in the *Guide for the Care and Use of Laboratory Animals* (now in its eighth edition) published by the Department of Health and Human Services, and the *Public Health Service (PHS) Policy on Humane Care and Use of Laboratory Animals* (Public Health Service 2002). The current version of the *Guide for the Care and Use of Laboratory Animals* is available at the following website: oacu.od.nih.gov/regs/guide/guidex.htm. Moreover, the Animal Welfare Act of 1985 established assurance procedures to monitor compliance with federal regulations for conducting research using animals. The American College of Sports Medicine (ACSM) has promulgated a policy statement on research with experimental animals, while the American Psychological Association (APA) has developed standards for ethical conduct in the care and use of animals in research and testing (www.apa.org/science/anguide.html). For further information, readers contemplating research involving animals are advised to consult the sources named above as well as their local IRB.

INSTITUTIONAL REVIEW BOARDS

Institutional Review Boards (IRBs) have been established by federal mandate to ensure compliance with governmental regulations pertaining to research involving human research participants as well as animals. The "Common Rule" (45 C.F.R. 46) requires that all research protocols involving human research participants be reviewed by an IRB to ensure compliance with the requirements set forth in this policy. IRBs have the authority to approve, require modifications in, or disapprove the research. In addition, local IRBs have the authority to grant waivers or alter certain requirements as specified in federal guidelines. Although regulations specify the general requirements for IRB membership, function, and operation, IRBs vary considerably from institution to institution. Therefore, it is important that a researcher review IRB guidelines pertinent to his or her institution.

For research involving human participants, the "Common Rule" specifies that the following criteria must be met in order to obtain IRB approval for the research:

1. Risks to subjects are minimized.
2. Risks to subjects are reasonable in relation to anticipated benefits, if any, to subjects, and the importance of the knowledge that may be expected to result.
3. Selection of subjects is equitable in relation to the purposes of the research and its setting. Special attention is given to vulnerable groups such as children, prisoners, pregnant women, mentally disabled persons, or those economically or educationally disadvantaged.
4. Informed consent will be sought from each prospective subject or the subject's legally authorized representative.
5. Informed consent will be appropriately documented as required by federal statute.
6. When appropriate, the research plan makes adequate provision for monitoring the data collected to ensure the safety of subjects.
7. When appropriate, there are adequate provisions to protect the privacy of subjects and to maintain the confidentiality of data.

In addition, if the research involves vulnerable populations, such as prisoners, children, human fetuses, neonates, or persons with physical handicaps or mental disabilities, additional safeguards shall be included in the research plan to protect the rights and welfare of these subjects. Subparts B-D of the federal regulations (45 C.F.R. 46 and 21 C.F.R. 56) provide the special protections that are prescribed.

IRB approval is required before any aspect of the research that involves human participants may commence. Institutions develop procedures that all researchers, from graduate students to full professors, must follow to obtain IRB approval. Typically, this includes completion of a standardized form and/or checklist that describes the proposed research and identifies the research participants, types of data to be collected, methods to be used, inherent risks and anticipated benefits, and procedures to assure confidentiality. Example 6.3 provides an example of such a checklist. If appropriate, an informed consent statement and, in some

Protection of Human Research Participants

DIRECTIONS: This form is to be completed and submitted to the Committee when the investigator plans a research project which, in the investigator's judgment, requires expedited or full Committee review. Items 1–13 are the categories which may qualify for expedited review. *If "yes" is the response to any of items 14–17, the study does not qualify for expedited review (full Committee review will be required).*

STUDIES INVOLVING MINORS AND ECONOMICALLY OR EDUCATIONALLY DISADVANTAGED PERSONS <u>MAY</u>, IN THE DISCRETION OF THE CHAIR, REQUIRE FULL COMMITTEE REVIEW.

STUDIES INVOLVING PREGNANT WOMEN, FETUSES, ABORTUSES, PRISONERS, OR PERSONS WITH MENTAL DISABILITIES <u>WILL</u> REQUIRE <u>FULL COMMITTEE REVIEW.</u>

Yes   No

____ ____   1.   Collection of hair and nail clippings in a nondisfiguring manner; collection of deciduous teeth and permanent teeth if patient care indicates a need for extraction.

____ ____   2.   Collection of excreta and external secretions including sweat and uncannulated saliva; collection of placenta at delivery; collection of amniotic fluid at the time of rupture of the membrane before or during labor.

____ ____   3.   Recording of data from research participants 18 years old or older using noninvasive techniques such as measurements, weighing, electrocardiography, echocardiography, or thermography. Research involving radiation outside the visible range, i.e., x-ray, must receive full Committee review.

____ ____   4.   Collection of blood samples by venipuncture, in amounts not exceeding 450 milliliters in an eight-week period and no more than two times per week from subjects who are 18 years of age or older and who are in good health and not pregnant.

____ ____   5.   Collection of both supra- and subgingival dental plaque and calculus, provided the procedure is not more invasive than routine prophylactic scaling of the teeth, and the process is accomplished in accordance with accepted prophylactic techniques.

EXAMPLE 6.3
Concluded

Yes   No

____ ____ 6. Voice recordings made for research purposes such as investigations of speech defects.

____ ____ 7. Moderate exercise by healthy volunteers.

____ ____ 8. The study of existing data, documents, records, pathological specimens, or diagnostic specimens.

____ ____ 9. Research on individual or group behavior or characteristics of individuals, such as studies of perception, cognition, game theory, or test development, where the investigator does not manipulate participants' behavior and the research will not involve stress to the participants.

____ ____ 10. Research on drugs or devices for which an investigational new drugs (IND) exemption or an investigational device exemption (IDE) is not required.

____ ____ 11. Videotaping, filming, or audio taping (other than 6 above).

____ ____ 12. Use of minors under age 18, or economically or educationally disadvantaged persons.

____ ____ 13. Use of deception.

____ ____ 14. Use of prisoners, pregnant women, fetuses or abortuses, the seriously ill, or persons with mental disabilities, or incompetent individuals.

____ ____ 15. Collection of information or recording of behavior which, if known outside of the research, could reasonably place the participant at risk of civil or criminal liability or damage the individual's social standing, financial standing, or employability.

____ ____ 16. Collection of information regarding sensitive aspects of the subject's behavior such as: drug and alcohol use, illegal conduct, or sexual behavior.

____ ____ 17. This project includes procedures that present more than minimal risk to the subject.

____ ____ 18. The participants are free to withdraw from the study at any time without prejudice.

cases, copies of research instruments (e.g., questionnaires, inventories, interview schedules) may also be required by the local IRB.

Guidelines set forth in the code of federal regulations (45 C.F.R. 46) establish three categories of review, depending upon the amount of risk present to the research participants: exempt, expedited, and full review. DHHS regulations describe six categories of research that may qualify for exempt status.

Research activities in which the only involvement of human participants will be in one or more of the following categories may qualify for exempt status:

1. Research conducted in established or commonly accepted educational settings, involving normal educational practices, such as (i) research on regular and special education instructional strategies, or (ii) research on the effectiveness of or the comparison among instructional techniques, curricula, or classroom management methods.

2. Research involving the use of educational tests (cognitive, diagnostic, aptitude, achievement), survey procedures, interview procedures or observation of public behavior, unless: (i) information obtained is recorded in such a manner that human subjects can be identified, directly or through identifiers linked to the subjects; and (ii) any disclosure of the human subjects' responses outside the research could reasonably place the subjects at risk of criminal or civil liability or be damaging to the subjects' financial standing, employability, or reputation.

3. Research involving the use of educational tests (cognitive, diagnostic, aptitude, achievement), survey procedures, interview procedures, or observation of public behavior that is not exempt under paragraph (b)(2) of this section, if: (i) the human subjects are elected or appointed public officials or candidates for public office; or (ii) federal statute(s) require(s) without exception that the confidentiality of the personally identifiable information will be maintained throughout the research and thereafter.

4. Research involving the collection or study of existing data, documents, records, pathological specimens, or diagnostic specimens, if these sources are publicly available or if the information is recorded by the investigator in such a manner that subjects cannot be identified, directly or through identifiers linked to the subjects.

5. Research and demonstration projects which are conducted by or subject to the approval of department or agency heads, and which are designed to study, evaluate, or otherwise examine: (i) Public benefit or service programs; (ii) procedures for obtaining benefits or services under those programs; (iii) possible changes in or alternatives to those programs or

procedures; or (iv) possible changes in methods or levels of payment for benefits or services under those programs.

6. Taste and food quality evaluation and consumer acceptance studies, (i) if wholesome foods without additives are consumed or (ii) if a food is consumed that contains a food ingredient at or below the level and for a use found to be safe, or agricultural chemical or environmental contaminant at or below the level found to be safe, by the Food and Drug Administration or approved by the Environmental Protection Agency or the Food Safety and Inspection Service of the U.S. Department of Agriculture.

Please note that "exempt" does not mean that the researcher can simply ignore IRB guidelines and not submit required forms; it means that the proposed research is exempt from the full review process established by the IRB. Many institutions actually extend their requirement for IRB review beyond that specified by federal regulations, another reason to become familiar with local IRB policies. Expedited review pertains to research in which there is no more than minimal risk to the participants and the IRB review of the proposed research is conducted by the chair of the IRB or a designated member or members of the committee. Regulations define minimal risk to mean that "the probability and magnitude of harm or discomfort anticipated in the research are not greater in and of themselves than those ordinarily encountered in the daily life or during performance of routine physical or psychological examinations or tests." Moreover, minimal risk is determined to be relative to the daily life of a normal, healthy person. Full IRB review is required in instances in which the proposed research project involves more than minimal risk to the participants.

DISCLOSURE OF RESEARCH FINDINGS

The culmination of a research project generally results in the disclosure of the results in one form or another. Usual methods of disclosure include publication in a professional journal in one's field, presentation at a professional conference, report to a sponsoring organization, a news release, and, for student researchers, completion of a thesis or dissertation. Chapter 17 provides additional information on disseminating the results of a research study. It is through the disclosure of research findings that the scientific method furthers our knowledge, thus affecting professional practices and personal choices. In order for research to be viewed as a credible source of knowledge, the honest and accurate disclosure of research findings is essential. According to Monette, Sullivan, and DeJong (2001), the preeminent ethical obligation of the researcher (in terms of reporting the results of research) is to not disclose inaccurate, deceptive, or fraudulent results. So doing would undermine the very nature of the scientific process.

Scientific misconduct has been defined by the U.S. Public Health Service (1989) in the following statement:

> "Misconduct" or "Misconduct in Science" means fabrication, falsification, plagiarism, or other practices that seriously deviate from those that are commonly accepted within the scientific community for proposing, conducting, or reporting research. It does not include honest error or honest differences in interpretations of judgments of data.

Meanwhile, the National Science Foundation (2002) provided a similar definition of research misconduct:

> "Misconduct" means (1) fabrication, falsification, plagiarism, or other serious deviation from accepted practices in proposing, carrying out, or reporting results from activities funded by NSF; or (2) retaliation of any kind against a person who reported or provided information about suspected or alleged misconduct and who has not acted in bad faith.

It is clear from these definitions that "fabrication, falsification, and plagiarism" serve as the underlying elements of scientific misconduct, at least as defined by these federal agencies. While the notion of fabricating or falsifying research findings is foreign to the principles underlying the scientific method, there have been a number of reported instances in which researchers have made up or altered data or otherwise misrepresented the true findings of the study. Examples of scientific misconduct are regularly reported in publications such as the *Chronicle of Higher Education* as well as the *ORI Newsletter.*

The Office of Research Integrity (ORI) (ori.dhhs.gov/) is responsible for developing policies, procedures, and regulations related to the detection, investigation, and prevention of scientific misconduct in biomedical and behavioral research conducted or supported by the U.S. Department of Health and Human Services (DHHS) or its agencies. Considerable resources to improve the integrity of research and reduce research misconduct are available at the ORI website, including reports documenting incidents of misconduct that have been reported.

Severe penalties are usually imposed on those researchers who are found guilty of scientific misconduct. Drowatzky (1996) provides an extensive listing of possible penalties, which may include letters of reprimand, salary freeze, reduction in professorial rank, prohibition from obtaining outside grants, fines, dismissal from university, and referral to legal system for further action. Student researchers caught falsifying research findings could possibly receive a failing grade, be placed on probation, suspended, or even expelled, depending upon the regulations at the given institution. For example, a graduate student in kinesiology at the home institution of one of the authors of this textbook received a grade of "F" for nine hours of thesis credit and was suspended from school for fabricating data in research undertaken for the thesis requirement. The penalty could have been even more severe.

Plagiarism is frequently recognized as a problem with student papers or reports, but we also see plagiarism by professionals and students alike in scientific

Plagiarism
The presentation of ideas or the work of others as one's own; the absence of proper credit.

writing. Plagiarism is simply the presentation of the ideas or works of others as your own without giving proper credit. The ethical principle to follow here is merely to give proper credit to those whose work you borrow or cite. This is done through appropriate documentation in accordance with the chosen style manual. Sometimes plagiarism is accidental; the writer is either unfamiliar with the rules for correctly paraphrasing or quoting sources, or is careless in recording and citing sources. A number of universities have established websites that provide tips on avoiding plagiarism. Following are two such examples:

Northwestern University:
www.writing.northwestern.edu/avoiding_plagiarism.html

Indiana University:
www.indiana.edu/~istd

Authorship is the primary method through which researchers receive recognition for their research efforts. Authorship should be limited to those who have made a significant contribution to the research. In fact, it is generally recommended that the order of authorship be based upon the magnitude of one's contribution to the research. The researcher who is primarily responsible for conceptualizing the problem and developing the research plan is usually listed as first author. Additional authors are listed in order of their contributions. Moreover, all co-authors should have agreed to be listed as such. It is also noted that inclusion of a co-author strictly on the basis of the position of authority they hold (e.g., departmental chairperson) is inappropriate. It is recommended that all issues about authorship be resolved early on in the research process and certainly prior to commencing the publication/reporting phase. Publication of student research undertaken for a thesis or dissertation requirement poses special problems. Our viewpoint is that the student should always be listed as first author; the faculty chair of the thesis or dissertation committee may be included as a co-author, as well as other faculty, depending upon their contribution to the research. The ethical principles published by the American Psychological Association and the American Education Research Association both include standards pertaining to authorship and should be consulted for further information.

The financial support provided by corporations, agencies, and foundations has provided many researchers with the means to conduct research activities and thus further the body of knowledge. Without this support, it is quite likely that the magnitude and quality of research would be different from what we see today. Yet *sponsored research* poses particular ethical concerns. Who owns the data? Who controls the release of the research findings? Are there limitations placed upon subsequent publication of the results when they are unfavorable to the sponsor? Is it appropriate to withhold sponsorship information when obtaining informed consent? Controversy over matters such as these can often be resolved through contractual agreement with the research sponsor. It is important for the researcher to carefully read such contracts prior to signing and to understand the rights and responsibilities articulated therein. Violation of contractual agreements is not only unethical, it also

Authorship
The primary method through which researchers receive recognition for their research efforts.

constitutes a breach of law. A specific standard concerning the ethical integrity associated with sponsored research is included in the ethical standards of American Education Research Association.

Summary of Objectives

1. **Discuss various instances of ethical misconduct in research involving humans.** The atrocities associated with human experimentation by Nazi scientists during World War II shocked the world and served as the impetus for the development of ethical codes of conduct for biomedical and behavioral research. Revelations of scientific misconduct in the United States, including the Tuskegee Syphilis Study, prompted further reforms.

2. **Identify ethical codes and federal regulations that serve to guide research in the United States.** The international outrage over Nazi experimentation led to the development of the Nuremberg Code, a set of basic principles that govern research involving human participants. In the United States, federal policies and regulations now provide ethical guidelines for human participants as well as animals.

3. **Understand the importance of informed consent in research involving human participants.** The key provision of the Nuremberg Code demands that research participants are made fully aware of the nature and purpose of the project in which they will be participating, that they voluntarily give consent, that they are legally capable of giving such consent, and that the researcher is responsible for obtaining the participants' consent. Many professional associations have also promulgated ethical standards that serve to guide research activities of their members as well as the disclosure of research findings.

4. **Understand the role and function of Institutional Review Boards in approving research activities.** Institutional Review Boards have been established to provide a mechanism for the protection of research participants and to ensure compliance with federal policy.

5. **Explain ethical considerations involved in the disclosure of research results.** When publishing or reporting the results of their research, researchers are responsible for ensuring that their findings have not been falsified, fabricated, or plagiarized. Severe penalties are usually imposed on those who are found guilty of scientific misconduct.

7

Selection of Research Participants: Sampling Procedures

OBJECTIVES

While all steps in the research process are important, perhaps the most crucial to a successful investigation are the procedures used in the selection of research participants. The researcher first identifies and defines the population from which information is to be obtained. To study an entire population is difficult, if not impossible, hence the use of the sampling process. Considerations are given to such factors as sample size, how representative of the population is the sample, and the appropriateness of the participants to the various research methods and tests. The process of sampling permits the researcher to generalize the results from a study of the sample to the larger population.

After reading Chapter 7, you should be able to

1. Identify and define a population from which a sample of research participants is to be selected.

2. Explain the importance of randomization in sample selection.

3. Know the various methods of selecting samples.

4. Know the various factors that are used to determine sample size.

The needs of the research problem usually dictate the type of participants who will be selected for study. Quite frequently, the research purpose statement indicates what participants will be used in an experimental or descriptive study. It is imperative that the researcher have a carefully thought-out plan for selecting the participants.

The participants must be appropriate to the methods, techniques, and instrumentation that will be incorporated in the study so they can produce the needed research data. Participants should be selected who may be expected to be available throughout the duration of the study. The number should be large enough to (1) ensure reliability of the research results and (2) permit a reasonable number of participants to be available to produce data in the event of subject mortality (e.g., injury, absence, dropout for any reason).

Obviously, the realities of the research setting and the practical needs of the researcher often affect the research participant selection process. A physical fitness study involving children may need a large number of participants, whereas a mountain climbing study on the relationship of nutrition and altitude may involve few participants. A researcher studying selected mechanical aspects in pole vaulting cannot select just any pole vaulter. The objective would be to study the high-level, world-class vaulters; the availability of these athletes is very likely to present a problem for the researcher.

POPULATION AND SAMPLE

Population
An entire group or aggregate of people or elements of interest from which a sample will be selected.

Element
The basic unit from which data or information is collected; normally the research participant.

The term **population** refers to an entire group or aggregate of people or elements having one or more common characteristics. Often, a population is the focus of a research effort. Populations can be made up of people, animals, objects, organisms, institutions, attributes, materials, or any other defined **element.** We can talk about a population of fitness test scores, organizations, and personality traits. All four-year colleges and universities in the United States, all fourth-grade teachers in Iowa, all adolescents in Battle Creek, Michigan, all NCAA Division III basketball coaches, and all health education majors at the University of Georgia can be referred to as populations. The point is, researchers can define or describe a population any way they choose to suit the particular research purpose. The variable of self-efficacy, for example, could be studied among older Americans, athletes, the mentally disabled, various socioeconomic groups, teenagers, and many other populations.

Populations, then, can be defined in numerous ways. They can be quite large, theoretically infinite, as would be the case of the fitness test of all high school students; or they can be finite, such as the number of dance majors at a particular college. As a general practice, populations are considered finite.

A major reason for doing research is to obtain information that can be generalized to a population of interest. This could be accomplished by studying an entire group, but this is often impractical, if not impossible, to do. For example, if we really wanted to know the physical fitness status of all preadolescent children in the United States, we could fitness test all members of that group. However, this would not be possible in terms of the number of researchers needed to collect the data, the tremendous amount of money needed to finance the project, and the exorbitant time and energy the project would require.

Sampling
The process whereby a small proportion or subgroup of a population of interest is selected for scientific study.

Sample
A subgroup of a population of interest from which data are collected.

Because it is often difficult, if not impossible, to study an entire population, the process of sampling is undertaken. **Sampling** is the process whereby a small proportion or subgroup of the population is selected for scientific observation and analysis. A **sample,** then, is a subgroup of a population of interest that is thought to be representative of that larger population. The researcher observes and analyzes certain characteristics of the sample to get an idea of what those characteristics may be like in the entire population. From the information (data) obtained from the sample, the researcher then makes inferences about the population. The mean blood pressure score for a sample of cardiac rehabilitation participants is used to approximate the mean blood pressure for the entire population of such participants enrolled in a rehabilitation program. These statistics, then, are used to estimate the population information (parameters). The extent to which the results of a study can be generalized from the sample to the population of interest is referred to as *population validity*. The concept of population validity is particularly important in quantitative research.

The first step in the sampling process is the identification of the target population. Since it is often not realistic to work with the entire target population, it is usually necessary to identify that portion of the population that is available to the researcher, the *accessible population.* This accessible population actually represents the **sampling frame,** or collection of elements, from which the sample is actually taken. Obviously, the accessible population should closely resemble the target population. The researcher then determines the desired sample size (e.g., the number of research participants) and chooses the method of sampling that best meets the needs of the research in terms of feasibility and the ability to select an appropriate sample. Lastly, the sampling plan is implemented and the research participants are selected. It is important to note that the sampling process described here follows a logical, top-down approach, whereby the population of interest is first determined and then the sample is selected. It is all too common for the beginning researcher to use the opposite approach, selecting the research participants first and then trying to retrofit this sample into some population. The recommended steps in the sampling process are summarized below.

Sampling frame
The accessible population or collection of elements from which the sample is drawn.

1. Identify the target population.
2. Identify the accessible population.
3. Determine the desired sample size.
4. Select the specific sampling technique.
5. Implement the sampling plan.

The crucial element in the selection of a sample from a population is that the sample be **representative** of, or similar to, the population on the characteristics being investigated. If a researcher uses just a few health promotion majors to find out what may be true about a very large number of health promotion majors, then it is imperative that the researcher be as certain as possible that the small group of majors is representative of the total population of health promotion majors. Said another way, whatever variable is being studied in a particular population (e.g., attitude, behavior, self-concept, fitness, motivation) should be present in the sample drawn from that population.

Representative sample
A sample or subgroup of a population that is similar to the population on the characteristics of interest.

RANDOM PROCESSES

Randomization in sample selection is important to the quality of the research for three reasons: first, to help ensure the representativeness of the sample to the population about which generalizations will be made; second, to show that the researcher was unbiased as to which members of the population were selected for the study; and third, to equalize characteristics among groups in research studies requiring multiple groups, such as experimental and control groups. If each group is representative of the population, the groups will start the research equal in ability, and the research will be safe from criticism about which research participants were selected and placed in each group. Furthermore, random sampling is a basic requirement underlying inferential statistical tests.

Before discussing specific sample selection techniques in more detail, it is important that a clear distinction be made between **random selection** of research participants and **random assignment** of research participants. While both utilize random processes to achieve their goals, the underlying purposes are very different (Drew, Hardman, and Hosp 2008). As we have already seen, the purpose of random selection is to select a sample that is representative of the population. This is important for generalizing the results of the study and enhancing the external validity (i.e., population validity) of the study. Meanwhile, the purpose of random assignment is to establish group equivalence by randomly assigning research participants to treatment conditions or comparison groups. It is especially desirable that groups are equivalent prior to the introduction of a treatment condition, thus providing greater confidence in attributing posttreatment differences to the treatment. Random assignment is important to the internal validity of a study, particularly in experimental research. In Chapter 8, we provide further discussion of both internal validity and external validity. Since the use of random selection or random assignment procedures will increase your ability to generalize to a population and to reduce the chances of extraneous variables affecting your results, researchers are advised to use randomization procedures whenever possible (Harris 1998).

SAMPLE SELECTION METHODS

There are two primary types of sampling procedures, each of which has several different techniques. **Probability sampling** involves using selection techniques wherein the probability of selecting each participant or element is known. These techniques all rely on random processes in the selection of the sample. In **nonprobability sampling,** meanwhile, random processes are not used in the selection of the sample, thus making it impossible to know the probability of selecting a given participant or element from the population. As a result, it is more difficult to claim that the sample is representative of the population, thus limiting the ability of the researcher to generalize the results of the study. We discuss both types of sampling procedures in the following sections.

Random selection
Technique of using random processes for the selection of a sample that is thought to be representative of the population of interest.

Random assignment
Technique of using random processes to assign research participants to treatment conditions or comparison groups.

Probability sampling
A sampling technique based upon random processes in which the probability of selecting each participant or element is known.

Nonprobability sampling
A sampling technique such as convenience sampling in which random processes are not used and the probability of selecting a given sampling unit from the population is not known.

Probability Sampling

As previously described, probability sampling utilizes random processes or chance procedures to derive the sample. A key characteristic of probability sampling is that every element within the population, more precisely the sampling frame, has a known probability of being selected for the sample. Furthermore, when random processes are used to select a sample, it is possible to estimate **sampling error,** or the chance variations that may occur in the sampling process. Conceptually, you can think of sampling error as the deviation of the sample mean (or other statistic) from the population parameter. Sampling error is not indicative of mistakes in the sampling process, but merely describes the inevitable chance variations that occur when a number of randomly selected sample means are computed (Best and Kahn 2005). Although no sampling technique, including probability sampling, can guarantee a sample that is representative of the population, probability sampling is generally recognized as an efficient method of drawing a representative, unbiased, sample from a population.

Simple Random Sampling.   A **simple random sample** is obtained when every individual or element in the population has an equal chance of being selected, and the selection of one person does not interfere with the selection chances of any other person. This process is considered to be bias-free because no factor is present that can affect selection. The random process leaves subject selection entirely to chance.

Several different procedures may be used to obtain a random sample—the fishbowl technique, a table of random numbers, and computer-generated random numbers. In the **fishbowl technique,** the names of every individual in a population are written on a piece of paper. The pieces of paper are placed in a bowl, box, hat, or similar container, and the number of pieces of paper corresponding to the number of participants needed in the sample is drawn from the container one at a time. If we wanted to study 50 students from a population of 300 fourth-grade students, we would place the names of the 300 students in a container. One name at a time would be drawn until the sample of 50 was filled. This technique can be accomplished in two ways. If, after each name is selected, it is put back into the container, the method is called *random selection with replacement.* If the names are not replaced after they are drawn, this is called *random selection without replacement.* There is not a lot of difference between the two procedures when the population size is large, but selection without replacement does not strictly meet the definition of the random selection process. In the example above, each student has 1 chance in 300 of being selected. If the names are not replaced, the probability of each subsequent name being drawn increases (1 in 299, 1 in 298, etc.). So, if a name is selected, it should be replaced. If it comes up again, put it back into the container. Each person in the population then continues to have the same opportunity, or percentage of chance, to be selected. Despite the statistical correctness of random selection with replacement, most researchers sample without replacement since an individual cannot be used as a research participant again after once being selected.

Sampling error
The extent to which sample values (statistics) deviate from those that would be obtained from the entire population (parameter); difference among groups means because the samples are not 100 percent representative of a population.

Simple random sample
A type of probability sample in which every element in the population has an equal chance of being selected and the selection of one element does not interfere with the selection chances of any other element (i.e., equal and independent).

Fishbowl technique
Simple random sampling technique by which the names of all members of a population are placed in a container (such as a fishbowl) and then randomly drawn from the container one at a time.

TABLE 7.1 Excerpt from a Table of Random Numbers

014	801	501	101	536	020	118	164	791	646
223	684	657	325	595	853	933	099	589	198
241	304	836	022	527	972	657	639	364	809
421	679	309	306	243	616	800	785	616	376
375	703	997	581	837	166	560	612	191	782
779	210	690	711	008	427	527	756	534	981
995	627	290	556	420	699	949	887	231	016
963	019	197	705	463	079	721	887	620	922
895	791	434	263	661	102	811	745	318	103
854	753	685	753	342	539	885	306	059	533

Table of random numbers
A table (or book) consisting of numbers arranged in a random order that may be used to select a random sample or to assign research participants to groups.

Perhaps a more convenient and sophisticated way to select a random sample, or to assign participants to groups, is to use a **table of random numbers.** Many tables have been produced in which the numbers (0–9) are randomly ordered. Table 7.1 is an excerpt from a table of random numbers. Such tables are relatively simple to use. Just assign a number to the members of the population, then use the columns of numbers to pinpoint those members of the population who will be selected for the sample. For a more complete random number table as well as for guidelines for its use, you may wish to consult a basic statistics textbook such as Harris (1998).

There are a variety of computer programs, SPSS among them, that can generate a set of random numbers and greatly aid the sample selection process. Moreover, there are websites available that are specifically designed to assist researchers in randomly selecting research participants as well as randomly assigning them to experimental conditions. One such site is the Research Randomizer, located at www.randomizer.org.

Stratified Random Sampling. A big help in ensuring a representative sample is the process of *stratification.* A **stratified random sample** is achieved by dividing the population into various strata or subgroups, based on some characteristic that is important to control in the study, and then selecting a set number of research participants from each strata. The following is an example from a study of how the high schools in a given state financed the girls' athletic programs.

Stratified random sampling
A type of probability sampling in which the population is first divided into specific strata or subgroups and then a set number of research participants are randomly selected from each strata.

SCHOOL SIZE		
SMALL	**MEDIUM**	**LARGE**
0–499 pupils	500–999 pupils	>1000 pupils

Let's say that there are 400 schools in the state and the researcher decides to study financing practices in a sample of 100, or 25 percent of the schools, and randomly selects that number. There are many more small schools than medium or large ones, and just by luck the selected sample contains 80 small schools, 15 medium schools, and 5 large schools. The resultant data on how schools in the state finance the girls' athletic programs would probably be unbalanced in favor of the small schools and would not fairly represent the financing strategies of the medium and large schools. This problem could be overcome, or at least minimized, by first stratifying the schools by size, then taking a proportional random number of schools from each stratum. In our example above, there are 250 small schools, 125 medium schools, and 25 large schools. Since the researcher wants a final sample of 100 schools (25%), proportional stratified random sampling (taking .25 $\times$ the number of schools in each stratum) would yield, roughly, 63 small schools, 31 medium schools, and 6 large schools. Thus, the final sample of 100 schools is quite representative of the total population of 400 schools. Any generalizations or inferences from the sample to the population stand a better chance of being more valid than if proportional stratified random sampling had not been used. While not completely foolproof, this procedure is considered to be the most efficient way to achieve representativeness.

In some studies, however, the primary focus is on the differences among the various strata or subgroups in the population. In these situations, nonproportional stratified random sampling should be used to select equal-sized samples from each stratum, thus making group comparisons easier. If the focus of the research question is on differences among the strata, the researcher should select an equal number of participants (elements) from each stratum; if the characteristics of the entire population are the main focus, proportional sampling is more appropriate (Ary, Jacobs, and Sorensen 2010).

Systematic Sampling.   When some "system" is applied to the selection of research participants, we call the procedure **systematic sampling.** More precisely, systematic sampling involves drawing a sample by selecting every kth element from a list of the population, where k is a constant representing the sampling interval. For example, in a study of a population of 200 public and private schools in a large city, the researcher obtained an alphabetized listing of the schools from the state's department of education. The researcher then determines there is a need to draw a 20 percent sample from the population; thus 40 schools will be selected. The sampling interval is determined by dividing the population size by the desired sample size: $k = 200 \div 40 = 5$. The starting point would be randomly selected among the first five schools on the list, and then every fifth school thereafter would be selected. In another situation a researcher may decide to select every one-hundredth person listed in a telephone directory. In this case, $k = 100$. Another version of systematic sampling is illustrated by a researcher who is situated at a particular location and stops every fifteenth person who passes by and asks each a series of questions. In each of these examples, some "system" was applied to the selection of the sample.

Systematic sampling
A type of probability sampling in which the sample is drawn by choosing every kth element (research participant) from a listing of the population, where k is a constant representing the sampling interval.

If the listing of the population elements is in random order, which is rarely the case, systematic sampling is a good approximation of random sampling. However, systematic sampling does not strictly satisfy the definition of random sampling and, hence, is not entirely bias-free. Once the first element is selected, all the remaining cases in the sample are automatically determined, while others have no chance of being selected. Thus, all members of the population do not have an independent chance of being selected for the sample. In the schools example above, if every fifth school is selected, schools 4 and 6 have no chance of being selected. Subtle biases may also be present in systematic sampling, particular when the population listing is not in random order. Many parochial schools, because their names begin with *S*, cluster together near the bottom of an alphabetized listing. As a result, they would probably not be adequately represented in a sample chosen through systematic sampling.

Systematic sampling is quick, efficient, and saves time and energy. This is particularly true when populations exist on a definitive list or roster. In this instance, it is simply convenient to select every *k*th element of the population, as opposed to using a table of random numbers, which usually is a little more time consuming. The resultant sample will provide a good estimate of the population of interest, particularly if the sample is relatively large.

Cluster sampling
A type of probability sampling in which the sampling unit is a naturally occurring group or cluster (such as classrooms) of members of the population.

Cluster Sampling.   Also referred to as area sampling, **cluster sampling** is particularly appropriate in situations where the researcher cannot obtain a list of the members of a population and has little knowledge of their characteristics, where the population is scattered over a wide geographic area, and in situations where it is impractical to remove individuals from a naturally occurring group. Cluster sampling is a type of probability sampling in which the sampling unit is a naturally occurring group or cluster of members of the population. Thus, instead of sampling individual members of the population, clusters are selected. Examples of clusters particularly applicable to kinesiology research include schools, classrooms, city blocks, hospitals, and worksites. Let's say that a researcher wants to survey 1,000 teachers out of a population of 4,600 teachers in 46 schools in a large city. Each school has approximately 100 teachers. If the teachers were selected at random, the chosen participants would be scattered all over the city. The expense in time, money, and energy in designing a plan to get information from the 1,000 randomly selected teachers is enormous. The researcher decides to randomly select 12 schools from the population of schools, and then survey all teachers in each school. The teachers in each school comprise a cluster. Allowing for certain factors of subject mortality, the researcher reasonably expects approximately 1,000 teachers to respond. In this example, the random selection is of the schools not of the teachers, who are of interest in the investigation. The schools are the sampling unit because they are what were sampled. Conclusions and inferences are always stated in terms of the **sampling unit.** Since schools are the sampling unit, the mean score of the teachers in a school represents the score for a school, with a sample size of 12, not 1,000.

Sampling unit
The element or group of elements (cluster) that is selected during the sampling process.

In general, cluster sampling is more practical and less costly than simple random sampling, but it does hold the possibility of greater sampling error, particularly if the number of clusters is small. Furthermore, if clusters are not of equal size, there is also the possibility of introducing sample bias. An alternative to the cluster sampling procedure described above would be the process of **multistage sampling** which involves successive selection of clusters within clusters. In multistage sampling, the researcher will frequently perform one or more rounds of cluster sampling and then, in the final stage, randomly select elements (research participants) from the chosen clusters. For example, a researcher interested in investigating the health behaviors of high school students in Illinois could not reasonably expect to obtain a listing of all high school students in the state. It is simply not feasible to utilize simple random sampling procedures in this case. However, through the use of multistage sampling, the researcher could first randomly select school districts within the state, then schools within the selected districts, and finally classrooms within schools. If the researcher did not want to utilize all students within the selected classrooms, in a final sampling stage he or she could randomly select students (after all, that is really what we are interested in) from the chosen classrooms.

Multistage sampling
A type of cluster sampling technique which involves the successive selection of clusters within clusters and/or elements within clusters.

Nonprobability Sampling

As indicated earlier, if a researcher is to justify generalizations about the population from which the sample is drawn, the sample must be selected at random. The random sample is a chance sample and follows the laws of probability. Some samples do not.

Samples not selected at random are called nonprobability samples. Examples are intact classes, volunteers, a typical group, or a typical person. The results of these kinds of samples frequently do not reflect accurately the traits of the population in which the researcher is interested. They may not, then, be representative of the population and can lead to faulty conclusions.

Suppose a researcher wants to study fifth-grade pupils on some physical fitness variable. These students belong to a class made up of four sections of 30 pupils each for a population of 120 prospective research participants. The researcher's plan is to select 30 participants from the 120 at random. However, the school principal says, "No, the random selection would mean that some pupils from each section might be selected in the sample, and if you indiscriminately pull them out of their respective sections for testing purposes you will disrupt the school schedule. Instead, select just one section, intact, and make arrangements to do your testing before or after the school day." The question is, how representative of the characteristics of all of the fifth graders in the school is this one fifth-grade section? How representative is it of similar fifth-grade populations? The point is, intact or available groups impose a serious restriction on the researcher's ability to generalize the data obtained to the larger population from which the sample was drawn.

The use of volunteers can introduce an element of bias into an investigation. Say a researcher visits four college personal health classes and asks the students to volunteer to be in a study on the sexual behavior and characteristics of undergraduate college men and women. Twenty-five of the 150 students volunteer. How representative are four classes of a population of undergraduate men and women? Maybe the population should be the 150 students in the four classes. How representative of the 150 are the 25? The sample of 25 volunteers may be biased. What caused 25 students to accept the invitation to participate in the study and 125 to decline? The problem with volunteers is that they may be different from the nonvolunteers on the characteristics that are the focal point of the study. They usually possess special kinds of characteristics, which permit them to volunteer and which tend to bias the sample. Similarly, the selection of one individual elite swimmer or one group of elite swimmers, based upon the assumption that they are typical of all elite swimmers, provides for an element of bias also. Selecting research participants in this manner does not permit all elite swimmers an equal chance to be studied; the law of probability, or chance, has not been permitted to operate. To generalize from the "typical" subject to, perhaps, several hundred, would be stretching a point, to say nothing about the limits it would place on the researcher's ability to gain statistical significance when generalizing from the "sample" of one (or one "typical" group) to a larger population.

Purposive Sampling.   With this method, the researcher knows that specific characteristics exist in a certain segment of a population. Since these traits are extremely critical to the results of the investigation, the researcher using *purposive sampling* selects those research participants who contain the characteristics. Biomechanics researchers often purposely select excellent performers in a sport when they are trying to determine correct kinetic and kinematic parameters. Such factors are found in the top gymnasts, swimmers, basketball players, and other athletes, but they are probably absent in beginners or lower-level performers. Purposive sampling is the primary method of selecting research participants in qualitative research. Here the researcher will generally select participants because they possess certain characteristics or satisfy specific criteria that the researcher sets. Patton (2002) provides additional information about purposive sampling and discusses a variety of purposive sampling strategies that have particular application to qualitative research.

Convenience Sampling.   Convenience sampling, as the name suggests, is selecting the research participants on the basis of being accessible and convenient to the researcher. This approach to sampling often involves the use of volunteers and those individuals in existing groups who are handy to the researcher. This could be, for example, students who are enrolled in a class taught by the researcher, fellow graduate students, participants in a health promotion program that is administered by the researcher, or members of a sport team that the researcher coaches.

However, volunteers are known to be different from nonvolunteers. Yet the use of convenience samples in research, particularly that conducted by graduate students, is commonplace. The major problem with a study using this approach to selecting research participants is that the results are not likely generalizable beyond the participants in the study. This does not mean that the study should not be conducted or that the results are not accurate or credible; it simply means that the researcher should be cautious in generalizing the findings. In an attempt to justify the use of a convenience sample, researchers generally attempt to show that the characteristics of the sample are similar to those of the population. Nevertheless, a wise researcher should recognize the limitations of using a convenience sample and point this fact out in the written report of the study.

SAMPLE SIZE

Often the first question that a beginning researcher asks is, "How many subjects do I need?" **Sample size** is difficult to determine with any degree of certainty. Beginning researchers, particularly students, often believe that a large sample will produce better data and more valid conclusions based upon these data. Regardless of size, the crucial factor is whether or not the sample is representative of the population. A well-selected and controlled small sample is better than a poorly selected and poorly controlled large sample. Sample size is influenced by population size. Fifty subjects out of 100 may be representative, but 50 subjects from a population of 1,000,000 would not be representative.

Sample size
The number of elements or research participants in a sample selected for scientific study.

In the 1936 presidential election, the *Literary Digest Magazine* predicted that the Republican candidate, Alfred Landon, would defeat the incumbent Democrat, Franklin Roosevelt. The prediction was based on responses to the magazine's survey of 10 million United States voters, 2 million of whom responded. President Roosevelt won the election in a landslide, carrying forty-six of the then forty-eight states. While one might say that 2 million respondents is a large sample, it is obvious that the majority opinion of these people did not represent the entire population of eligible voters. The sample was drawn from telephone and automobile registration lists. In 1936, in the depths of an economic depression, a lot of people did not have telephones or automobiles. Those who did possess them had money and probably aligned themselves with the Republican party. The sample was biased and unrepresentative of the political leanings of most U.S. citizens.

In contrast, in 1988 George H.W. Bush was predicted to be the presidential victor with less than 5 percent of the votes cast. The sample on which the prediction was based was obtained through careful stratification of the voting population on several characteristics previously known to be related to voting practices, followed by proportional random sampling. This sample was unbiased and representative.

The size of the sample does become important in the statistical applications used to analyze the data produced by the sample, and in making inferences from the

Statistical power
The probability that the statistical test will reject the null hypothesis when, in fact, the null hypothesis is false.

sample to the population. The **power** of a statistical test is the probability that the test will reject the null hypothesis when, in fact, the null hypothesis is false. A powerful statistical test is one that can detect even small differences or a small effect. One of the factors that influence the statistical power of a test is sample size. In general, the larger the sample size, the more statistical power generated by the statistic being used. A long-standing convention in experimental research is to consider 30 per group as the minimum acceptable sample size. Another guideline is that sample size never needs to exceed 50 percent of the population. Conducting a prospective power analysis before a study has started can help a researcher determine the sample size needed to detect a difference that is considered important. For more information about statistical power and conducting a power analysis to determine sample size, the interested reader may wish to consult other research and statistics books, such as Thomas, Nelson, and Silverman (2005), Kraemer and Thiemann (1987), and Cohen (1988).

Sample size will also depend on the research approach utilized. Experimental studies will typically employ fewer research participants than will descriptive studies. Samples in experimental research are usually quite "captive" and, depending on the data-collecting demands, result in less subject mortality than in descriptive research. In the descriptive approach, especially when sending survey instruments through the mail, subject mortality, or attrition, can be quite large. The practice in descriptive research is to select a large enough sample so that if attrition does take place (i.e., people fail to return a completed survey instrument or questionnaire), an ample amount of data will still be produced.

Nonresponse in questionnaire studies must not be taken lightly. If 500 questionnaires are sent and only 100 are returned, what does this mean? How representative is the sample of 100 of the larger population from which the participants were drawn? What selective or systematic factor is operating to cause 400 people to decline the opportunity to participate?

The method of selecting the sample is probably just as important as sample size. Random sampling, as indicated earlier, is the best approach to sample selection because the laws of probability operate in such a way that sampling error in both large and small samples can be estimated. Utilizing random sampling, however, does not guarantee that the sample will be representative of the population. As previously noted, *sampling error* is the variation due to chance that exists between a population parameter and a sample statistic. This should not be considered a mistake or carelessness in the sampling process, but rather it is the expected random variation that a researcher would expect when using random processes for selecting the sample. Estimates of sampling error give researchers a gauge of the confidence they should place in their findings (Best and Kahn 2005). The selection process, the types of variables being studied, how the data on those variables are collected, the proposed statistical procedures, and elements of public relations may all operate to dictate sample size.

Whenever a sample is used, it is logical to wonder what the results might have been if all of the people in the population had been included. An appropriate sample usually provides a good estimate of what the results would have been. All estimates involve some degree of error; the goal is to minimize that error. The researcher never knows exactly how much error is present, but it can be at least partially controlled by obtaining a sample that is in proportion to the total number of people in the population. Let's say, for example, that a researcher wants to survey parental opinion on whether or not sex education should be taught in the elementary school. The percent of "yes" responses will be determined. The researcher wants to be able to say with 90 percent certainty that the sample percent comes within 5 percentage points of what the findings would be if all of the parents had been surveyed. Although the researcher knows there will be some variation in the percent of "yes" opinions from the sample to the population, if there is high confidence (90%) that this variation is small ($\pm.05$), faith in the sample percentage increases.

In this example, if 3,000 parents made up the population, the sample would have to include 341 parents. While several attempts have been made to develop a foolproof computational formula for determining the exact size of a sample, none presently exists. However, many statistics books do present various procedures for determining the sample size needed based on the confidence limits set by the researcher. Table 7.2 presents a table that was developed by Krejcie and Margan (1970) for determining sample size. It is based on 90 percent certainty (confidence) that the sample and population percentages do not differ more than .05. Tables for other situations can be found in books devoted to statistics or sampling procedures. In addition, there are numerous resources on the Internet that provide online calculations for determining sample size. The following are examples of such sites:

Sample Size Calculator: www.stat.ubc.ca/~rollin/stats/ssize

Creative Research Systems: www.surveysystem.com/sscalc.htm

As we have seen, a variety of factors affect sample size determination. The following guidelines, adapted from Best and Kahn (2005), summarize key considerations for determining sample size:

1. Sampling error is inversely related to sample size. That is, the larger the sample size, the smaller the sampling error and the greater likelihood that the sample is representative of the population.

2. Descriptive and correlational research typically should have larger samples than are required for experimental studies.

3. Sample size should increase as variability within the population increases. In other words, larger samples are needed with a heterogeneous population as compared to a population that is more homogeneous in nature.

4. When samples are to be divided into smaller groups to be compared, the initial sample size should be large enough that the subgroups are of adequate size to make meaningful comparisons.

TABLE 7.2 Determining Sample Size from a Given Population

N	S*	N	S	N	S
10	10	220	140	1,200	291
15	14	230	144	1,300	297
20	19	240	148	1,400	302
25	24	250	152	1,500	306
30	28	260	155	1,600	310
35	32	270	159	1,700	313
40	36	280	162	1,800	317
45	40	290	165	1,900	320
50	44	300	169	2,000	322
55	48	320	175	2,200	327
60	52	340	181	2,400	331
65	56	360	186	2,600	335
70	59	380	191	2,800	338
75	63	400	196	3,000	341
80	66	420	201	3,500	346
85	70	440	205	4,000	351
90	73	460	210	4,500	354
95	76	480	214	5,000	357
100	80	500	217	6,000	361
110	86	550	226	7,000	364
120	92	600	234	8,000	367
130	97	650	242	9,000	368
140	103	700	248	10,000	370
150	108	750	254	15,000	375
160	113	800	260	20,000	377
170	118	850	265	30,000	379
180	123	900	269	40,000	380
190	127	950	274	50,000	381
200	132	1,000	278	75,000	382
210	136	1,100	285	1,000,000	384

Note: N is population size.
   S is sample size.
* Sample size for 90% confidence that the difference in the population and sample percentage is no more than .05.
Source: Krejcie, Robert V. and Margan, Daryle W. (1970). Determining sample size for research activities. *Educational and Psychological Measurement*, 30, 607–610. Reprinted by permission.

5. Practical factors such as subject availability and costs are legitimate considerations in determining appropriate sample size.

6. The power of the statistical test needed to detect a meaningful effect or relationship is a factor related to sample size determination. The larger the sample size, the greater the statistical power, all other factors remaining constant.

Summary of Objectives

1. **Identify and define a population from which a sample of research participants is to be selected.** The identification of the target population is the first step in the sampling process. The goal of sampling is to identify a subgroup of the population of interest that is thought to be representative of that larger population.

2. **Explain the importance of randomization in sample selection.** Randomization is crucial in ensuring that the sample is representative of the population about which generalizations will be made. It also helps eliminate researcher bias from the research process and helps equalize characteristics among groups in studies involving more than one group.

3. **Know the various methods of selecting samples.** There are two primary types of sampling procedures. Probability sampling relies on random selection techniques in which the probability selecting each participant or element is known; techniques include simple random sampling, stratified random sampling, systematic sampling, and cluster sampling. Less reliable for the purpose of generalization are nonprobability sampling procedures—such as purposive sampling and convenience sampling.

4. **Know the various factors that are used to determine sample size.** Sample size is dependent upon factors such as: research approach utilized, population size, variability within population, statistical power needed, desired sampling error, as well as practical considerations. Regardless of sample size, the crucial issue is whether the sample is representative of the population.

Part Two

Types of Research

Research can be classified or typed in a variety of ways. Some authors use a three-classification system: experimental, descriptive, and historical. Other authors use a system with more than three classifications, which essentially splits into more parts the three classifications previously mentioned. Classifications can be developed based on a variety of criteria, such as the methods used, the intended use of the research, and the type of setting in which the research takes place. More than anything else, classifications of research serve as a convenient way of presenting research. Many research studies do not fit neatly under one research classification but have characteristics of several research classifications. The point to remember is that all well-conducted research is good research. There is no hierarchy to these research classifications.

In this book, types of research are discussed under five chapter headings. In Chapter 8, "Experimental Research," we deal with a type of research that is traditional and commonly conducted. It is research to find new ways of doing things in the future. In Chapter 9, "Descriptive Research," we cover many different research approaches. These also are traditional and commonly conducted types of research to describe the present situation. In Chapter 10, "Qualitative Research," we describe a common type of research in the social sciences though a relatively new type of research in kinesiology. The methods in qualitative research differ considerably from the methods commonly found in experimental research. In Chapter 11, "Meta-analysis," we deal with a reanalysis of many research studies already conducted in an attempt to draw conclusions which are supported by many studies. It is a type of research which has become commonly used in some areas of kinesiology. In Chapter 12, "Historical Research and Action Research," we consider two other approaches to conducting research. Historical research describes research conducted to show what happened in the past. It is not a common type of research in kinesiology but is slowly becoming more prevalent. "Action research" is conducted in the natural setting where it will be applied. It is a type of applied research which is conducted to try to find an answer to a problem that exists in the local or natural setting.

8

Experimental Research

OBJECTIVES

This chapter contains information concerning experimental research. You should be familiar with how experimental research is conducted and the major issues in conducting this type of research.

After reading Chapter 8, you should be able to

1. Understand what experimental research is and how it is conducted.
2. Know the threats to validity and how to control them.
3. Recognize the types of designs commonly used in experimental research.
4. Identify common errors of interpretation in research findings.

Experimental research is a traditional type of research and is conducted in most disciplines. It is virtually the only type of research performed in the sciences. In all cases, experimental research is conducted to increase the body of knowledge in the discipline and to suggest what procedures should be followed in the future. For example, a researcher who compares the effectiveness of two or more teaching or training methods, drugs, or techniques is trying to determine if there is one that is best and should be used in the future. The scientific method discussed in Chapter 1 is always followed in experimental research. Finally, experimental research always involves manipulation of the experimental unit (e.g., human participants, animal participants). Consider the typical methodological study where each group of participants receives a different treatment. The treatment received by a participant has the potential to change (manipulate) the participant. Isaac and Michael (1995) state that the purpose of experimental research is to investigate cause-and-effect relationships by subjecting experimental groups to treatment conditions and comparing the results to control groups not receiving the treatment.

PROCEDURE IN EXPERIMENTAL RESEARCH

In order to conduct a research study in a systematic manner, the researcher should follow a definite, orderly procedure, starting with initiating a problem area and ending with dissemination of the research findings. The five Ps, *prior planning prevents poor performance*, really apply here. Recall the 12 basic steps in the research process presented in Chapter 2. The procedure outlined below applies specifically to experimental research and provides researchers with 14 systematic stages.

1. *State the research problem.* Clearly identify both the problem to be researched and the purpose of the research. The research should not continue without a clear statement of the purpose because all subsequent steps and the entire conduct of the study are based on the statement of purpose.

2. *Determine if the experimental approach is appropriate.* Experimental research is conducted for the future and involves some manipulation of the participants by applying an experimental treatment. Not all aspects of the research have to be experimental, but the major thrust and conduct of the research is experimental.

   It is interesting to note that a study comparing existing groups (e.g., physical fitness differences between boys and girls) is often considered experimental research, but there is no manipulation of the participants. However, if the difference between boys and girls in terms of leisure time pursuits is being studied, the research is more apt to be classified as not experimental. In these two situations, the research will be conducted the same way no matter how it is classified.

3. *Specify the independent variable(s) and the levels of the independent variable(s).* As explained in Chapter 2, an *independent variable* is used to form the experimental groups and is unaffected by the experimental treatment. The levels of the independent variable are the number of different values it will take in the research study. For example, if four treatment groups are used in a study, the independent variable is treatment, and there are four levels. If the independent variables are training days with three levels and training time with four levels, the design is two-dimensional and each of the 12 groups receives a different combination of the two treatments, as presented in Table 8.1. Group 1 trains three days a week for 30 minutes each training day, while group 12 trains five days a week for 60 minutes each time.

   Essentially, it is at this point that decisions are made concerning the basic design of the study.

4. *Specify all the potential dependent variables. Dependent variables* are the variables that could be measured during the research study to generate the data for analysis. Scores of participants on these variables are dependent on

TABLE 8.1 Example Two-Dimensional Design

		MINUTES OF TRAINING TIME PER DAY			
		30	40	50	60
NUMBER OF TRAINING DAYS PER WEEK	3	Group 1			
	4				
	5				Group 12

the treatment they received. One or more dependent variables are identified at this step. The number and type of dependent variables are influenced by the statement of the research problem mentioned earlier.

5. *State the tentative hypotheses.* Experimental research requires a written *research hypothesis* that is either accepted or rejected based on the findings of the research study. The hypothesis is based on personal belief, presently accepted beliefs, and/or what the research literature supports. Since the researcher is supposed to be unbiased as to the outcome of the study and, in many cases, has no special insight as to outcome of the study or present beliefs, the research hypothesis is often one of equality. That is, the research hypothesis states that all groups are equal in ability at the end of the study, or, if a single group is measured before and after the experimental treatment, the hypothesis states there is no change in the ability of the group. However, a research hypothesis of inequality is also common. For example, if the research is comparing a traditional method with a new method and the researcher thinks the new method is better, the research hypothesis will be stated accordingly.

This statement is considered tentative because hypotheses very often have to be modified as the planning of the study progresses. Further, tentative hypotheses need to be established at this early stage because they influence some of the later steps in the research process.

6. *Determine the availability of measures for the potential dependent variables,* which were identified in number 4. These measures must have acceptable validity and reliability. Ideally, these measures already exist and are easily identified based on the researcher's knowledge and/or review of the literature. Often, the researcher will have to modify an existing measure to meet the needs of the study and to make the measure appropriate for the participants in the study. Such modification is acceptable as long as the measure, as

changed, remains valid and reliable. Sometimes the researcher will have to develop an entirely new test, instrument, or procedure to obtain the measure for a dependent variable. This is time-consuming since validity and reliability of the new measure must be determined before it is used. If the researcher decides a measure neither exists nor can be developed, the potential dependent variable is eliminated from further consideration.

7. *Pause to consider the success potential of the research.* Based on all numbers 1 through 6, does it seem that the research can be successfully conducted? If the research has little success potential, the project should be dropped before considerable time and energy is invested. Many things can be considered here. Certainly the time, expense, and difficulty of doing the research are concerns, and availability of participants is often a major consideration. The possibilities for establishing the levels of the independent variable(s) (see number 3) realistically and ethically must be taken into account. Also, the availability of measures for the dependent variables influences the success potential of a study.

8. *Identify the full potential of intervening variables.* Variables should be classified into the following groups: (1) should be controlled; (2) can be permitted to vary systematically; (3) can be ignored because of their relationship to variables classified as (1) or (2); and (4) can be left alone. Variables that can affect the outcome of the study must be controlled. Ways of controlling variables are discussed in this chapter. Systematic variables are not a danger to the outcome of the study because they vary in a known manner or in the same manner for all participants and groups in the study. Maturation of the participants is an example. If two variables are highly related, controlling one of them will control the other. Height and weight are an example. Variables that the researcher does not believe can affect the outcome of the study can be left alone. Care should be exercised to make sure that all important intervening variables are identified and that they are not misclassified as unimportant.

9. *Make a formal statement of the research hypotheses.* This is a refinement of number 5 based on information gained and changes made in the study during numbers 6 through 8. Issues related to stating hypotheses are addressed under number 5 and should be reviewed here. The research hypotheses stated at number 9 are important because the execution of the whole study is geared toward eventually providing the researcher with evidence for accepting or rejecting the hypotheses.

10. *Design the experiment.* This is usually a time-consuming step in experimental research because it involves considerable planning and identification of procedures for conducting the study. Even the smallest details of the day-to-day conduct of the study must be carefully considered. Insufficient planning at this point is the downfall of many experimental research studies. Planning for data collection, sample selection, and data analysis all take place here.

Before any data collection takes place, it is important that each research hypothesis be stated and that analysis techniques for all the data to be collected are known to exist. The value of conducting a pilot study at this step cannot be overemphasized.

11. *Make a final estimate of the success potential of the study.* It is good to pause before the experiment begins and check whether all stages of planning have been conducted adequately. Are there any aspects of the research study that could seriously limit the quality of the experiment in terms of potential conclusions? Particularly, are the procedures and controls in the potential study going to produce valid results addressing all of the research hypotheses?

12. *Conduct the study as planned in numbers 1 through 11.* There are likely to be aspects of the study that could be improved, but if the planning of the study has been thorough, no major problems will compromise the quality of the study. During the implementation of the study, constantly verify that the integrity of the experiment is being maintained. This continues through the final data collection.

13. *Analyze the data according to the data analysis plan.* The need for some analysis not in the original plan may arise during the course of the data analysis. This additional analysis is acceptable as long as it does not seem to be an effort to obtain findings in support of what the researcher wants to prove.

14. *Prepare a research report.* This report should, at minimum, contain the procedures used in the study as well as the major findings of the study. The report may be little more than a record of the research that the researcher will later use for reference when the memory of the details of the research is less clear. On the other hand, the report could be as extensive as a master's thesis.

INTERNAL AND EXTERNAL VALIDITY

Internal validity
Validity of the findings within or internal to the research study.

External validity
Validity of generalizing the findings in a research study to other groups and situations.

Validity was defined and discussed in Chapter 5 in terms of a measurement. Experimental research involves two other important classifications of validity. The first classification is **internal validity.** Internal validity deals with how valid the findings are within, or internal, to the study. Did the experimental treatments make a difference in the study in that the treatments caused the participants in the study to change in ability or are the changes in the ability of the participants due to other factors (see "Threats to Internal Validity" later in this chapter)? If the treatments caused the change in the ability of the participants, then internal validity can be claimed.

The second classification, **external validity,** is the degree to which findings in a research study can be inferred or generalized to other populations, settings, or experimental treatments. Particularly, external validity is concerned with whether the findings for the sample of participants in the study can be inferred to the population they represent and to other populations. In other words, are the findings in the research study unique to the participants in the study, or do the findings apply to other groups? If the findings in a research study can be inferred or generalized to other populations, settings, or experimental treatments, external validity can be claimed. A study using inmates in a prison might lack in external validity. Good internal validity is required to have good external validity, but good internal validity does not guarantee good external validity.

Control of all variables operating in an experimental research study is highly desirable but seldom, if ever, accomplished. The researcher would like all participants to be treated the same in terms of all variables (e.g., sleep, food, exercise) except for the experimental or treatment variable, which is allowed to vary among participants. Too much control can harm external validity, but not enough control destroys internal validity. Having so much control that the research setting is unique or totally removing the research from the setting where it will be applied destroys external validity. Excellent control is possible in prisons and military installations, but findings on participants in these places may not apply to participants in other situations.

CONTROLLING THREATS TO VALIDITY

Campbell and Stanley (1963) discuss 12 factors that can threaten the validity of an experimental research study. Isaac and Michael (1995) also discuss these potential threats in detail. The first eight factors threaten internal validity, and the last four factors threaten external validity. Obviously, a researcher tries to control as many of both types of these factors as possible in an experimental research study.

Threats to Internal Validity

History.   History refers to specific things that happen while conducting the research study that affect the final scores of the participants in addition to the effect of the experimental treatment. Suppose that participants participate in an activity or program outside of the research study but that this activity is very similar to the experimental treatment. If this outside participation increases their final scores, it makes the experimental treatment seem more effective than it really is. A second example is the atypical occurrence, such as an epidemic, local disaster, or one-time emphasis on the research topic in the community, that occurs in the lives of the participants during the research study and that affects their final scores.

Maturation.   Because the participants grow older during the experimental period, their performance level changes and this change is reflected in their final scores. For example, as young participants grow older during the 15-week experimental period, their physical performance level changes no matter what the effect of the experimental treatment. Similarly, as elderly participants grow older over the course of a six-month fitness program, their physical performance level decreases no matter what the effect of the fitness program.

Seasonal changes might also be considered here. For example, between September when the research study begins and December when the study ends, participants become less physically fit due to less daily activity because they are in school all day and the weather is bad. This loss of fitness counteracts the effect of the experimental treatment. A control group (group receiving no treatment) can be an effective check on the maturation threat.

Testing.   The act of taking a test can affect the scores of the participants on a second or later testing. For example, participants are pretested, then the experimental treatment is administered, and finally the participants are posttested. One reason why participants do better on the posttest is because they learn from the pretest. The pretest is like a treatment. This poses a real problem if the pretest and posttest are the same knowledge or physical performance test. Baumgartner (1969) tested participants with several physical performance tests, retested them two days later, and found that scores had improved from the initial test to the retest.

Instrumentation.   Changes in the adjustment or calibration of the measuring equipment or use of different standards among scorers may cause differences among groups in final score or changes in the scores of the participants over time. This suggests that researchers need to check the accuracy of their measuring equipment regularly and frequently and make sure a standard scoring procedure is used. Any difference in the test scores of several treatment groups or change in the test scores of the participants in a group over time (pretest to posttest) must be due to differences among groups or a change in the participants over time and not due to changes in the calibration of the equipment or scoring procedure. Testing equipment and scoring procedures must be held constant for each participant in research environments involving multiple pieces of the same equipment, multiple scorers, or multiple days of data collection.

Statistical Regression.   The tendency for groups with extremely high or low scores on one measure to score closer to the mean score of the population on a second measure is called statistical regression. This tendency may be mistaken for experimental treatment effect. For example, a high IQ and a low IQ group are formed. An experimental treatment is applied to both groups for 12 weeks. Then a physical ability test is administered to both groups, and it is found that they are equal in physical ability. This equality may be due to the regression effect or to the treatment effect. Using random sampling procedures to form groups eliminates the threat.

Research studies in which the research question is whether groups that differ in one attribute differ in terms of another attribute may have similar problems. For example, does a population of individuals with disabilities differ from a population of individuals without disabilities in their beliefs concerning use of leisure time?

No treatment is applied in this example, so random samples from the two populations are obtained and a score for beliefs about the use of leisure time is obtained for each participant. The finding that the two populations do not differ in their leisure-time-use beliefs is due to the regression effect.

Selection.   The way participants are selected or assigned to groups can be biased. This may result in groups that are not representative of a population, groups that are not equal in ability at the beginning of the experiment, and/or groups that differ at the end of the experiment for reasons other than differences in the integrity of the experimental treatments. Random selection of participants and random assignment of participants to groups usually controls this threat. Thus, following the random sampling techniques outlined in Chapter 7 and using sample sizes that are sufficiently large for the research situation will control this threat. When participant selection is a threat it is often due to small sample size per group and/or failure to use one of the necessary alternatives to simple random sampling when required for the research setting.

Experimental Mortality.   This particular threat to internal validity is created with the excessive loss of participants so that experimental groups are no longer representative of a population or similar to each other. Some participant loss is to be expected in a research study, but if many participants of the same type drop out of a group it can considerably change the characteristics of the group and the outcome of the study.

Also, this applies to disproportional participant loss among the groups. Usually groups are about the same size at the start of the research study, but if at the end of the research study they are considerably different in size, this is a concern.

Interaction of Selection and Maturation or History.   The maturation effect or history effect is not the same for all groups selected for the research study, and this influences final scores. This problem may arise when each group is an intact preexisting group rather than a randomly formed group. For example, if the groups differ considerably in age or background, this may affect how they respond to the experimental treatments. Also, if groups start out unequal in ability due to maturation or history, they may not have the same potential for improvement as a result of the experimental treatments.

Threats to External Validity

Interaction Effect of Testing.   This effect occurs when the pretest changes the group's response to the experimental treatment, thus making the group unrepresentative of any particular population and certainly unrepresentative of a population that has not been pretested. There is always the danger that administering a test before the experimental treatment (pretest) changes the participants. For example, the pretest may make the participants more aware of the need to increase their knowledge or performance level, causing them to respond to the experimental treatment more positively than they otherwise would.

Interaction Effects of Selection Bias and Experimental Treatment. The participants or groups selected in a biased manner react to the experimental treatment in a unique way so they are not representative of any particular population. High IQ or high skill level or metropolitan participants may not react to a particular treatment in the same way as low IQ or low skill level or rural participants and, thus, are not representative of them. If the population is well defined before the sample is drawn, this threat should be minimal. The problem (threat) can easily occur when a convenient group is used in the research and an attempt is made to define a population that fits the group.

Reactive Effects of Experimental Setting. The experimental setting is such that the experimental treatment has a unique effect on the participants or groups that would not be observed in some other setting. Thus, the results of the study are not representative of any particular population. If any element of the experimental procedure alters the normal behavior of the participants, then the effect of the experimental treatment may be altered and it will not have the same effect on a different group of participants. For example, participants may think the experimental treatment or drug is supposed to cause a change in their behavior or performance, so they react or perform differently for reasons that are not due to the treatment. Participants who react to the researcher in a unique manner provide another example. Conducting the research in a lab rather than in the natural setting is a third example.

Multiple-Treatment Interference. Multiple-treatment interference is the effect of prior treatments on the response of the participants or groups to a present treatment. This makes their response to the present treatment unique and not representative of the way any other population would respond to the present treatment. This effect can occur when the same participants are used in several related studies. For example, the same high performance level runners are used in three different studies dealing with the physiological responses to running. Are their responses in the third experiment influenced by participating in the two previous studies? Researchers should check on the background and experiences of potential participants to control this threat to external validity.

TYPES OF DESIGNS

Designs
The ways a research study may be conducted.

Designs are the variety of ways a research study may be structured or conducted. Campbell and Stanley (1963) present the advantages and disadvantages of many types of design in terms of how each controls the threats to validity. They classify designs as being either preexperimental, true experimental, or quasi-experimental. Only a few representative designs are presented here since it is impossible to present all the designs that the reader may encounter.

The **preexperimental designs** are weaker than true experimental designs in terms of control. Preexperimental designs have no random sampling of participants, are usually one group or two unequated groups, control few threats to validity, and have many definite weaknesses. The one-group pretest/posttest design is an example. It requires that a group be tested before the experimental treatment is administered and again after the experimental treatment has been administered. For example, 50 participants are administered an initial (pretest) fitness test. Then the participants are administered the experimental treatment which, in this case, is doing prescribed exercises one hour per day, three days per week for 18 weeks. Finally, the final (posttest) fitness test is administered. This is the same fitness test used for the pretest. If the group improved in fitness from the pretest to the posttest, the experimental treatment is judged to be effective. But all of the change from the pretest to the posttest may not be due to the experimental treatment. The change could be partially or totally due to the threats to validity of history, maturation, testing, instrumentation, selection and maturation or selection and history interaction, interaction effect of selection bias and experimental treatment, or interaction effect of testing. Only the threats to validity of selection and experimental mortality are definitely controlled in this design. Another example is the use of intact classes. All pupils in one class receive treatment A, and all pupils in another class receive treatment B. There is no random sampling of participants or random assignment of participants to treatments, so it is not known if the two treatment groups started the study equal in ability. If the treatment groups are unequal at the end of the study it may be because (1) the treatments were not equally effective, (2) the groups were unequal at the start of the study, or (3) some combination of the two previous reasons.

Preexperimental designs
Designs that have poor control often due to no random sampling.

The **true experimental designs** are recommended over other classifications of designs because they offer good control. True experimental designs always have random sampling of participants, random assignment of participants to groups, and all threats to internal validity controlled. The pretest/posttest control group design is an example. It is an extension of the preexperimental design just presented. Here, the experimental group is tested before and after the experimental treatment is administered. The **control group** is tested at the same times as the experimental group, but receives no treatment that should change its ability. Each group is a random sample from a population. Provided the experimental and control groups are equal in ability on the pretest, if the experimental group performs better than the control group on the posttest, the result should be due to the experimental treatment. This design controls the eight threats to internal validity but does not control the interactive effect of testing. Another example is the use of two experimental groups and a control group. From a population some members are randomly assigned to each of the three groups, but all members of the population are not selected as participants. Further, the two experimental and one

True experimental designs
The best type of design because there is good control with sufficient random sampling.

Control group
In a research study, the group which received no treatment which should change its ability.

control treatments are randomly assigned to groups. Assuming the three groups are equal in ability at the beginning of the study, differences among the three groups at the end of the study should be due to differences in the effectiveness of the three treatments.

Many times, the researcher will conduct the research in the setting where the research will actually be applied, but the situation will lack the control required for the true experimental design. The researcher quite often controls the data collection times and who is tested, but does not totally control when and to whom the experimental treatment is administered. Further, random assignment of participants to groups is not always possible. These situations lead to quasi-experimental designs.

Quasi-experimental design
An acceptable design but with some loss of control due to lack of random sampling.

The **quasi-experimental designs** are fine as long as the researcher understands what the designs do not control. These designs lack either random sampling of participants or random assignment of participants to groups. Quasi-experimental designs are much better than preexperimental designs. The nonequivalent control group design is an example. It is just like the pretest/posttest control group design except participants are not assigned to groups by using random sampling procedures. Instead, the experimental and control groups are existing groups, like classes or facilities, that are similar in characteristics and may be equal in ability. The pretest will indicate how similar they are before the experimental treatment is administered to the experimental group. This design controls the threats to validity of history, maturation, testing, instrumentation, selection, and experimental mortality; but it does not control threats to validity of the interaction effects of maturation and history, or the interaction effect of testing. Thus, this design does not have as much control as the true experimental design—the pretest/posttest control group design.

Designs have been discussed in terms of how they control the threats to validity. Also, designs can be discussed in terms of their complexity and ability to answer research questions. Simple designs answer one research question and more complex designs answer several research questions. To present various designs in an abbreviated form, X is used to represent a treatment is administered and O is used to represent data is collected. For example, $O_1 \, X \, O_2$ indicates that the participants are tested initially (O_1), a treatment is administered (X), and participants are tested once again (O_2). Presented in Table 8.2 are examples of designs ranging from simple to complex. In designs 1 and 2, the research question is simply whether some treatment will cause a change in the scores of a group; design 2 is the better design because it uses a control group. Designs 2 and 3 are both two-group designs but have different research questions. The fourth design is a combination of designs 2 and 3. Design 5 is essentially design 3 extended to three or more groups. Design 6 is presented primarily as a lead-up to design 7. Design 7 is superior to design 6 because more information is obtained in the form of combinations of A and B treatments. The A treatment and B treatment in designs 6 and 7 are two different treatments. For example, A treatment is three methods of instruction, and B treatment is two different number of weeks of instruction. In this example, design 7 is used because combinations of treatments A and B are possible. However, if A treatment

TABLE 8.2 Example Research Designs in Ascending Order of Complexity

DESIGN	RESEARCH QUESTION	DESIGN*	REMARKS
1	Is treatment effective?	O_1 X O_2	A group is tested before and after a treatment; compare means for O_1 and O_2 to see if O_2 is better.
2	Is treatment effective?	O_1 X O_2 O_3 O_4	Treatment group gets X and control group gets no treatment; sometimes O_1 and O_3 not collected; if means for O_1 and O_3 are equal, groups started equal; compare means for O_2 and O_4 to see if O_2 mean is better.
3	Which treatment is better?	X_1 O_1 X_2 O_2	One group receives X_1 and another group receives X_2; compare means for O_1 and O_2 to see if equal.
4	Is each treatment effective? Which treatment is better?	O_1 X_1 O_2 O_3 X_2 O_4	One group receives X_1 and another group receives X_2; if means for O_1 and O_3 are equal, groups started equal; compare O_1 and O_2 means and compare O_3 and O_4 means to see if treatments are effective; compare means for O_2 and O_4 to see if one treatment is better.
5	Which treatment is better?	X_1 O_1 X_2 O_2 X_3 O_3	Same as design 3 but more than two groups; compare means of O_1, O_2, and O_3.
6	The two questions are: (1) Which A treatment (A_1, A_2, A_3) is best?	A treatment X_1 O_1 X_2 O_2 X_3 O_3	See design 5; compare means of O_1, O_2, and O_3.
	(2) Which B treatment (B_1, B_2) is better?	B treatment X_1 O_1 X_2 O_2	See design 3; compare means of O_1, and O_2.
7	The three questions are: (1) Which A treatment (A_1, A_2, A_3) is best?	X_{11} O_{11}[†] X_{12} O_{12} X_{21} O_{21}	A treatment: Compare means of $(O_{11} + O_{12})$, $(O_{21} + O_{22})$, $(O_{31} + O_{32})$.
	(2) Which B treatment (B_1, B_2) is better?	X_{22} O_{22} X_{31} O_{31} X_{32} O_{32}	B treatment: Compare means of $(O_{11} + O_{21} + O_{31})$, $(O_{12} + O_{22} + O_{32})$.
	(3) Which combination of the A and B treatments $(A_1B_1, A_1B_2, A_2B_1, A_2B_2, A_3B_1, A_3B_2)$ is best? There are six groups, each receiving one of the six combinations of A and B.		Combinations: Compare means for O_{11}, O_{12}, O_{21}, O_{22}, O_{31}, O_{32}. See designs 3, 5, and 6.

$$\begin{array}{c|cc} & B_1 & B_2 \\ \hline A_1 & A_1B_1 & A_1B_2 \\ A_2 & A_2B_1 & A_2B_2 \\ A_3 & A_3B_1 & A_3B_2 \end{array}$$

* X = treatment is administered O = data is collected
[†] X = the treatment for the A B treatment group

is three ways of teaching first aid and *B* treatment is two ways of teaching sex education, the two treatments cannot be combined, so design 6 is used.

A design must control the major threats to validity and allow the researcher to answer the research questions. However, the KISS principle (*keep it simple, stupid*) should not be overlooked. The design must be adequate, but don't make the design any more complicated than it has to be.

In the previous section we learned that random selection and random assignment of research participants influence how a design is classified. So random selection of participants should be strived for in a design. Sometimes using an alternative to simple random sampling will enable the researcher to achieve random selection of research participants and random assignment of research participants to groups for a true experimental design. (Simple random sampling and alternatives to simple random sampling are discussed in Chapter 7.) From the design standpoint if there are two or more groups, the basic procedure is (1) define the target population, (2) identify the accessible population, (3) randomly select participants, and (4) randomly assign participants to groups.

> *Example:* A therapist (athletic trainer or physical therapist) wants to compare the effectiveness of two different exercise programs for people with a certain injury. Because it is unlikely that at any given time the therapist would have access to a large number of people with this specific injury, she cannot simply randomly select 30 or more individuals for each treatment group. However, she does have several options for alternative sampling.
>
> The therapist could contact colleagues at several locations to request that they systematically use the two exercise programs on their clients who have the injury. This would essentially give her a larger sample on which to test the two programs. Alternatively, the therapist could conduct the research study on her own clients over several years until she has enough research participants. In either case, when a client has the injury, the client should be randomly assigned—perhaps by flipping a coin—to one of the two exercise program treatments.
>
> It is important to note that with this procedure, all clients who have the injury are used in the research study, so there is no random selection of research participant resulting in a preexperimental design.
>
> A true experimental design can be achieved if the therapist is willing and able to use a random selection of clients from her pool of clients with the particular injury in question. This would give her a smaller sample, as not every client with the injury would be considered a research participant. For example, every fifth client with the injury would be eliminated from the study.

VALIDITY IN SUMMARY

Two classifications of validity and the threats to each classification have been discussed. In many research studies maximum internal and external validity cannot be obtained due to constraints on finances, time, participants, the research setting, or other resources. The researcher must decide what is most important, internal or external validity, and which threats to validity are more important to control than others.

As indicated earlier in the chapter, good internal validity is required to have good external validity. Campbell and Stanley (1963, 5) indicate that internal validity is the basic minimum for an experimental design. Thus, a research study must be designed in a manner that establishes good internal validity.

A researcher must consider the threats to validity while designing the study. After selecting a tentative design of the study, the researcher should determine which of the threats to validity exist, the seriousness of these threats, and how easy it is to control each threat. It is impossible to generalize to all research situations, but the strategy to follow is to modify the tentative design of the study to control the major threats to validity and those that are easy to eliminate. Minor threats and threats that are hard to eliminate may have to be uncontrolled. This strategy is much harder to accomplish when a major threat is hard to eliminate.

Cook and Campbell (1979) subdivide internal validity into statistical conclusions validity and internal validity, and subdivide external validity into construct validity of cause or effect and external validity. Discussion of statistical conclusion validity and construct validity of cause or effect requires background beyond the scope of this book. Advanced students may appreciate a discussion of the four types of validity.

METHODS OF CONTROL

Control is vital in experimental research. The researcher wants to control the effect of all variables except the experimental variable. Although ideal, this degree of control is seldom if ever achieved in kinesiology research. Nevertheless, the researcher must control the effect of the variables that could have a major impact on the study. Control of variables can be obtained in several ways.

The best way to control the effect of variables is by **physical manipulation.** The researcher physically controls all aspects of the participants' environment and experience throughout the experimental period. Thus, the amount of sleep, food intake, drug use, stimulation, stress, exercise, practice, or training is the same for all participants unless one of these variables is the experimental treatment. For example, if each of four groups is being taught by a different method, teaching method is the experimental treatment. The method varies from group to group, but the researcher tries to keep all other variables constant for all groups. Controlling all variables except the experimental treatment is difficult unless the participants happen to be prisoners, military recruits, or animals. The researcher tries to be sure each group receives the designated teaching method without any additional benefit from the method outside the experiment and without opportunity to benefit from the teaching method of another group. Since

Physical manipulation
Method of gaining control by the researcher physically controlling the research surroundings.

some variables cannot be physically controlled, the researcher might resort to other control methods.

Selective manipulation
Method of gaining control by selectively manipulating certain participants or situations.

Selective manipulation is commonly used to gain control and can take many forms. The intent of selective manipulation is to increase the likelihood that treatment groups are similar in characteristics and/or ability at the beginning of an experiment. By selecting only certain participants, the researcher manipulates the treatment groups to gain control. **Matched pairs** and **block designs** are forms of selective manipulation. The population to which the results of the research study are inferred or applied is defined. Accessible members of this population are tested on one or more variables that the researcher wishes to control in the study. Based on this variable(s) participants with similar scores are matched into pairs if two groups are needed or into blocks if more than two groups are needed in the research study. The same number of participants is randomly assigned to each treatment group from each pair or block. This procedure produces groups that start the experiment basically equal in terms of the variable(s) used for matching.

Matched pairs design
A form of selective manipulation by which participants are matched to gain control.

Block design
An extension of matched pairs design for three or more groups.

The variable(s) used for matching should be ones the researcher feels must be controlled because the variable(s) can have a major effect on the outcome of the study. Some common matching variables are initial ability, age, height, weight, gender, and IQ.

Example 1: The researcher wants to compare two teaching methods. She believes that gender may influence the effectiveness of a teaching method. So, the researcher assigns 20 boys and 20 girls to each teaching method using random sampling procedures.

This is different from subject pairing as presented earlier because it equates or balances the two treatment groups in terms of gender. If the researcher is willing to match participants based on both gender and IQ, 20 pairs of boys and 20 pairs of girls could be formed with the two participants in a pair basically equal in IQ score. From each pair, a participant is randomly assigned to each teaching method group. The groups are taught by the teaching method assigned to them, and then a test is administered to all participants. Differences between groups are checked based on test scores.

Example 2: The researcher is going to compare three different methods of developing strength in college males. Ninety-eight students are administered a strength test. Based on these initial test scores 13 blocks with six students of similar strength in a block are formed. Two students from each block are randomly assigned to each group. Participants train for 10 weeks with the method assigned their group. Then the strength test is administered again to each participant. Based on this final test score, differences among groups are determined.

Counterbalanced design
Method of gaining control by all participants receiving all treatments but in different orders.

Another common form of selective manipulation to gain control is the **counterbalanced design.** These designs require that all participants receive all treatments, but in different orders. However, these designs are limited to situations where it makes sense for participants to receive all treatments. Counterbalanced designs are an alternative to designs where each group receives one of the treatments, and differences among groups are examined to see if all treatments are equally effective. Campbell and Stanley (1963) and statistics books like Winer, Brown, and Michels (1991) and Keppel and Wickens (2004) discuss counterbalanced designs.

A simple example of a counterbalanced design is the comparison of the effectiveness of two drugs, A and B. To conduct the study a sample of participants is randomly drawn from a population. One-half of the participants receive drug A first and drug B later, while the other half of the participants receive drug B, then A. The process sequence is the same in both cases: A drug is administered, the participants are tested to determine the effect of the drug, a period of time passes to allow the drug to wear off and the participants to return to normal, the other drug is administered, and the participants are tested to determine the effect of the drug. Each participant receives a score under both drug A and drug B, so a comparison between the two drugs is possible. If there is an order effect so that the first drug taken influences the response of a participant to a second drug, the order effect is neutralized by counterbalancing.

Sometimes researchers conduct a study using only participants of one rather than both genders, or participants very similar in age or experience rather than more heterogeneous in terms of these attributes. For example, rather than use college undergraduate students as participants, the researcher uses 18- or 19-year-old freshmen. These techniques might be considered selective manipulation.

Often, **statistical techniques** are used to gain control in an experimental research study. Statistical techniques are applied when physical manipulation or selective manipulation of variables is not possible. The researcher knows, at the beginning of the study before the treatments are administered, that the experimental groups differ in terms of one or more variables that must be controlled in the study. If these variables are not controlled, the integrity of the research study is seriously compromised. Sometimes the variables that must be controlled are the same ones that would be used to form blocks in the block design discussed under selective manipulation techniques. In this situation, the research setting is such that the participants are already in groups so a block design cannot be used. The following is an example of the use of a statistical technique.

Treatment groups in the research study very often differ in initial ability. If the groups differ in ability at the end of the experiment, it is not known whether this is due to the initial inequality or difference in effectiveness of the treatments. A statistical technique commonly used in this situation is **analysis of covariance (ANCOVA).** Basically, the ANCOVA technique adjusts the differences among the groups in scores at the end of the study based on differences in initial ability among the groups. If differences among the groups are found after final scores are adjusted, the researcher concludes that all experimental treatments are not equally effective.

Statistical techniques
Method of gaining control if other control techniques are not possible.

Analysis of covariance (ANCOVA)
A statistical technique to gain control by adjusting for initial differences among groups.

Covariate
Score used to adjust for initial differences among groups in ANCOVA.

Variate
The score adjusted in ANCOVA.

In the ANCOVA technique, one or more scores called the **covariates** are obtained at the beginning of the study. Covariates are used to adjust differences among groups in terms of a score called the **variate,** collected at the end of the study. A statistical test of the differences among the groups in terms of the adjusted data is provided as part of the ANCOVA technique. The ANCOVA technique can be used with a variety of research designs and with as many covariates and types of covariates as the researcher desires. Extensive discussion of ANCOVA is found in Huck (2008), Winer, Brown, and Michels (1991), and Keppel and Wickens (2004).

In Chapter 14 there is a discussion of effect size, and statistical power. Some of this discussion relates to the issue of control.

COMMON SOURCES OF ERROR

Many possible sources of error can cause the results of a research study to be incorrectly interpreted. When error is present, the outcome of the study is not totally due to the experimental treatment. These sources of error are more specific than the threats to validity discussed earlier in the chapter. All sources of error are not a concern in every research study. Those sources of error discussed in this section of the chapter do not cover all potential sources.

Hawthorne Effect

This source of error is named for a research study that was conducted at the Hawthorne Electric Plant in the 1920s. It was observed that having a group of workers participate in a research study caused them to feel special so they acted differently from the typical worker. The research study was conducted to determine how changes in the working environment would affect productivity. Results of the study showed that productivity increased no matter whether the change in the working environment was supposed to increase or decrease productivity. This points out that participants in an experiment may perform in an atypical manner due to the newness or novelty of the treatment and because they realize that they are participating in an experiment. This suggests that, as much as possible, the participants should be unaware that they are participating in an experiment and also unaware of the hypothesized outcome of the study. Particularly in studies comparing new and traditional methods (e.g., teaching, training), the researcher does not want the new method to seem superior to the traditional method due to the Hawthorne effect.

Placebo Effect

The participants in an experimental treatment may believe the treatment is supposed to change them so they respond to the treatment with a change in performance. In a typical study to determine the effect of a drug, participants are pretested, administered the drug, and posttested. The researcher wants any change in the performance of the group from pretest to posttest to be due to the drug and not due to the fact that the participants think the drug is effective. In this example, the researcher has a second group (control group) that goes through the same procedure (pretest, drug, posttest) as the experimental treatment group, except the drug the control group receives is a **placebo,** a drug that can have no effect on the participants. Assuming the experimental and control groups were equal in pretest scores and that the psychological response to a drug is the same for both groups, superiority of the experimental group in posttest scores is due to the positive effect of the drug.

Placebo
A treatment that can have no effect on any dependent variable of participants in a control group.

In some studies the experimental group receives a treatment and the control group receives nothing. This seems like a poor research technique since the control groups should be receiving some placebo if psychological response to a treatment is to be the same for both groups. The treatment for the control group should be one that cannot affect the test score used to compare groups at the end of the study.

"John Henry" Effect

In studies with an experimental group and a control group, the control group knows it is not supposed to be better than the experimental, so it tries harder and outperforms the experimental group. This might be called the "Avis effect" after Avis Cars—we are number two, but we try harder. Of course, there could be a reverse "John Henry" effect where the control group gives up. It is also possible for the experimental group to improve due to the treatment and for the control group to improve due to the "John Henry" effect, thereby making the groups equal in performance at the end of the study. Again, it seems better to keep the design and expectations of the study unknown to the participants if possible.

Rating Effect

Several kinds of rating errors can occur. The **halo effect** is the tendency to let initial impressions or ratings of a participant or group influence future ratings. The halo effect can cause *overrater error* and *underrater error* to occur, in which the researcher tends to overrate or underrate participants. Finally, there is **central tendency error** where the researcher tends to rate most participants in the middle of the rating scale. Also, these rating errors can occur when participants are asked to rate statements about beliefs, practices, or problems (see Chapter 9). For example, each participant rates each of 25 statements about health practices on a 1-to-5 scale, with 5 being important and 1 being not important.

Halo effect
The tendency to let initial impressions influence future ratings or scores of a participant.

Central tendency error
A tendency to rate most participants in the middle of the rating scale.

Rating errors can be minimized by not looking at previous ratings. Also, a rating scale with 4 (e.g., excellent, above average, below average, terrible) to 7 (e.g., very strongly agree, strongly agree, agree, neutral, disagree, strongly disagree, very strongly disagree) well-defined different values can minimize rating errors. Rating errors can be minimized if the researcher develops the rating process properly.

Experimenter Bias Effect

The bias of a researcher can affect the outcome of the study. Experimenter bias may influence methodology, treatment, and data collection. This bias is often in favor of the experimental treatment the researcher believes is best.

Some people believe the researcher should not be involved in administering any of the treatments or collecting any of the data in methodological studies where each group receives a different method, such as teaching or training, over many weeks. This brings up an interesting dilemma when there are two or more groups in a methodological study. Should the same person administer the methods to all groups, or should different people administer the methods? If the same person administers all methods, the study could be criticized because the person may have biases and may not be equally effective with all methods. If different people administer each method, the study could be criticized because all people may not be equally effective with their methods. So the situation is a no-win situation (similar to a "heads I win, tails you lose" coin flip). None of this discussion addresses whether the researcher is administering any methods. In many studies the researcher does not have a choice who administers the methods, but if choices exist, the researcher selects the best procedure for the research setting. Usually the researcher is involved in administering the treatments and collecting the data because it is the researcher's study and there is no one else to do these tasks.

When possible, the researcher keeps the participants unaware of the purpose of the study and of their role in the study in order to eliminate any possible participant-caused error. Specifically, the participants are unaware of whether they are receiving the experimental or control treatment. This study is referred to as a **single-blind study.** The research setting and procedures used in many studies often preclude the single-blind study. When both the participants and those conducting the study (administering treatments and collecting data) are unaware of the purpose of the study and the way in which participants are grouped, the study is referred to as a **double-blind study.**

Single-blind study
A study in which participants are unaware of the purpose of the research study and their role in the study.

Double-blind study
A study in which participants and those conducting the study are unaware of the purpose of the study and group membership of participants.

Participant-Researcher Interaction Effect

Do participants respond better to researchers of the same gender, do they respond better to researchers of the opposite gender, or does it make any difference? It is reasonable to assume that, in some research settings, gender of the participants and researcher is influential and therefore contributes to error. What is important in any study is that the difference among groups in the research study and the effectiveness of the treatments in the study are not due to a participant-researcher interaction. The participant-researcher interaction effect should be minimal if the researcher functions with all groups in the same professional manner.

Post Hoc Error

This type of error is introduced by assuming a cause-and-effect relationship between two variables when such a relationship does not exist. For example: More people die in bed than any other place; therefore, beds are dangerous.

MEASUREMENT IN EXPERIMENTAL RESEARCH

Experimental research almost always requires measuring the participants involved with some test or procedure. Thus, questions like, What tests or procedures are available? How are the reliability and validity of these measures determined? How are these tests or procedures administered? commonly arise. Guidance in answering these questions is often found in measurement books. Researchers collecting physical performance data should consult measurement books in physical education and exercise science like Baumgartner, Jackson, Mahar, and Rowe (2007). If using some paper-and-pencil test or instrument to collect data, researchers might read measurement books in education and psychology such as Thorndike et al. (1991). Two excellent measurement books in health, which also contain considerable information on measurement in research, are Green and Lewis (1986) and McDermott and Sarvela (1999).

The newest tests, procedures, and techniques may not yet be in the measurement books, so they must be found in the research journals. Measurement specialists tend to conduct research dealing with improving or developing measurement tests, procedures, and techniques. Some researchers in all areas do measurement research on occasion.

Summary of Objectives

1. **Understand what experimental research is and how it is conducted.** Experimental research is conducted for the purpose of increasing the body of knowledge in a particular discipline; it is virtually the only type of research performed in the sciences. Experimental researchers use the scientific method (presented in Chapter 1) to prove or disprove particular hypotheses.

2. **Know the threats to validity and how to control them.** Researchers in kinesiology can take several steps to ensure

the validity of their findings. Maintaining good control is a crucial part of experimental research. Several methods of control can be used when designing experiments in health and human performance, including random selection and assignment, physical manipulation, selective manipulation, counterbalanced design, and statistical techniques.

3. **Recognize the types of designs commonly used in experimental research.** The variety of ways in which a research study can be conducted are called designs. Designs commonly used in experimental research include preexperimental designs, true experimental designs, and quasi-experimental designs.

4. **Identify common errors of interpretation in research findings.** Many possible sources of error can result in skewed interpretations of research findings. Among these are the Hawthorne effect, placebo effect, "John Henry" effect, rating effects, and central tendency error.

Descriptive Research 9

OBJECTIVES

This chapter contains information about descriptive research. You should become familiar with the various types of descriptive research and the techniques commonly used in conducting descriptive research.

After reading Chapter 9, you should be able to

1. Identify the common types of descriptive research.
2. Explain several types of survey methods.
3. Evaluate the quality of a research questionnaire.

Whereas in the last chapter we found that experimental research focuses on the future, descriptive research is oriented toward the present. Descriptive research is conducted to describe a present situation, what people currently believe, what people are doing at the moment, and so forth.

Descriptive research is a broad classification of research under which many types of research are conducted. Some people mistakenly believe that experimental research is the only approach. Others mistakenly think that descriptive research is easier to conduct than experimental research. Any type of research is good if it is conducted properly, and all research is demanding. For the study to be conducted well, the researcher needs to have some formal training and practical experience in the research area. It is foolish to try to conduct a research study in physics without sufficient formal training. Likewise, it is an error to try to use on elementary school-aged children the same techniques that are used on adults.

Descriptive research is conducted by collecting information and, based on this information, describing the situation. Descriptive research can, but does not have to, include a research hypothesis. Consider a study in which 10,000 high school seniors are selected from a population and surveyed as to whether they smoke tobacco, and 38 percent indicate they do. The researcher reports that 38 percent of high school seniors in the population smoke tobacco. Using the same research procedures, the researcher could have hypothesized prior to conducting the study that 30 percent of high school seniors in the population smoke tobacco. In this case, the researcher reports the 38 percent and whether the research hypothesis is accepted or rejected.

Descriptive research is commonly conducted in physical education and may be the predominant research approach in health, recreation, and sports management. Descriptive research is conducted in exercise science, but not as commonly as in the other disciplines mentioned.

TYPES OF DESCRIPTIVE RESEARCH

The types of descriptive research are briefly described in this section to provide a general awareness of and broad appreciation for them. The types of descriptive research discussed are survey, developmental, case study, correlational, normative, observational, action, and causal-comparative. Isaac and Michael (1995) offer a useful overview of descriptive research and the types of descriptive research.

Survey

Survey research is the most common type of descriptive research. It involves determining the views or practices of a group through interviews or by administering a questionnaire. The questionnaire may be administered to a group by the researcher or mailed to the members of the group for them to complete and mail back to the researcher. Survey research will be discussed in detail later in this chapter.

Developmental

Developmental research usually deals with the growth and development of humans over time. For example, what are the growth and developmental changes each year from age 6 to age 18? More accurately, what are the growth and developmental attributes of each age group? Other developmental research might examine how organizations or professional groups develop over time.

Longitudinal approach
Method by which a group is measured and observed for years.

There are two approaches to developmental research. One is the **longitudinal approach** in which a group is measured and observed on a regular basis for multiple years. For example, twice a year from age 6 to age 18 a large group of children is fitness tested. Based on this information, fitness standards are developed for each age level. The problem with this research approach is that it takes many years to complete, and it is difficult to keep track of the participants over the many years that the study lasts. However, such studies are tremendously valuable. Presently, many epidemiologists wish there were more fitness data available on middle-aged adults as children—to be able to answer questions concerning how fit children need to be in order to be fit as adults. As valuable as longitudinal studies may be, they are not a good choice for master's theses or doctoral dissertations due to the vast length of time involved.

The other approach to developmental research is the **cross-sectional approach.** Taking the earlier example of developing fitness standards for age groups with the cross-sectional approach, large samples of each age group are tested at the same time, and standards for each age group are developed. The assumption underlying this research approach is that each age group is representative of all other age groups when they will be or were that age. If this assumption is true, cross-sectional research will yield the same results as longitudinal research, but in a shorter time period. Cross-sectional research cannot always answer questions that longitudinal research answers. The earlier question by epidemiologists about fitness in children as an indicator of fitness in adults can be answered only with a longitudinal study.

Cross-sectional approach
Method for testing many groups and assuming each group is representative of all other groups when they are at the point in time.

Case Study

Case study research typically involves studying a person or event in great detail and describing what is found. A study of the training techniques or performance techniques of a highly skilled athlete is an example of a case study. It is assumed that less-skilled performers should use techniques of the highly skilled. A study of the way the Boston Marathon is organized and conducted for use as a model for how to organize and conduct a marathon is another example of a case study.

Being highly organized and very systematic in collecting the information needed to write the report is vital in this research approach. Essential to case study research is preparation by looking at literature on how to conduct case study research and at actual case studies for the techniques used.

Correlational

The purpose of correlational studies is to determine if a relationship exists between variables. The statistical techniques used in correlational research are discussed in Chapters 13 and 14. To determine if a relationship exists between two variables, each participant must be measured on both variables. For example, to determine if a relationship exists between time spent practicing a task and ability in performing the task, a practice time and task ability score must be obtained for each participant. If the data analysis shows that the longer a participant's practice time, the better the participant's task ability score tended to be, the researcher concludes that a relationship exists and that practicing a task is beneficial.

Usually the variables in a correlational study are not ones that the researcher tries to manipulate as in an experimental study. In the previous example, the researcher just determined how much each participant practiced and how well each participant performed the task. Many correlational studies deal with the relationship between a participant classification variable (e.g., height, weight, gender, age, income, education) and a variable of interest to the researcher. For example, what is the relationship between age and beliefs concerning use of leisure time?

Sometimes correlational studies involve three or more variables, and the purpose of the research is to determine how well one of the variables can be predicted by some combination of the other variables. For example, how well can college grade point average be predicted by high school grade point average and SAT scores?

Correlational studies can be conducted to try to explain why participants differ on a variable. This is a regression approach to a correlational study. Why don't all dancers execute a dance move with equal skill? Part of this difference in ability among dancers is explained by differences in amount of training, percent body fat, flexibility, and leg length to body height ratio. Wouldn't it be interesting to find that the leg length to body height ratio explained much of the difference among dancers in executing a move and that ability had little to do with things like amount of training, percent body fat, or flexibility?

Normative

Norms are standards of performance. The purpose of normative research is to develop performance standards. Performance standards are developed on a large representative sample from a population; these standards then are applied to other samples from the population.

Norm-referenced standards
Standards to rank-order individuals from best to worst.

Percentile ranks
A descriptive value that indicates the percentage of participants below a designated score; used in norm-referenced standards.

Standards can be *norm-referenced* or *criterion-referenced.* The majority of standards have been norm-referenced, but this discussion will consider normative research contributing to the development of either type of standard. **Norm-referenced standards** are designed to rank order individuals from best to worst and are usually expressed in **percentile ranks.** Test scores commonly achieved are presented in charts; for each test score there is a percentile rank indicating the percent of the participants in the norming group who scored below that test score. An example of norm-referenced standards is presented in Table 9.1. The percentile rank for the test score 4 is 42, indicating that 42 percent of the participants scored below the test score of 4. Standards published with most physical fitness tests prior to 1980 and many other nationally distributed tests are norm-referenced. Measurement books such as Baumgartner, Jackson, Mahar, and Rowe (2007) detail how to develop norm-referenced standards.

TABLE 9.1 Example of Percentile Rank Norms for a 10-Point Test

TEST SCORE	0	1	2	3	4	5	6	7	8	9	10
PERCENTILE RANK	3	8	15	30	42	55	65	74	80	91	100

Criterion-referenced standards are a minimum proficiency or pass-fail standard. Drivers license test standards and Red Cross lifesaving and first aid certification standards are criterion-referenced. Many physical fitness tests now have criterion-referenced standards. For example, if the criterion-referenced standard for passing the written drivers license test is 70 percent, the examinee must answer at least 70 percent of the test questions correctly to pass. Any percentage from 0 percent to 69 percent is failing, and any value from 70 percent to 100 percent is passing.

Criterion-referenced standards
Minimum proficiency or pass-fail standards.

Observational

This is research where the data are observations of people or programs. For example, five days a week for 18 weeks a researcher observed a community recreation program and wrote down everything he observed. At the end of the 18 weeks, the researcher wrote a report based on those recorded observations.

With this type of research, data collection and analysis are quite time-consuming and involve considerable technique. Formal training and practical experience are necessary before this type of research can be attempted.

Observational research has gained in popularity within kinesiology since 1980. It is discussed in detail in Chapter 10.

Action

Action research is conducted in the natural setting where it will be applied. Thus, it lacks some of the control possible with other types of research, but the results of the research are certainly correct for the setting. Action research is always conducted to try to find an answer to a problem that exists in the natural setting. Practitioners who constantly strive to do a better job are actually performing an informal type of action research. An example of action research could be the testing of a new approach to interest students or adults in starting a fitness program. Isaac and Michael (1995) contrast formal research, action research, and the casual approach to solving problems; they characterize action research as less precise and demanding than formal research, but superior to the casual approach.

Causal-Comparative

Also called *ex post facto,* **causal-comparative research** is research conducted using data that were generated before the research study was ever conceived. It is *"after the fact" research,* looking for relationships or explanations for certain things that presently exist by looking at data from the past. For example, looking at differences between heavy drinking and nondrinking 18-year-olds based on

Causal-comparative research
Research that seeks to investigate cause-and-effect relationships that explain differences that already exist in groups or individuals; also called *ex post facto research.*

information kept on file about these individuals over the last eight years is ex post facto research.

Isaac and Michael (1995) present a thorough discussion of this research method, also referring to it as causal-comparative research. Best and Kahn (2005) warn that just because two variables are related does not mean that a cause-and-effect relationship exists, with one variable causing an effect on the other variable. Several research books in education (Wiersma 1991; Best and Kahn 2005) discuss this research approach in detail.

SURVEY RESEARCH

Survey research is the most common type of descriptive research performed in the kinesiology area. For this reason, survey research is discussed further in this section of the chapter. The information presented in Chapter 5 under "Measurement Techniques" and "Questioning Techniques" should be reviewed at this time. Particularly the information concerning scaling techniques (rating scales, semantic differential scales, and Lickert scale) and structured questionnaires applies to the discussion at this time concerning questionnaire construction and use.

In survey research, information concerning opinions or practices is obtained from a sample of people, representing a population, through the use of interview or questionnaire techniques. This information provides a basis for making comparisons and determining trends, reveals current weaknesses and/or strengths in a given situation, and provides information for decision making.

As with most types of research, information obtained by a survey has limitations. Survey information reveals, at best, what the situation *is,* not what the situation *should be.* Surveys that deal with behaviors or attitudes do not reveal the factors that cause or influence the behaviors or attitudes. Further, a survey cannot be used to secure all the information sometimes needed for decision making. Surveys are quite often limited by the sample used and the information obtained. Finally, the information obtained may be inaccurate or misinterpreted.

The many survey methods and techniques used with them make it impossible to discuss all methods and techniques in detail. The authors' intent in this section of the book is to provide an overview of the methods and to discuss some of the more common techniques. Books are available on the survey method and the techniques involved with it. Bradburn, Sudman and Wansink (2004) have written a practical guide to questionnaire design. Sage Publications (2011) and Lawrence Erlbaum Associates (2011) list in their catalogs many excellent publications dealing with survey research, survey construction, phone interviews, personal interviews, attitude measurement, and much more. Recently, Web-based surveys have been used (Cronk and West 2002; Daley, McDermott, Brown, and Kittleson 2003; Pealer and Weiler 2000; Riva, Teruzzi, and Anolli 2003; Sills and Song 2002; Simsek and Veiga 2000; Vispoel 2000; Dillman, Smyth, and Christian 2008).

Preliminary Considerations in Planning a Survey

As in all types of research, the objective in planning the survey is to try to ensure that the data collected will be pertinent to the research question or problem. Survey research is performed no more easily or quickly than any other type of research. Sufficient training and experience in doing survey research, plus considerable planning, are necessary.

One consideration is whether the survey method is the most appropriate way to investigate the research problem. Survey research can be very time-consuming and financially expensive, so estimates of the time and cost should be made early in the planning stage. Finally, survey research can be conducted by phone interview, personal interview, administered questionnaire, or mailed questionnaire; planning should involve consideration of which survey method is best.

Survey Methods

Phone interviews are not often used by researchers in kinesiology as the primary data collection method. Personal interviews are becoming more prevalent. Administering a questionnaire to a group of participants is a technique commonly used in the field. However, the mailed questionnaire to a sample of participants is the method more often used than any other.

Phone Interview.   Marketing research, a form of survey research, and product sales commonly take place over the phone. Why do people in marketing research always call you at dinner time? Because you are likely to be home and probably have not been home all day. This is a phone interview technique: Call when people are home and are probably willing to talk to you. Don't call at 3:37 A.M., although people are usually home. When the phone is answered, the caller has about 10 seconds to say something to get the person's attention, or the individual is likely to hang up. This is also a technique: What questions do you ask the person, and in what order do you ask the questions? How long can you hold a person's attention on the phone? Ask questions that require a short answer, and plan how to record the person's answers. So there is considerable planning and technique in doing a phone interview. Much of the planning and technique for doing a phone interview is the same as that for doing a personal interview.

What are the advantages of a phone interview over other survey techniques? Phone interviews are quick and inexpensive when the sample is spread over a wide geographical area. But the method does not allow for very many questions to be asked, and recording the answers may be difficult. Talk to the survey researchers in business and sociology on campus who do phone interviews. Read the literature on phone interviews. Many of the educational research books address the topic. Babbie (2004) discussed phone surveys and noted that not all people have phones and listed numbers. This may bias phone survey results. However, Babbie indicated that random-digit dialing overcomes this problem and that this technique has gained popularity.

Personal Interview.   In the personal interview the researcher meets with each member of the sample, and based on their conversation, the needed information is obtained. If the sample is small and accessible, this is a feasible technique. When the information the researcher desires cannot be collected by asking a series of questions on paper (questionnaire), the personal interview must be used. For example, an interview is probably necessary to obtain information from a senior citizen about how things were 50 years ago.

What are some things to consider if the personal interview is selected as the data-gathering technique? One issue is how to contact potential participants for an interview time. Another is the decision whether to use a **structured interview** (asking each participant the same specific questions), a **semistructured interview** (asking each participant the same general questions), or an **unstructured interview** (just letting the conversation develop). The decision is dependent on what information the researcher needs, whether questions can be formulated in advance, and what the participant is comfortable with or will tolerate. Still another decision is how to record the information provided by the participant. Tape recording the interview may be best because every word is permanently saved. An alternative is to take notes during the interview. Both approaches may be unacceptable to the participant or be so intimidating that the participant will not be open or totally truthful with the researcher. A sufficiently experienced or skilled interviewer may be able to just talk to people, and then write everything down after the interview is over and the participant is no longer present. The point is, personal interviews require much more planning and technique than many people realize.

Some of the advantages of the personal interview are completeness of response, ability to clear up misconceptions, opportunity to follow up responses, and increased likelihood that the respondent will be more conscientious with the interviewer present. Isaac and Michael (1995) favor the structured interview because it requires less training of the researcher and is more objective than the unstructured or semistructured interview. They also present some guidelines for interviews. Other useful references for those who desire additional information are Wiersma (1991), Rubin (1983), Babbie (2004), and Gall, Gall, and Borg (2010).

Administered Questionnaire.   For a variety of reasons, the majority of survey research conducted in kinesiology uses a questionnaire as the data-gathering technique. A questionnaire is a series of questions or statements on paper. Each participant is given a copy of the questionnaire. The participant responds to the questionnaire and then returns it to the researcher. If the researcher can meet with the participants, the questionnaire will probably be administered to all the participants at one time or to several groups of participants at several times. However, the most prevalent procedure is to mail or distribute the questionnaire to the participants,

---

Structured interview
Interview for which each participant is asked the same specific questions.

Semistructured interview
Interview for which each participant is asked the same general questions.

Unstructured interview
Interview for which no questions have been prepared for a participant; a conversation.

who complete the questionnaire on their own, and then return it to the researcher. Since the majority of procedures are the same no matter whether the researcher administers the questionnaire or distributes it for completion, the majority of information about questionnaires is discussed in the section on distributed questionnaires. Information specific to administered questionnaires is presented here.

If the researcher is unable to get the participants together at one time or in several groups to administer the questionnaire, the researcher may as well distribute the questionnaire. Often, a researcher seeks permission to administer a questionnaire to an intact group such as a class, school, agency, or exercise program. The other possibility is to organize the participants so they come together in one or more groups to complete the questionnaire. In either case, a room or facility must be secured for administering the questionnaire. The facility must be large enough to easily accommodate the largest possible group and conducive to completing a questionnaire (i.e., is quiet, contains desks or tables providing a writing surface, has adequate seating, etc.). Some thought should be given to whether pencils and other materials need to be provided. Certainly, what to say to the participants about the purpose of the questionnaire and how to complete it needs to be planned. How to pass out and receive back the questionnaires has to be thought through. The larger the group, the more important these plans become, particularly if the researcher has access to the room or facility for only a limited amount of time. A common pitfall is to think that a questionnaire that typically takes 45 minutes to complete can be administered in 60 minutes. All participants will not arrive on time, giving the verbal directions and distributing and receiving the questionnaire will take time, and some participants will take more than 45 minutes to complete the questionnaire.

Distributed Questionnaire.   When the sample is geographically spread or cannot be brought together as a group, the distributed questionnaire is used. Distribution may be by mailing it to the participants or putting it in their mailbox at work, by handing it to the participants in class or at work or in some location where they gather, or by having another person distribute the questionnaires for you in classes or on job sites. This will include some planned procedure for having participants return the completed questionnaire to the researcher. Researchers distribute more questionnaires by mail than by any other method.

Good questionnaire research requires considerable planning and technique and is not something that just anyone can throw together quickly. Professional pollsters and marketing research experts conduct outstanding questionnaire research. Graduate students often do a poor job with questionnaires due to lack of knowledge and sufficient planning.

Everyone receives many questionnaires in the mail each year. The good ones are often completed and returned; the poor ones usually go in the trash. By way of example of the latter, the authors once received a poorly xeroxed copy of a questionnaire. One question asked, "Do you belong to TAHPERD?" First, was the question referring to the Tennessee or Texas Association of Health, Physical Education, Recreation and Dance? Second, why would a person living in Georgia belong to either one? The questionnaire was a xeroxed copy of one that another researcher had developed for use in Tennessee. The questionnaire went in the trash.

The following discussion of questionnaire research assumes that the questionnaire is distributed and returned by mail. Questionnaire development, format, distribution, return, and examples are treated separately.

Questionnaire Development. Questionnaires are used for a variety of purposes, and very often the purpose dictates the type of items (i.e., question or statement) used in the questionnaire. So item type is one decision to be made in questionnaire development. An item is classified as **open-ended** if participants have the freedom to respond however they choose. For example, the question "Why did you enroll in this adult fitness program?" is open-ended. A second type of item is **completion;** the subject fills in the blank. For example, "What is your age in years to the last year?" is a completion item. The third type of item is **multiple choice** or closed-ended; the possible responses to the item are provided and the participant selects the most appropriate response(s).

Following are two examples of a closed-ended item:

Open-ended item
Question for which no potential response is provided; participants respond however they choose.

Completion item
Question for which answer is left blank and participant fills in the blank.

Multiple-choice item
Question for which responses are provided and the participant selects the most appropriate response(s).

1. Select the response below that best reflects your feelings about the research course you are presently taking.

1. Great   4. Below average

2. Above average   5. Terrible

3. Average

2. Of the vehicles listed, check the ones you own.

———— 1. Car   ———— 4. Motorcycle

———— 2. Truck   ———— 5. RV

———— 3. Jeep   ———— 6. Van

Commonly, questionnaires are used to determine opinions or attitudes. Here is an example:

Indicate your degree of agreement or disagreement for each of the following items.

1. Being the best in a group is very important to me.

1. Strongly agree   3. Disagree

2. Agree   4. Strongly disagree

Each item must be carefully written so it is easy to understand and not ambiguous. This takes considerable time if done correctly since the questionnaire must be read and edited several times. Rules and hints on writing knowledge tests generally apply here. The reading level as well as the attention span of the participants must be considered. Directions for responding to the questionnaire must be presented at the top of the first page of the questionnaire. An example question and response are often provided right after the directions. If the questionnaire is supposed to cover a content area or be all-inclusive, then care must be taken to develop items that cover the necessary area.

Reliability and validity of the questionnaire must be determined *before* it is used in the research study. Validity (discussed in Chapters 5 and 15) is the degree to which the interpretations of the questionnaire data are correct. Thus, it is assumed that the questionnaire measures what it is supposed to measure. Just because you developed the questionnaire does not make it perfect. Validity is usually estimated by a jury of experts. The jury should have representation from content experts, questionnaire construction experts, and questionnaire use experts. Hopefully, the jury will find the questionnaire to be well constructed, covering the necessary content, and ready for use. Based on the input from the jury, the questionnaire may be revised and evaluated by the jury again, depending on the extent of the revisions.

Reliability (see Chapters 5 and 15) is consistency of response. The researcher wants to be assured that the responses of the participants to the questionnaire would not be different if the questionnaire were administered to them at some other time. As ideal as it might be to administer the questionnaire to some participants on two different days to check for consistency of response, this is rarely done. Instead, researchers put several pairs of items in the questionnaire with items in a pair either similar or opposite. Items 6 and 33, below, provide an example of paired opposite items.

6. I like candy.　　　**33.** I don't like candy.

  1. Agree　　　　 1. Agree

  2. Disagree　　　 2. Disagree

The questionnaire is administered and the responses to paired items are examined to see whether they are as expected. No matter whether the questionnaire is administered on two different days or on one day with paired items, an intraclass R can be obtained as an estimate of reliability, either for each item administered twice or for each pair (see Chapter 15 or Baumgartner, Jackson, Mahar, and Rowe 2007).

The goodness of the questionnaire should be determined before it is used to collect the research data. This is always the case with the reliability and validity of a questionnaire just discussed. Some researchers determine reliability or validity using data from the research study. The problem with this is that if the reliability or validity is poor, it is too late to make changes in the questionnaire to improve reliability or validity. Unreliable or nonvalid data are no good, so all unreliable or nonvalid data should be discarded.

As discussed in Chapter 5, under "Instrument Development," a pilot study is the best solution to this possible problem. The questionnaire is administered to a small number of individuals similar to the participants who will take part in the research study, and the reliability and validity for their data are estimated. As part of the pilot study, it is a good idea to keep track of such things as how long it takes individuals to complete the questionnaire, whether the questionnaire appears to contain any ambiguous items, and any other factor that could affect the successful administration of the questionnaire. Based on the pilot study, the questionnaire is revised as needed.

Questionnaire Format.   The appearance and layout of the questionnaire is as important as the content. The questionnaire must be professional in the way it is typed, and in the quality of the paper and reproduction, or people will not complete it. Items need to be arranged in rows or columns for a neat appearance, ease of completing the questionnaire, and ease of data entry into the computer, if necessary, for analysis. Demographic information such as age, gender, education, and income are often requested on the questionnaire. Since questions about age and income sometimes irritate people, demographic questions should be placed at the end of the questionnaire. Irritating questions at the end of a questionnaire are often left blank, but if they appear at the beginning of a questionnaire it may cause the entire questionnaire to go into the trash. In fact, any controversial item should be placed at the end of the questionnaire for the same reason (e.g., "Have you gained a lot of weight in the last five years?").

Answers to closed-ended items that will be computer-analyzed need to be numerically coded. Participants should be asked to check the appropriate item or circle the appropriate number.

EXAMPLE:

Poor format
What is your gender? _____

Good format
Circle the number for your gender.
1. Female   2. Male

or
Check the number for your gender.
_____ 1. Female
_____ 2. Male

Closed-ended items are preferable to completion items. Also, it is better to provide choices in the form of nonoverlapping intervals rather than specific values, particularly on items that may have a large number of different values, for which the participant may not know the exact value, where the researcher does not need the exact value, or which may irritate the participant.

EXAMPLE:

Poor format

What is your income? _____

Good format

What is your income?

_____ 1. Less than $12,000

_____ 2. $12,001 to $18,000

_____ 3. $18,001 to $27,000

_____ 4. $27,001 to $40,000

_____ 5. More than $40,000

Inform the participant whether one answer is desired or whether multiple answers to an item are desired (see the earlier example in this chapter on vehicles owned). This is particularly important when the data are going to be computer-analyzed, because sufficient space must be allowed to accommodate all answers. When multiple answers are possible, each answer choice is treated as if it were an item: A one (1) is entered into the computer if that answer is checked, and zero (0) if it is not checked.

Questionnaire Distribution.   The biggest concerns with distribution are controlling the cost of getting the questionnaire to the participants and trying to obtain a high rate of questionnaire return. The researcher can influence both. For example, the fewer the pages in the questionnaire, the less expensive it is to mail and the shorter it looks to the participant, the more likely that it will be returned. Generally, there is a tendency to have too many items on a questionnaire. No matter what the number of items, reproduce the questionnaire on both sides of the page and use the smallest readable print size. Even the weight of the paper used can sometimes influence mailing rate.

The researcher is expected to provide a self-addressed stamped envelope for returning the questionnaire. Failure to do so will almost certainly decrease the rate of return. To minimize the postage on the return envelope, ask participants to respond to all closed-ended items on a standardized answer sheet rather than on the questionnaire and to just return the answer sheet. Standardized answer sheets are often an efficient tool for organizing the data to be entered into a computer. However, if groups are not familiar with standardized answer sheets, their use will decrease questionnaire return rate or result in such poorly erased or completed answer sheets that data will be lost.

A good mailing list is an essential component of distributing a questionnaire. Lists are not always highly accessible. Lists with the name of a person rather than a title (e.g., "department head") are generally desirable. However, if the questionnaire is going to the person presently in the position and there is considerable turnover in the position, a title may be better than a personal name. Check into the advantages and disadvantages of bulk mail in comparison to first- and second-class mail in terms of cost, speed of delivery, and forwarding, because considerable cost reduction is possible with bulk mail.

Researchers can do a number of things to try to improve the percentage of questionnaires returned. To give some idea of the extent of this problem, the expected rate of return is 50 percent; perhaps an 80 percent return may be expected from professional participants who have an interest in the questionnaire results; but only a 10 percent return is likely when surveying the general public. For this reason researchers tend to send out enough questionnaires to ensure a desired number of returns. However, a small percentage of returns makes the goodness of the results questionable. Are the participants who returned the questionnaire really a representative sample of the target population? Would the results have been different if more people had returned the questionnaire? It is important to motivate people in every way possible to return the questionnaire. A cover letter with the questionnaire explaining why the study is being conducted and its importance to humanity will improve the return rate. A cover letter signed by an influential person also increases the return rate. Offering to share the results, giving money, a catchy saying ("a penny for your thoughts," and enclose a penny) all help to motivate people to return the questionnaire.

Sending the questionnaire out at a time when people are likely to have time to complete and return it is good strategy. Sending questionnaires to coaches in the middle of their season or to anyone just before Christmas is not wise. Also, one to three follow-up letters sent at two- to three-week intervals after the first mailing, reminding people to return their questionnaire, increases the percentage of returns. Having participants put their name on the questionnaire before they return it makes follow-up easier and is to the advantage of the researcher. However, some participants will not return the questionnaire or will not be totally truthful in completing it if they have to put their name on it. If there are any highly personal items on the questionnaire or any items dealing with illegal activities, do not request the participant's name on the questionnaire.

EXAMPLE:

How often do you smoke pot?

1. Weekly
2. Monthly
3. Several times a year
4. Never

Law enforcement agencies have been known to confiscate questionnaires dealing with illegal activities. Generally, it is better not to ask for names on questionnaire returns unless you really need them.

Questionnaire Return.   Most survey studies require the use of a computer to analyze the volume of scores. A 50-item closed-ended questionnaire returned by 350 participants generates 17,500 scores. So when questionnaires are returned, scan them to be sure they are ready for data entry. Even if names are on the questionnaires, give each questionnaire an identification number, enter that number and questionnaire data into the computer, check the information for data entry error, and then destroy the questionnaire. Of course, open-ended questions must be analyzed by hand.

Anticipate that some items on some questionnaires will not be answered because participants will accidentally skip or decline to answer certain items. This is acceptable as long as only a few items on each questionnaire are left blank and it otherwise seems that the participant completed the questionnaire accurately. Some researchers put items on a questionnaire to check for accuracy of participant response and reject those questionnaires that fail the accuracy check. For example, a drug use questionnaire includes a long list of drugs and requests participants to check the ones they use. Kerosene is on the list of drugs, and a participant checks it; the questionnaire is rejected. Unexpected responses to open-ended items are sometimes found. The same drug use questionnaire contained this item: "Is there a big drug problem on campus?" One participant responded, "No!! You can get it anywhere." The questionnaire was not rejected.

The accuracy of participant response to attitude scale questionnaires is usually checked by stating some items positively (e.g., smoking is okay) and some items negatively (e.g., drinking alcohol is evil) to produce a varied response to items within participants. In this case, a researcher rejects the returned questionnaire if visual inspection shows that the majority of the items are answered with the same response; it appears that the participant just checked answers without reading the items.

Questionnaire Examples

I. *Poor format*

Listed are activities taught in the physical education department. Please check the activities you have taken at the university. If you check an activity, then please check the skill level you presently have in the activity. "B" is beginner, "I" is intermediate, and "A" is advanced.

| ACTIVITY | TAKEN | SKILL LEVEL | | |
		B	I	A
Archery Bowling Golf Dance Swimming Tennis				

Note: This is a poor questionnaire because much space is wasted, and there is no numerical coding of responses.

Improved format

Listed are activities taught in the physical education department at the university. Please use the following code to indicate your status for each activity.

CODE: 0—Did not take activity

1—Took activity; presently have beginner level skill

2—Took activity; presently have intermediate level skill

3—Took activity; presently have advanced level skill

_____ Archery	_____ Dance
_____ Bowling	_____ Swimming
_____ Golf	_____ Tennis

II. *May I have about five minutes of your time?*

I need your assistance.

This is my dissertation research. The purpose of the study is to determine what faculty members think are important attributes in a department head. Using the scale shown below, please rate the importance of each attribute of a department head. Then return your ratings in the enclosed addressed, stamped envelope.

Importance Rating Scale

Extremely   Extremely
Unimportant _____ Important

       1   2   3   4   5   6   7

Attributes

_____ Friendly

_____ Professional

_____ Organized

_____ Good looking

III. *Using the key below, rate each task by putting an "X" in the face that best represents your feeling.*

KEY ☺ I know that I have the ability to perform the task.

☺ I am not sure that I have the ability to perform the task.

☹ I know that I don't have the ability to perform the task.

1. How do you feel about your ability to dribble a ball without your opponent getting it away from you? ☺ ☹ ☺

2. How do you feel about your ability to do a front roll? ☹ ☺ ☺

Note: This questionnaire can be scored 3–2–1 from smile to frown; the faces follow no pattern from item to item; faces can be used with young children.

IV. *What are the four biggest problems in our discipline today?*

    Note: This is an open-ended question because the researcher does not know all the problems and probably does not have enough space on the questionnaire to list all the problems.

V. *What was your undergraduate degree major?*

VI. *An example of a questionnaire is presented in Example 9.1.*

    Note: It is not the content but the form of this questionnaire which is important; the original questionnaire is for tests no longer used.

EXAMPLE 9.1
Example Questionnaire

The AAHPERD Fitness Tests Opinionnaire

The American Alliance for Health, Physical Education, Recreation, and Dance (AAHPERD) presently distributes the Youth Fitness Test (used by the President's Council on Physical Fitness and Sport) which was introduced in 1957 and the Health Related Physical Fitness Test which was introduced in 1980. AAHPERD must decide whether to continue to distribute the two tests, combine the two tests into one test, or discontinue one test. Numerous groups and committees have given AAHPERD their recommendations. However, public school physical education teachers have had very limited input on this important issue. This is your opportunity to make your views known. What AAHPERD does will influence what fitness tests are available to you in the future.

This opinionnaire is endorsed by the American Alliance for Health, Physical Education, Recreation, and Dance.

This opinionnaire should take less than 15 minutes to complete. Please complete each question and return it today in the stamped, self-addressed envelope.

1.   Are you aware of the Youth Fitness Test (due to college classes, reading, workshops, etc.)? (circle number)   1. Yes   2. No

2.   Have you administered the Youth Fitness Test within the last three years? (circle number)   1. Yes   2. No

3.   Does your school or school system require that you administer the Youth Fitness Test on a regular basis? (circle number)   1. Yes   2. No

4-a.   If you were given the choice, would you administer the Youth Fitness Test on a regular basis? (circle number)   1. Yes   2. No
    3. I do not have enough information about the test to decide.

(Continued)

EXAMPLE 9.1
Continued

4-b. If you answered *no* above, circle *one* or *more* reasons why you would not plan to use the test. [circle number(s)]

1. Too time-consuming   2. Too unfamiliar
3. Lack of equipment   4. Not in line with program objectives
5. Not sufficiently motivating 6. Not valid
7. Not enough space   8. Other (specify) _____

_____

[*Note:* Questions 1 through 4-b were repeated here for the Health Related Physical Fitness Test (questions 5 through 8-b).]

9. Do you administer some kind of fitness test in your physical education program at least once a year? (circle number)

1. Always   2. Usually
3. Seldom   4. Never

For each fitness test item listed below, please indicate if you feel the item should be part of a fitness test battery. (circle a number under *Yes, No,* or *No Opinion*)

	YES	NO	NO OPINION
10. Distance run	1	2	3
11. Sit-ups	1	2	3
12. Pull-ups (boys)	1	2	3
13. Flexed-arm hang (girls)	1	2	3

[*Note:* Questions 14–18 are not listed to save space.]

Finally, we would like to ask a few questions to help us interpret the results and to give you a chance to make comments and suggestions.

[*Note:* Several of the original nine questions are included.]

3. What is your school called? (circle number)

1. Elementary school   2. Middle school/Junior high school
3. Senior high school   4. Other (specify grade levels) _____

4. What percent of your teaching time is spent teaching physical education, *not* health education or other subjects? (circle number)

1. 0–20   2. 21–40   3. 41–60   4. 61–80   5. 81–100

EXAMPLE 9.1
Concluded

5.   What is your age? (circle number)

   1. 20–29 years   2. 30–39 years
   3. 40–49 years   4. 50–59 years   5. 60 years or older

6.   What is your gender? (circle number)   1. Female   2. Male

9.   Is there anything else you would like to tell us with regard to fitness testing? If so, please use the space below.

The questionnaire presented in Example 9.1 has a number of desirable features. The cover page includes an introduction to the opinionnaire, an estimate of the amount of time needed to complete the opinionnaire, and instructions for returning it. For each question, the number of answers which may be circled is identified. All answers are number-coded. Participants are allowed to answer "no opinion" for questions 10 through 18. Finally, the opinionnaire ends with some demographic questions.

Questionnaire Summary.   Research using a questionnaire as the data-gathering instrument is quite common in kinesiology. Considerable information has been presented concerning construction and use of a questionnaire. For people who will seldom use a questionnaire, it may be too much information. But for people who will use a questionnaire in their research, it is probably not enough information. A number of excellent sources are available for those who desire more information. All of the following are enlightening: Isaac and Michael (1995); Wiersma (1991, chap. 7); Best and Kahn (2005, chap. 5); and Neutens and Rubinson (2002). Books specific to survey methods and mail surveys such as Babbie (1990), and Weisberg and Bowen (1977) are excellent sources.

Summary of Objectives

1.   **Identify the common types of descriptive research.** The most common and familiar type of descriptive research is the survey. Other types of descriptive research include developmental research, case studies, correlational studies, normative research, observational research, action research, and causal-comparative, or "after the fact," research.

2.   **Explain several types of survey methods.** Surveys can be conducted as phone interviews, or personal interviews, which can vary in structure from very specific to very

general. Surveys can also be conducted through the use of administered questionnaires. Questionnaires can include multiple-choice or closed-ended questions, which are easy to compare, as well as open-ended questions that allow more varied responses.

3. **Evaluate the quality of a research questionnaire.** To be a useful research tool, a questionnaire must meet several criteria. The survey itself must be carefully designed and administered to a randomly chosen but appropriate population, and should be easy to read, complete, and submit. Questions should be unambiguously written and should extract the desired information in a consistent manner. Validity and reliability of surveys should be judged by a panel of experts.

Qualitative Research 10

Jennifer Waldron
University of Northern Iowa

OBJECTIVES

This chapter contains information regarding qualitative research. After reading this chapter you should understand the distinct role of the six qualitative research traditions in kinesiology. Further, you should understand how data collection and data analysis in qualitative research are woven together.

After reading Chapter 10, you should be able to

1. Identify the constructivist paradigm and characteristics of qualitative research.
2. Name and explain the six qualitative traditions.
3. Articulate the process of data collection via interviews.
4. Understand a basic method of data analysis.

The majority of this textbook is devoted to quantitative methodology; however, research in kinesiology has increasingly used qualitative methodology to expand the knowledge base about human movement. Similar to quantitative research, **qualitative research** is an umbrella term describing multiple methodologies, strategies, approaches, and data analysis techniques (Merriam 2009). Qualitative researchers examine a phenomenon (i.e., observable circumstance) comprehensively and in detail (Henderson 2006; Patton 2002). Alternatively, quantitative research attempts to quantify and generalize phenomenon. Because quantitative and qualitative methods examine different facets of an issue, they are not interchangeable and cannot be substituted for each other (McCracken 1988). Examining a similar issue, a quantitative study may measure and examine heart rate to determine exercise intensity during a spinning class, whereas a qualitative study would inquire about the experiences people had with their heart rate and exercise intensity in the spinning class. Therefore, during the early phases of research development, researchers must determine whether qualitative or quantitative research methods are most appropriate. Because qualitative research is much more complex than this chapter is able to present, it is recommended that students planning to use qualitative

Qualitative research
Research based upon nonnumerical data obtained in natural settings through extensive observations and interviews whose primary aim is the interpretation of phenomena and the discovery of meaning.

methodology in their research enroll in a qualitative research methods and/or analysis course.

The qualitative research process occurs in five, interrelated phases (Denzin and Lincoln 2000). The first phase is the researcher as a multicultural subject. As the primary instrument of data collection, researchers approach the research setting based on their own social class, gender, racial, cultural, and ethnic community perspective (Denzin and Lincoln 2000). Throughout the research process, researchers are using their own perspectives to understand and explain the experiences of participants. In a systematic, rigorous manner, qualitative research blends the researchers' observations with the meaning participants give to the phenomenon of interest (Denzin and Lincoln 2000). Therefore, researchers' awareness of their multiple identities continues throughout the entire study. The additional four phases of the qualitative research process are theoretical perspectives and paradigms, research traditions, methods of collection and analysis, and the practices of interpretation and evaluation. Specifically, this chapter will examine these four phases of the qualitative research process. In order to highlight examples of the behind-the-scenes processes and decisions of qualitative research, we will include examples from four published studies of our own work (Krane, Waldron, Michalenok, and Stiles-Shipley 2001; Kowalski and Waldron 2010; Waldron and Dieser 2010; Waldron and Kowalski 2009). The studies included use focus group and individual interviews to examine (1) the body image of female exercisers and athletes, (2) the perceptions of health and fitness in physically active college students, and (3) the hazing experiences of former and current athletes.

THEORETICAL PERSPECTIVES AND PARADIGMS

Paradigms are beliefs, values, and techniques shared by a community of scholars to conduct research (Kuhn 1962) or "a basic set of guidelines that guides action" (Guba 1990, 17). Although multiple paradigms are used in qualitative research (e.g., critical, postmodern), the focus of this chapter is on the extensively used, interpretive or constructivist paradigm (Creswell and Miller 2000; Merriam 2009; Miles and Huberman 1994). A constructivist paradigm significantly differs from a positivist or post-positivist paradigm used in quantitative research (Creswell 2007; Henderson 2006; Merriam 2009; Silk, Andrews, and Mason 2005). Whereas research from a post-positivist paradigm uses deductive techniques to produce an objective, generalizable finding, the constructivist paradigm uses inductive techniques to understand the multiple realities of participants.

When using a constructivist paradigm, a researcher assumes that reality is socially constructed and centers on relationships and wholeness (Creswell 2007; Henderson 2006; Merriam 2009). Multiple realities exist because people define and understand their own reality based on their own historical, social, and temporal environment. The importance of the social environment, specifically Western culture, was important in understanding both the culturally ideal body and body image concerns of female exercisers and athletes because women in different cultures may experience different expectations about their bodies (Krane et al. 2001). Because reality, knowledge, and behavior are created from the experiences and interactions of individuals (Henderson 2006; Merriam 2009; Patton 2002; Silk et al. 2005), the qualitative researcher is interested in the relationships participants have. A major aspect of the study by Krane and colleagues was how relationships with peers, teammates, and the media influenced how women felt and thought about their bodies. Finally, researchers using constructivist paradigms assume that the phenomenon of interest is a complex system, which cannot be simplified into separate parts (Creswell 2007; Patton 2002). To understand the complex experiences female athletes have with their bodies, their experiences and perspectives in both social and athletic situations had to be considered (Krane et al. 2001). In summary, a constructivist paradigm underscores the meaning people have constructed about a phenomenon and highlights the importance of the context.

Emerging from the constructivist paradigm are many characteristics common to qualitative research. All qualitative research focuses on meaning and understanding and is presented using rich, thick description (Creswell 2007; Merriam 2009; Patton 2002). Rich description includes "statements that produce for the readers the feeling that they have experienced, or could experience, the events being described in a study" (Creswell and Miller 2000, 129). Qualitative data analysis uses inductive processes in order to uncover themes and concepts and to build theory (Creswell 2007; Henderson 2006; Merriam 2009; Patton 2002). Using theory, researchers approach a topic with curiosity and remain open to the unfolding of more specific research questions. Additionally, inductive processes move from the specific, individual cases to the general (Berg 2004). By examining individual experiences of the phenomenon and then creating themes, qualitative researchers work to apply the findings to people in similar situations.

Researchers typically use purposeful sampling to obtain participants who can speak directly about a phenomenon of interest (Patton 2002). Additionally, most qualitative research happens in the natural setting of the participants (Creswell 2007; Patton 2002; Pitney and Parker 2009). Researchers go to the participants to collect data. Because reality is constructed, it is impossible for researchers to remain objective during the research process (Henderson 2006). Researchers are not separate from the research process. Instead, researchers are multicultural subjects who are part of the data collection process and as such, must be aware of and acknowledge their multiple identities and their experiences of the phenomenon.

Most qualitative studies use a research design that is emergent and flexible (Creswell 2007; Merriam 2009; Patton 2002; Pitney and Parker 2009). One way that qualitative research is emergent and flexible is through the interconnection of data collection and data analysis. For instance, data analysis starts after the first or second interview in order to gain an appreciation of the data, to start initial work on creating themes, and to modify the interview guide as needed (Amis 2005). For example, after completing and transcribing two interviews with athletes about their hazing experiences, we began to read and reflect on the interviews. We realized when asked about long-term effects of hazing, participants only responded with negative effects. This analysis allowed us to modify the interview guide and inquire about both positive and negative long-term effects of hazing.

RESEARCH TRADITIONS

There are multiple traditions of qualitative research, which share the aforementioned characteristics. Each approach has different assumptions, emphases, purposes, and techniques of analysis. When starting a qualitative research project, it is important to determine which approach best suits the purpose of the research. This section will focus on six common qualitative traditions to inquiry (Creswell 2007; Merriam 2009; Patton 2002). Readers are directed to the Creswell book for further information about research traditions.

A narrative tradition is "the interpretation of stories" (Smith and Sparkes 2009, 10), which occurs through a narrative analysis or a specific narrative form (Creswell 2007). During narrative analysis, researchers collect descriptions of events or phenomena and create stories from these descriptions with a plot line that has a beginning, middle, and end (Merriam 2009). This technique was used to report the findings of focus group interviews with men who had been hazed in sport (Waldron, Lynn, and Krane 2010). Specific narrative forms include biography, **life history,** or oral history where researchers work with a few participants who share life experiences about a phenomenon (Creswell 2007). Sparkes and Smith (2002) used life histories of four rugby players with spinal cord injuries to understand their ongoing experiences with their bodies. During the multiple interviews of two to five hours each, participants shared the lived experiences of their bodies pre-injury and post-injury.

Phenomenological research is interested in the common and shared experiences of people (Creswell 2007). Using phenomenology, researchers assume there is an **essence** (i.e., core meaning) of the shared experience and attempt to experience the phenomenon through in-depth interviews or observations (Patton 2002). During this process, researchers explore their own personal beliefs about the phenomenon and bracket them so that personal beliefs do not interfere with the data collection and analysis (Creswell 2007; Merriam 2009). Started in the field of anthropology, the ethnographic tradition focuses on understanding cultures. The researcher is immersed in the day-to-day lives of an entire cultural group via participant observation. (See Example 10.1.)

Life histories
Studies that cover the lives of individuals or that result from one or more individuals providing stories about their lives. Also known as *narrative research* or *biographical research*.

Phenomenological research
Identifies the "essence" or core of human experience.

Essence
Core meaning of an experience.

> An ethnographic approach was used to determine factors influencing team cohesion during a soccer season (Holt and Sparkes 2001). Participant observation helped establish long-term relationships and show commitment to understanding the social world of soccer. Using this approach, the researchers were able to discover how team cohesion fluctuates during a competitive season. Not only were environmental, leadership, athletic, and team factors highlighted, their ethnographic work also revealed how willingness to make personal sacrifices and role acceptance influenced cohesion.

EXAMPLE 10.1
Ethnographic Study on Team Cohesion
From Holt, N. L., and Sparkes, A. C. (2001). An ethnographic study of cohesiveness in a college soccer team over a season. *The Sport Psychologist, 15,* 237–259.

When using **grounded theory,** researchers create and generate theory from the data. The foundation of this approach is that "theory emerges from systematic comparative analysis and is grounded in fieldwork so as to explain what has been and is observed" (Patton 2002, 125). The theory generated is typically a substantive theory, meaning it is specific and for everyday situations (Merriam 2009). Theoretical sampling typically occurs and a specific data analysis technique, the constant comparative method of data analysis, is used (Glaser and Strauss 1967). (See Example 10.2.)

Grounded theory
Derivation of a theory from the views of the participants in a study; develops theories that are "grounded" in real-world experiences.

> One study using grounded theory created a theoretical model of how African American women adopt and maintain physical activity (Harley, Buckworth, Katz, Willis, Odoms-Young, and Heaney 2009). After coding the data from the interviews with 15 physically active women, the researchers developed the Physical Activity Evolution Model (see p. 102) to explain both the physical and psychological changes needed to adopt and maintain physical activity. This model represents a substantive theory and future research can build on this initial model.

EXAMPLE 10.2
Grounded Theory Study on Physical Activity Participation
From Harley, A. E., Buckworth, J., Katz, M. L., Willis, S. K., Odoms-Young. A., and Heaney, C. A. (2009). Developing long-term physical activity participation: A grounded theory study with African American women. *Health Education Behavior, 36,* 97–112. DOI: 10.1177/1090198107306434.

Qualitative case studies explore a singular case or bounded system (e.g., person, program, event; Creswell 2007; Merriam 2009). Merriam (1998, 27) asserts that a bounded case can be determined by asking if "there is a limit to the number of people involved who could be interviewed." If the answer is yes, then the phenomenon is bounded and a case study would be appropriate. When undertaking **case study** research, in-depth data collection typically occurs with multiple sources of information (Creswell 2007). For example, case study of an elite gymnast highlighted why she engaged in excessive practice, competed while injured, and experienced unhealthy eating patterns (Krane, Greenleaf, and Snow 1997).

Case study
Study that provides an intensive, holistic, and in-depth understanding of a single unit or bounded system. Also involves studying an event, activity, program, process, or one or more individuals.

BOX 10.1
Basic Qualitative Study
on Fitness and Health

Working to understand the perspectives of fitness and health in college men and women, Waldron and Dieser (2010) utilized a basic qualitative approach. Participants were interviewed and emerging themes, including the importance of competence, the difficulty of healthy eating at the university, and physical appearance being intertwined with health and fitness, were uncovered via inductive analysis. Using a basic qualitative approach, the researchers were able to gain a deeper understanding of the phenomenon of interest. These findings can be used to assist universities in developing campus-wide health strategies.

Many times in the field of kinesiology researchers are interested in understanding and describing experiences people have with movement without using one of the aforementioned traditions and, thus, are conducting basic qualitative research (Merriam 2009). Basic qualitative research uses the interpretive paradigm and specific characteristics of qualitative research to descriptively explore and understand a phenomenon. (See Box 10.1.)

DATA COLLECTION

After choosing a research tradition, researchers need to consider a number of research design issues. During this process, researchers establish methodological congruence, where the research purposes, questions, and methodology are integrated together to create a cohesive study (Richards and Morse 2007). Therefore, when designing the study, the researcher must always consider the research purpose and questions. Because of the flexible and emergent design, data collection and data analysis are intertwined; however separating these pieces of conducting research is useful for understanding each. Data collection design issues include: (1) locating and accessing the data site, (2) determining the sampling technique, (3) collecting and recording the data, and (4) maintaining ethics and confidentiality (Creswell 2007; Patton 2002). Each of these issues will be considered further in the following sections.

Accessing the Data Site and Sampling

Without access to the data site, researchers will be unable to conduct their study. Therefore, locating and accessing the data site is an important component of the research process. When contemplating the data site, it is important to consider how observable demographics (e.g., gender, age, race) may influence recruiting potential participants (Berg 2004). Researchers may be more successful when they possess similar characteristics of the participant (Henderson 2006). For example, because hazing is a sensitive topic with participants potentially sharing sexually explicit behaviors, same-sex interviews were used in order to optimize recruitment and create a trusting environment (Waldron and Kowalski 2009; Kowalski and Waldron 2010).

Accessing data sites takes research, patience, persistence, and some luck (Amis 2005). Often, researchers find and contact a gatekeeper (e.g., athletic director, coach, program coordinator) who has entry to the desired site and participants (Amis 2005; Krane and Baird 2005). Researchers may already know a gatekeeper, resulting in easier entrance to the data site. In cases where a relationship has to be established with a gatekeeper, gaining access to the data site may be a process that takes time (Krane and Baird 2005). It is also common for researchers to find a sponsor or key informant, who typically has status within the data site, to help persuade others to participate in the study (Amis 2005; Krane and Baird 2005). Being able to create relationships with gatekeepers and sponsors takes times and energy, but is necessary to gain entrance to the environment of interest.

After gaining access to a data site, researchers decide on a purposeful sampling technique (see Miles and Huberman 1994, 28, or Patton 2002, 243–244, for specific sampling techniques). Researchers need to consider the information they want to obtain, the purpose of the research, the number of participants needed for credibility, and time and resource constraints (Patton 2002). No definitive rules exist for determining sample size. A typical guideline is that the sample size is sufficient when the research reaches saturation or redundancy in the data (Pitney and Parker 2009). That is, when the researcher is consistently hearing similar information and no new themes are emerging, sample size is likely sufficient.

Methods to Collect Data

There are a number of methods used to collect or discover qualitative data. Although not widespread in kinesiology, one method of data collection is examining documents and audiovisual materials such as photographs, videos, personal letters, public documents, photographs or videos taken by participants, and medical records (Creswell 2007). (See Box 10.2.)

BOX 10.2
Data Collection Via
Photographs

A special edition of *Qualitative Research for Sport and Exercise* (Phoenix 2010) focused on visual methods in physical culture and featured research using photographs, videos, maps, diagrams, symbols, and other visual documents as the means of data collection. One featured study was examining how female college athletes portrayed themselves in photos (Krane et al. 2010). The participants in the study selected the attire, location, and pose of their photo shoot and were asked to discuss their favorite photo. When portraying themselves in the photos, each female athlete incorporated a signifier of their athletic identity.

Another means of qualitative data collection is observation. Qualitative observation requires researchers to "observe social interactions and patterns, conversations, events, and all the seemingly mundane activities inherent to a particular setting" (Krane and Baird 2005, 95). These observations are recorded in detail in the form of field notes. One observational study examined pain and injury in a high school and a college rugby team (Fenton and Pitter 2010). One researcher, who was the athletic trainer, recorded field notes during each practice and competition. In this position, as participant observer, the researcher was able to observe injuries in the rugby players and decisions the players made while injured. As a qualitative observation, results were presented as in-depth, detailed, rich description.

Of the multiple techniques for data collection, the most common is interviewing. For example, within a ten-year period, 80 percent of the published qualitative work in sport psychology journals used interviews (Culver, Gilbert, and Trudel 2003). **Interviews** are purposeful conversations used to gather information and are the key means to collecting data when researchers are unable to observe the phenomenon (Amis 2005; Berg 2004; Creswell 2007; Merriam 2009). Although it is a conversation, the researcher's primary role is to allow the participants to converse and discuss, in detail, their experiences. Researchers may use individual interviews (i.e., interviewing one person at a time) or focus group interviews, where a group of participants are interviewed. Because interviewing is the most popular method of qualitative data discovery, the rest of this chapter will focus on this technique.

Interview
Face-to-face interaction (individual or group), telephone interaction (individual or group), or chat room discussion.

Interview Guides and Questions

As interviews are purposeful conversations, researchers must generate and structure questions to ask participants during the interview. Questions in interview guides should be based on the scholarly literature review and the purpose of the research study (Berg 2004; McCracken 1988). Further development of the interview guides comes from the researcher reflecting, understanding, and appreciating personal experience with the topic in order to consider areas not observed in scholarly literature (McCracken 1988). For instance, prior to forming the interview guide, each member of our research team discussed a specific situation where they were aware of their bodies, in either a pleasant or unpleasant way.

After considering these two sources, researchers should create an outline of the broad categories relevant to the study (Patton 2002). From this outline, questions are created. It is necessary for the guide to be critically examined by a colleague familiar with the topic (Berg 2004). Additionally, the researcher should carefully answer the questions in the guide (Henderson 2006). Changes can be made to the interview guide at this point in time. Many researchers recommend pilot testing the interview guide with participants (Berg 2004; Merriam 2009). Henderson, however, suggests that time is better spent collecting actual data than pilot testing. After the first interview, the effectiveness of the interview questions and guide are evaluated and changes are made. As part of the flexible and emergent research design, researchers continually evaluate the interview guide and adapt it as needed throughout data collection.

Interview Guides.   Different types of interview guides provide varying levels of structure and flexibility for the interview. Two classifications of interview guides, closed and standardized open-ended, do not conform to an interpretive paradigm and will not be explored. The most common type of interview guide is semi-structured (Amis 2005; Patton 2002). A semi-structured interview contains some structure, in that questions are based on predetermined topics, while maintaining flexibility by allowing researchers to reorder questions, add new questions, word questions differently, and add or drop prompts (Amis 2005; Berg 2004; Merriam 2009). Because flexibility is built into a semi-structure interview, the guide acts as a checklist to ensure the researcher is addressing the set of issues of interest (Patton 2002). Although researchers should be familiar with the language (e.g., slang, jargon, colloquialism) of participants prior to starting the interview, semi-structured interviews allows researchers to change the language in order to fit the needs of the participants (Amis 2005; Berg 2004). In my work with hazing, very few athletes used the word "hazing" to describe their behaviors; instead most used "initiation" or "ritual" (Kowalski and Waldron 2010; Waldron and Kowalski 2009). Therefore, during interviews, the researchers used the language of the participants in order to reflect their perspective.

The final guide type, the informational interview, is flexible, loose, and spontaneous, allowing researchers to understand complex topics without preconceived notions (Amis 2005; Patton 2002). This interview guide has no set order or wording to the questions and questions are added or dropped as needed (Berg 2004). Typically, this interview guide is for exploratory work when the researcher does not know enough about phenomenon to ask relevant questions (Merriam 2009). Informal interview guides are rarely the sole means of data discovery and often result in creation of a semi-structured interview guide (Amis 2005; Merriam 2009).

Interview Questions.   After choosing the appropriate interview guide, researchers develop and order the questions. Beginning questions should be neutral, noncontroversial, mild, nonthreatening, and broad (Berg 2004; Henderson 2006; Merriam 2009; Patton 2002). For example, if interviewing athletes, an effective first question is "tell me about your leadership experiences in sport." This allows participants to become comfortable discussing personal experiences with the researcher. Neutral questions are also closed, demographic questions, which often are asked at the beginning of an interview (Berg 2004; McCracken 1988). Patton, however, suggests these questions should be kept to a minimum at the beginning of an interview because they may bore the participant, resulting in loss of interest. Instead, researchers should either spread the demographic questions throughout the interview or save them to the end. Using noncontroversial and neutral questions at the beginning of the interview allows the participant to become comfortable with the researcher and helps establish rapport and trust. As the interview unfolds, researchers can ask more controversial and specific questions about the phenomenon. Finally, all interviews should end with a question, such as, "Anything you want to add?" or "What should I have asked you that I didn't think to ask?" (Patton 2002, 379). This concluding question allows the participant to expand on ideas or add relevant ideas not addressed in the interview.

Within the interview guide, researchers should create and use different types of questions (Berg 2004; McCracken 1988). Essential questions or grand-tour questions access information of central focus to the study and allow the participants to tell their story about a phenomenon on their terms (Berg 2004). A second type of question category, extra questions, parallels the essential questions but the questions are worded differently in order to check reliability of participant responses (Berg 2004). If discrepancies arise in response to essential and extra questions, researchers need to continue to question participants about their experiences. It is possible that the lived experiences of participants are contradictory and researchers have to accept that contradiction and ambiguity. Discussing their hazing experiences, many athletes were contradictory in their descriptions (Waldron and Kowalski 2009). As researchers, we presented their contradictions and explored how athletes grappled with the acceptability of their behaviors.

The menu of essential and extra questions that researchers can create is vast. These questions can inquire about (1) experience and behavior, (2) opinion and values, (3) feeling and emotion, (4) knowledge, and (5) sensory experience (Patton 2002). More specific question types query about hypothetical situations, address ideal positions, and suggest devil's advocate views (Strauss, Schatzman, Bucher, Ehrlich, and Sabshin 1981). With hypothetical questions, participants will answer questions beginning with "What if" or "Suppose," in order to provide a description of their experience. Ideal position questions address the positive and negatives of a phenomenon by asking about an ideal situation associated with the phenomenon (Strauss et al. 1981). Likely, some of the topics of the interview will be controversial or potentially threatening to the participants. One way to begin to address these controversial topics is via asking devil's advocate questions (Strauss et al. 1981). These questions typically start with "Some people would say. . . ." Although this mechanism depersonalizes the issue, the response typically reflects participants' opinion. Using this menu of questions, researchers can develop effective questions that invite participants to respond with valuable and constructive answers.

Interview prompts
Interpretive type questions used to seek more information or detail from the participant during an interview; also called interview probes.

Another category of questions used throughout the **interview are prompts** or probes. Prompts are interpretive questions used to seek more information, detail, and elaboration from the participant (Merriam 2009; Strauss et al. 1981). Prompts can be floating or planned (McCracken 1988). Floating prompts happen spontaneously and can include raising eyebrows at the end of a comment, repeating a key word, or asking the meaning of a specific word or phrase. These prompts happen spontaneously and will differ from interview to interview. Planned prompts are part of the interview guide and are used to encourage participants to discuss issues that do not readily come to their minds. Situational, transitional, reflective, and emotional prompts are commonly used (Henderson 2006). Situational prompts encourage the participants to provide further description of the phenomenon. Transitional prompts ensure the participants have finished discussing a topic before the researcher moves on to another area. For example, a researcher may ask if the participant would like to share other examples related to the current topic. Reflective prompts encourage the participant to discuss the meaning or importance attached to a phenomenon whereas emotional prompts inquire further about participants' feelings. Additionally, researchers can use auto-driving prompts by asking participants to comment on picture, video, or other stimulus (McCracken 1988). Auto-driving prompts were used in a study examining health and fitness. Participants were asked to respond to photos of healthy individuals with culturally ideal bodies and with nonculturally ideal bodies (Waldron and Dieser 2010).

There are multiple guidelines for creating and asking effective questions. First, effective interview questions are open-ended (Merriam 2009). Participants should be unable to answer questions with a single word, such as yes or no. Second, they should be neutral. Neutral questions do not lead the participant toward a particular, desired answer and are not affectively worded (Amis 2005; Berg 2004; Merriam 2009; Patton 2002). An example of a leading question might be "Why was hazing harmful to your team?" Here, it is assumed that hazing is harmful, although this view may not be held by the participant. The question is also affectively worded, which can produce negative emotional responses in the participant. Asking questions that start with "why" may produce an upsetting response in participants, possibly because it has a punitive connotation (Berg 2004). Therefore, researchers are encouraged to use questions asking "how come" as an alternative. Third, double-barreled and complex questions should be avoided (Berg 2004; Merriam 2009; Patton 2002). Double-barreled questions require response to two different issues in a single question. For example, asking college students "What does it mean to be healthy and fit to you?" contains two different topics of interest (i.e., health and fitness). It is more effective to separate these into two questions so that participants are able to respond successfully to each one. Finally, complex questions can confuse the participant so questions should be kept brief and concise so participants hear the question in its entirety.

Engaging in the Interview.   After accessing the data site and creating the interview guide, researchers need to contact potential participants. When contacting participants, researchers provide information about the purpose and the procedure (e.g., length) of the interview. Interviews are scheduled at a time and place that is convenient and comfortable for the participants. Additionally, the consent form, interview guide, audio or video recorder, and backup batteries and tapes are brought to the interview.

Not only does a fresh, hard copy of the interview guide ensure all categories of interest are examined during the interview, but it is also a place for strategic and focused note-taking (McCracken 1988). On the interview guide, researchers write notes about observations of interest including major discussion points, language use, and nonverbal cues (Amis 2005; Patton 2002). Taking these notes during the interview is essential to (1) assist with creating new questions to ask in future interviews, (2) help with the emergent quality of research, (3) facilitate later analysis, and (4) act as a backup in case of malfunctioning technology (Patton 2002).

Upon arrival at the interview site, researchers should immediately start building rapport (i.e., positive feelings and respect) with participants (Berg 2004; Henderson 2006; Patton 2002). It is important to be punctual for the interview, be courteous, and use accepting, positive body language (Henderson 2006; McCracken 1988). Prior to starting the actual interview, idle chatter about non-interview topics, including the personal background of the researcher, can help establish common ground (Berg 2004; Henderson 2006; McCracken 1988). Additionally, having participants ask questions about the research process can assist in building rapport (Henderson 2006).

As the interview unfolds, researchers continue to establish rapport with participants by maintaining neutrality. Maintaining neutrality occurs by creating an environment where participants are able to respond however they want without being worried about shocking, angering, or embarrassing the researchers (Amis 2005; Patton 2002). To preserve neutrality, researchers can provide illustrative examples of what others have stated about the phenomenon to show they have heard it all (Patton 2002). For example, in our hazing work, we want athletes to share potentially embarrassing situations. Therefore, we often highlight extreme hazing behaviors we have heard about to show we are not shocked by these situations. Other techniques to maintain neutrality are role-playing questions, which place the participants as the experts, as well as simulation questions where participants are asked to imagine themselves in a situation of interest (Patton 2002). A sample role-playing question might be "Suppose I was a new person on your sport team, what would you tell me about the hazing or initiation experiences?" A sample simulation question might be "Suppose I was present during a hazing activity, what would I see going on? Take me there." Another technique to sustain rapport throughout the interview is using support and recognition responses (Patton 2002). These include words of thanks, support, and praise, and also use of appropriate nonverbal feedback. Additionally, researchers can show they are listening by echoing back what they heard from the participant (Berg 2004).

Maintaining rapport also requires researchers to reduce their own chatter, avoid interruption, and be comfortable with silences (Amis 2005; Berg 2004; Henderson 2006). Some researchers are uncomfortable with silences and they automatically fill the space by talking; however, it may take time for participants to formulate a response, and by talking, the researcher may prevent a complete response from participants. If this happens continually, participants may no longer be engaged in the interview. Therefore, silences should be extended up to 45 seconds (Berg 2004). By counting slowly and making eye contact with the participant during this time, most participants will naturally respond to the silence.

At the conclusion of the interview, researchers debrief and thank participants, as well as answer any questions about the research study. Researchers provide the timeline for study completion and ask participants' consent to be contacted in the future to verify data analysis. Once the interview is over, the participant is assigned a pseudonym or fictitious name and the tape should be labeled with the pseudonym, date, and time of the interview. Field notes, containing information about where the interview occurred, the topics covered, the reaction of the participant, effective prompts, unfamiliar terminology, quality of rapport, and quality of information received, should be written without delay (Henderson 2006; Patton 2002). Generally speaking, researchers will create several single-pages of notes for each hour in the field (Henderson 2006). Field notes are a supplementary source of raw data that become part of the data collection and analysis process.

Transcription occurs as soon as possible after the interview. Interviews are transcribed verbatim and include pauses, laughter, and fillers (Henderson 2006). After transcription, if there are areas of the interview that are unclear or confusing, the researcher can contact the participant for clarification (Patton 2002). Transcription is a time-consuming process with a 5:1 ratio (Henderson 2006). That is, researchers typically complete five hours of transcription work for every hour of interviews. Taken together, from accessing the data site to transcribing interview, the data collection process is lengthy and researchers have to prepare themselves for the intense time commitment.

Confidentiality and Ethics.   Many similar issues of confidentiality and ethics arise during both qualitative research and quantitative research. Therefore, this section will highlight aspects of confidentiality and ethics unique to qualitative research (see Patton 2002, 408–409). Because researchers meet and establish rapport with participants, maintaining confidentiality is critical in qualitative work. In order to protect identity and dignity, participants should not be identified in any way possible, unless they provide permission (Amis 2005; Berg 2004; Patton 2002). This confidentiality extends to the family, friends, teammates, colleagues, and organizations of participants. Researchers maintain confidentiality by using pseudonyms and changing the names of places, locations, and other potential markers of identity. It is important that the pseudonyms reflect characteristics of the participant's identity and do not distort the data (Amis 2005). For example, a female Japanese American athlete should have a pseudonym, such as Akari, reflecting these characteristics. Researchers need to be clear about the parameters of confidentiality; for example, researchers are typically unable to guarantee confidentiality if there is evidence of illegal activities or abuse (Patton 2002). Another ethical issue related to confidentiality is whom researchers can talk to about how the interviews and observation are personally affecting them. Because researchers are the data collection instrument, they may have mental and emotional reactions during the data collection process (Patton 2002). Therefore, it is important to consider how researchers can discuss these issues with others, without breaching the confidentiality of participants.

Researchers should also consider ethical ways to collect data and the boundaries of their data collection. Specifically, researchers are challenged to respond ethically when pushing for information, particularly sensitive information, from participants by weighing the benefits (e.g., value of the response) and the risks (e.g., distress of the participant; Patton 2002). For example, in an interview with a female athlete, tears began to well up as she described her hazing experiences to us. At this moment, we made her a partner in the decision-making process (Patton 2002) by reassuring her that she was able to decide how much she was comfortable sharing. It is also possible that participants will request the tape to be paused during difficult parts of the interview (Henderson 2006). Researchers must respect the right of participants to decline being taped or audio recorded at any time.

DATA ANALYSIS

As data collection is unfolding, qualitative researchers are also engaging in data analysis. Data analysis consists of generating, developing, and verifying themes (Corbin and Strauss 2008) via inductive and comparative processes (Merriam 2009). The CREATIVE approach is a useful acronym to remember the process of data analysis: Consider the study's research question, Read through the transcripts, Examine the data for information related to the research question, Assign the labels to units to capture meaning, Thematize the data, Interpret emerging themes as they relate to the research question, Verification, and Engage in writing (Pitney and Parker 2009, 54). Furthermore, the movement of data analysis is in "analytic circles rather than using a fixed linear approach" (Creswell 2007, 150). In other words, researchers will move through the CREATIVE process repeatedly in order to credibly generate, develop, and interpret themes. Because considering the research question (C) is used throughout data analysis, this section will explore data reading (RE), data reduction and interpretation (ATI), and verification (V).

Data Reading

Data reading consists of reading and rereading the transcripts and examining the data for information related to the research question (Pitney and Parker 2009). As data familiarization is occurring, researchers will reflect on the data through writing memos (Creswell 2007). Memo writing allows researchers to examine and start to understand the information contained in the interviews as it relates to the research purpose and question.

Various types of memos are used during qualitative research. Memos store reflections of analytic thought and analytic ideas, including the connection between theory and the emerging data (Corbin and Strauss 2008). Personal memos highlight personal thoughts, feelings, and reflections about the phenomenon, interview, or method (Henderson 2006). Finally, summary memos work to synthesize the content from several memos and can include short quotes from raw data (Corbin and Strauss 2008). When creating memos, use a date and a heading (Corbin and Strauss 2008) and identify the information as a fact, quote, or interpretation (Henderson 2006). Both field notes and memos should be referred to throughout data collection and analysis to help understand and describe the phenomenon (Henderson 2006).

Data Reduction

Data reduction requires researchers to assign labels to capture meaning of the data and thematize the data (Pitney and Parker 2009). Data reduction describes, indexes, simplifies, and transforms raw data to be manageable via the technique of coding (Berg 2004; Creswell 2007; Huberman and Miles 1998). Coding is the process of investigating raw data, assigning shorthand designations, and raising it to the thematic level (Corbin and Strauss 2008; Merriam 2009). Although data reduction depends on the research tradition (e.g., narrative, phenomenological), a basic data reduction process will be presented here. Reducing the data and coding requires researchers to consider and examine multiple sources of material, including the research question, scholarly literature, personal experience, and observations during the interview (McCracken 1988). Researchers are cautioned, however, to "be prepared to use all of this material as a guide to what exists there [in the data], but he or she must be prepared to ignore all of this material to see what none of it anticipates" (McCracken 1988, 42). In other words, researchers are receptive to bracketing previous knowledge and experience about the phenomenon in order to understand the experiences of the participants.

After reading through the transcripts extensively and creating memos, researchers start an inductive, brainstorming process to break the data apart (Corbin and Strauss 2008; Merriam 2009). Researchers examine the *utterances* (i.e., data units) within the interview and separate the material relevant to the purpose of the study from the unimportant material (Corbin and Strauss 2008; McCracken 1988). Although not all raw data are used during this process, researchers must be open to all potentials and possibilities contained with the data (Corbin and Strauss 2008; Merriam 2009). It is imperative that researchers consider all material within the raw data and recognize when their own or participants' biases are intruding into analysis and be comfortable with the contradictions. During the coding process researchers continually ask "so what" and "what if," as well as examine language and emotions (Corbin and Strauss 2008). Researchers then cluster the utterances together and label the cluster with a code (McCracken 1988; Merriam 2009).

Data reduction
A process of investigating and transforming raw data, often using a coding technique, in order to make sense of and identify themes within the data; part of data analysis in qualitative research.

Again, codes will develop by themselves, by evidence in the transcript, by the literature, and by personal experience (McCracken 1988).

After spending sufficient time brainstorming, researchers work to relate the codes to each other (Corbin and Strauss 2008). The focus is on comparing the codes, relating them to each other, and creating higher-order themes (Corbin and Strauss 2008; McCracken 1988). Themes should be (1) responsive to the purpose of the research, (2) exhaustive in that all important themes are included, (3) mutually exclusive so that each utterance (data unit) belongs to only one theme, and (4) conceptually congruent, meaning that all categories are at the same conceptual level (Merriam 2009).

Interpreting Data

Interpreting the emerging themes as they relate to the research question helps researchers understand the larger meaning of the data based on hunches, intuition, and theoretical constructs (Creswell 2007; Pitney and Parker 2009). Interpreting the themes becomes a more deductive process as researchers determine if the theme exists and find evidence of the final themes (Merriam 2009). During this phase of data analysis researchers display the data in an organized, compressed manner to allow for drawing conclusions (Berg 2004; Huberman and Miles 1998). Data display can be a table, summaries of statements, matrices, trees, or propositions (Berg 2004; Creswell 2007). Because of the emergent design and interconnectedness of qualitative work, researchers are also determining if further data collection and analysis is needed during this phase.

Verification

Verification
Method for testing interpretations for plausibility, sturdiness, or confirmability.

The final piece of data collection and analysis is verification. **Verification** requires researchers to confirm the trustworthiness of the data. As Corbin and Strauss (2008, 302) state, "findings are trustworthy and believable in that they reflect participants', researchers', and readers' experiences with a phenomenon but at the same time the explanation is only one of many possible 'plausible' interpretations." This process ensures that conclusions are drawn from confirmable patterns in data and that the procedures to reach conclusions can be articulated (Berg 2004). Trustworthiness results in findings that are consistent (i.e., make sense based on the data collected), credible (i.e., plausible with a connection to the real world), and transferable (i.e., can be applied to similar environments; Lincoln and Guba 1985; Merriam 2009).

There are multiple strategies to validate findings and it is recommended that two validation strategies, at minimum, be used during a study (see Creswell and Miller 2000). Verification strategies should be considered during the planning phases of the study design. The strategy of prolonged engagement ensures (1) adequate time spent immersed in the data site building trust, learning the culture, and checking for misinformation; and (2) saturation of the data to allow for a full uncovering of the experience of the phenomenon (Creswell and Miller 2000; Lincoln and Guba 1985; Merriam 2009; Pitney and Parker 2008). Triangulation is using multiple methods to collect data (e.g., interview, observation, documents) to help ensure data reflect and represent the actual experiences of participants (Lincoln and Guba 1985; Merriam 2009; Miles and Huberman 1994; Patton 2002). Peer review or peer debriefing is an external check where a colleague, who has familiarity with the phenomenon, asks hard questions about the methods, meanings, and interpretations (Lincoln and Guba 1985; Merriam 2009; Miles and Huberman 1998; Pitney and Parker 2008). A fourth validation strategy is negative case analysis (Lincoln and Guba 1985; Miles and Huberman 1998; Patton 2002). When analyzing data, researchers must also explore cases that do not fit the analysis. This refines the working theme's hypotheses and ensures all cases and experiences are fitting the coding system.

Member checking is sending data analysis to participants to verify that the data analyses, interpretations, and conclusions ring true and allows for fine tuning to better reflect the experiences (Lincoln and Guba 1985; Merriam 2009; Miles and Huberman 1998). Another validation strategy, rich and thick description, is providing detailed information about participants' experiences so that the reader can transfer information and experiences to other settings (Lincoln and Guba 1985; Merriam 2009). Clarifying research bias requires that the researcher reflect on experiences, perceptions, and assumptions which may influence interpretation (Amis 2005; Creswell and Miller 2000; Henderson 2006; Merriam 2009). The final validation strategy is audit trails and external audits. Lincoln and Guba (1985) state that the audit trail consists of how the data were collected, how themes were derived, how decisions were made, and the tracking of memos. External audits, then, are a consultant examining the process and product of the study to assess accuracy (Creswell and Miller 2000).

Summary of Objectives

1. **Identify the constructivist paradigm and characteristics of qualitative research.** Using the constructivist paradigm in qualitative research, researchers assume that multiple realities exist and are socially constructed via interactions with others. Major characteristics of qualitative research include (1) a focus on meaning, (2) inductive processes, (3) purposeful sampling, (4) data collection in the natural setting, (5) identities and experiences of the researchers are integral to the research process, and (6) an emergent and flexible research design.

2. **Name and explain the six qualitative traditions.** Multiple qualitative research traditions exist. Each tradition has

different purposes and techniques of data analysis. The six qualitative traditions are narrative, phenomenological, ethnography, grounded theory, case studies, and basic qualitative research.

3. **Articulate the process of data collection via interviews.** When preparing to conduct a qualitative study, researchers should consider (1) access to the data site and sampling techniques, (2) methods to collect data, and (3) concerns related to ethics and confidentiality. Effective questions should be designed for the interview guide. During the interview, researchers need to establish and maintain rapport with participants. To maintain confidentiality, researchers need to mask all names and other identity markers of participants.

4. **Understand a basic method of data analysis.** Data analysis starts during data collection. The CREATIVE approach (Pitney and Parker 2009) represents a basic approach to data analysis: Consider the study's question, Read though the transcripts, Examine the data for information, Assign labels, Thematize the data, Interpret emerging themes, Verify data, and Engage in writing.

Meta-analysis 11

OBJECTIVES

In this chapter, we present information concerning the meta-analysis approach in research. You should become familiar with this approach and the terms and techniques used with it.

After reading Chapter 11, you should be able to

1. Understand why the meta-analysis approach is utilized.
2. Know how the meta-analysis approach is conducted.

Meta-analysis is a relatively new approach in kinesiology research. Although used in disciplines outside of kinesiology since the 1960s, it was seldom utilized or discussed in kinesiology until the 1980s. The tutorial on meta-analysis by Thomas and French (1986) certainly brought the meta-analysis technique to the attention of many people in kinesiology. **Meta-analysis** is the reanalysis of the results from a large number of research studies in an effort to draw conclusions which are supported by many research studies. Thus, meta-analysis is much more than a review of related literature, as a part of an experimental or descriptive research study; it is the major thrust of the research study since it is the research approach.

Meta-analysis
A research approach involving the reanalysis of the results from a large number of research studies.

META-ANALYSIS IN KINESIOLOGY

Let's take a situation where the meta-analysis approach might be used. The question to be answered is whether warm-up is necessary before participating in physical performance activities. A large amount of research has been done on this topic. The results of the research are inconclusive; some point toward yes, some no. There are so many research studies to consider that it is impossible to read and keep track of all the information; you can't see the woods for the trees. Based on all of this research it is impossible to say whether warm-up is or is not necessary before participating in physical performance activities. Furthermore, if we examine the available research more carefully, we will find that the various studies differ in terms of the way the research was conducted. Some studies were conducted to see if warm-up was beneficial for participants to obtain their best score, while other studies dealt with the effects of warm-up on injury prevention. Some studies were conducted on high performance level athletes and other studies were conducted on novice performance level individuals. Further, some studies were conducted with physical performance activities requiring quick maximum exertion movements for a short period of time (like sprinting), while other studies were conducted with physical performance activities requiring slow submaximal exertion movements for a long period of time (like distance running). In addition, participants in these research studies varied in age (from 14 to 35 years) and in gender. Also, some research studies were conducted with large numbers of participants while other studies were conducted with three to five participants. In some research studies, a small difference was noted between warm-up and no warm-up; in other studies a large difference was noted. Do you give the same importance to both outcomes? Last, but not least, some research studies were conducted with excellent procedures, and some research studies were conducted with marginally acceptable procedures. Do you give the same weight to both classifications of studies? What is the big picture here? The results obtained in a single research study may be dependent on one or more of the things just mentioned, and when all the research studies are considered, no conclusion can be drawn as to whether warm-up is necessary. It is much like mixing apples and oranges and getting fruit salad.

With meta-analysis the results from available research studies are reanalyzed, and, if necessary, allowances are made for the variables that need to be controlled because they may influence the findings in a research study. In the earlier example, these variables could be training level of the participants, type of physical activity, age, and gender. Further, studies judged to have too small a number of participants and/or marginally acceptable procedures may not be used in the meta-analysis. Certainly, meta-analysis is not using all of the research studies available and counting the number of research studies which support each position of a research question. Meta-analysis has definite procedures with systematic steps which assist the researcher in drawing defensible conclusions. It is an approach where the information from a large number of research studies can be handled in an economical manner, minimizing the chance that the volume of information will overwhelm the researcher and subjective judgments will cause the researcher to draw incorrect conclusions. Presently, meta-analysis studies are commonly conducted in many different areas in kinesiology to synthesize the results from a large amount of research available on a topic.

The meta-analysis approach can be studied from the standpoint of using it in your research or understanding it when another researcher uses it. Obviously, to *use* meta-analysis in your research requires more knowledge than is required in simply understanding the meta-analysis approach when used by another researcher.

In the Department of Kinesiology at the University of Georgia, a meta-analysis course is taught, and, in many universities, such a course is taught in kinesiology departments, in educational psychology departments, and elsewhere. A class seems to be the best way to learn about the meta-analysis approach. Books like Rosenthal (1991) are written about meta-analysis techniques. A discussion of meta-analysis may be included in some research books. Thomas, Nelson and Silverman (2005) devoted a chapter to the topic. Neutens and Rubinson (2002) devoted one page to the topic, in a chapter on analyzing and interpreting data. Tutorials in research journals and books (Thomas and French 1986; Lipsey and Wilson 2001; Rosenthal and DiMatteo 2001) and reading research articles in which meta-analysis is used are valuable in learning about the meta-analysis approach. A strategy in learning about the meta-analysis approach might be to read a short overview, like a book chapter or tutorial, concerning the meta-analysis approach to get a general knowledge of the approach and then read a research article in which the meta-analysis approach is used. Following this, if there still is an interest in and/or need to learn more about the meta-analysis approach, taking a meta-analysis course or reading a book dealing with the meta-analysis approach would be advantageous. The approach in this chapter is to provide a brief nontechnical overview of the meta-analysis approach so that you can understand it when another researcher uses it in a research study.

The first chapter in the Rosenthal (1991) book is a good introduction to the meta-analysis approach. Many of his other chapters are somewhat mathematically oriented. However, for the serious reader, his book is an excellent source. In chapter 1 he states that meta-analysis may be used to compare results from several research studies or combine results from many research studies. No matter whether the intent of the meta-analysis is to compare or combine research study results, the calculation of **effect size** is basic to the meta-analysis approach.

EFFECT SIZE

In Chapter 1 of this text, the concept of conducting the research on a sample selected from a population was introduced. In Chapter 14 dealing with inferential data analysis techniques, using information from a sample to estimate a population effect will be discussed. As presented in Chapter 14, a sample is selected from a population, and information obtained on the sample is used to estimate population information or effect. For example, if one sample from the population received training method A and another sample received training method B, and based on a statistical test, training method A was found to be superior to training method B, the researcher would infer that, for the population, training method A is superior to training method B. Although, based on the statistical test, the researcher concluded that training method A is superior to training method B, there is no guarantee that the difference between the two methods is large enough to be of practical importance. If the sample who received training method A are 10 pounds stronger than the sample who received method B, that may be a practical difference, but if the difference is only .5 pounds, this is not a practical difference. An effect size is calculated in an attempt to estimate

Effect size
An estimate of the practical difference between two means; used in meta-analysis as a standard unit of measurement.

whether a difference is a practical difference. Effect size (ES) can be calculated in a variety of different ways depending on the research design and the intent of the research. Here is a common way of calculating ES:

$$ES = \frac{\text{mean score of Group A} - \text{mean score of Group B}}{\substack{\text{standard deviation for one group or the standard deviation for} \\ \text{the combined (pooled) groups}}}$$

For example, if the mean score for sample A is 75 and the mean score for sample B is 65 and the pooled standard deviation is 10, ES = (75 − 65)/10 = 1.0. Cohen (1988) states that an effect size less than .20 is small, around .50 is medium, and greater than .80 is large. Thus, in the example, the ES of 1.0 is large and the difference (75 − 65) is probably a practical difference.

The inferential statistical test that a researcher uses to determine whether two samples differ in mean score is influenced by sample size (n). As sample size increases, the difference between the means to have a significant difference decreases. The sample size does not influence ES.

With the meta-analysis approach, an effect size is calculated for each research study used, so the same measurement or indicator is used for each research study when comparing or combining them. Thus, with the meta-analysis approach, each research study is like a human participant in experimental or descriptive research.

For example, a meta-analysis was conducted to determine if an exercise program was effective in increasing fitness. The researcher suspected that the number of weeks of exercise training would be an influencing factor and that there would be a large difference among studies in the number of weeks of exercise training. So he analyzed effect size by classifications of weeks of exercise training. Ninety-eight of the 121 identified research studies were used in the meta-analysis. His findings were as follows:

WEEKS OF TRAINING	NUMBER OF STUDIES	EFFECT SIZE
Less than 6 weeks	15	.01–.21
6–9 weeks	28	.19–.63
10–17 weeks	42	.51–.94
More than 17 weeks	13	.58–1.17

Mean ES = .61

In this example, if the analysis had not been conducted by weeks of training, the effect size would have been .61, which is medium size; whereas, from the analysis by weeks of training, large effect sizes were found, indicating practically significant differences. Further, if the meta-analysis had not been used, the researcher might not have been able to make any sense out of the 98 research studies.

As noted earlier, effect size can be calculated with a variety of different formulas. The formula presented where the difference (d) between the mean performance of two samples is used can have several different denominators, depending on the research design. Also, the d-formula is the one commonly used. However, there is another effect size procedure using a correlation coefficient (r). Correlation is introduced in Chapter 13. Each procedure for calculating effect size has advantages and disadvantages. When reading meta-analysis studies, you will find some where a correlation coefficient was used for effect size.

PROCEDURES IN META-ANALYSIS

As noted earlier, meta-analysis is often used within kinesiology, in many different areas. In some areas, you will see fewer meta-analysis studies than in other areas. If there are not many research studies available on a topic, there may not be enough research studies and/or a need to conduct a meta-analysis. Also, if the information needed to conduct a meta-analysis (means, standard deviations, correlation coefficients, and so on) is not published in research studies, a meta-analysis will not be possible. For example, this information is typically not published in a qualitative research study. As with all research approaches, a meta-analysis must be conducted in a systematic and carefully planned manner. The meta-analysis is only as good as the research studies and techniques used.

1. **Compile references.** Using several different literature search techniques, data bases referenced in Chapter 3, and so on, compile a list of all research studies pertaining to the research topic for the meta-analysis. You might find, on the topic, a review article that has a large bibliography. Probably the review article contains only good research studies selected by the knowledgeable author of the article. In addition, some earlier meta-analysis articles on the topic and/ or on a topic similar to your topic could yield a large list of references.

2. **Determine your criteria.** Make a basic list of things that must be in any research study before you review the studies extensively. Probably you will have a large number of research studies and there is no reason to extensively review a research study if later you will not use it in the meta-analysis. If there is not enough information in the research study to calculate effect size, there is no reason to extensively review the research study. If the knowledge base for the meta-analysis topic is changing rapidly, you might decide to not review any research study that is more than 10 years old. This decision might be the correct decision, but it might be perceived as an incorrect decision in that it eliminates any older classic studies and/or limits the generalizability of the meta-analysis study. Research studies not published in research journals or in books based on the research might be excluded from the meta-analysis. Theses and dissertations are unpublished and usually harder to

obtain than research journal articles. Some researchers believe that if the research was good, it has been published in a research journal—which suggests that unpublished research is not to be trusted. Again, excluding certain research studies may or may not be the correct decision. Research studies with small numbers of participants, maybe less than 30, might be excluded, in that the research findings may be unique to the participants. Of course, it would be nice to review only good research conducted by knowledgeable people and published in good journals.

3. **Review each study.** Review each research study carefully, taking good notes concerning the basic information (author, research article title, journal name, journal volume and pages, date the issue of the journal was published), the number and type of participants in the research study, the type of treatment(s) applied to the research participants, the length of time of the study, the quality of the procedures used in the research study, the findings, and the information needed for calculating effect size. Moderator variables are factors which influence the relationship between two variables or effect size. If the relationship between two variables or effect size is not the same for males and females, gender would be a moderator variable. Moderator variables need to be identified and coded at this step. You must have the expertise to evaluate whether a research study was well conducted, because you don't want to use weak research studies in the meta-analysis. Keep a list of research studies reviewed and a list of research studies not reviewed, so you don't go back to a research study twice. It is important to get the necessary information in a research study the first time and apply the same standards to all research studies. A purpose of meta-analysis is to remove subjectivity as much as possible.

4. **Decide which studies you'll use.** Make decisions concerning what studies will be used in the meta-analysis and whether moderator variables like gender, age, physical or health characteristics will be considered in the meta-analysis. It is important here, as in step 2, to list the criteria used for *not* using a research study in the meta-analysis and to apply the criteria equally to each research study.

5. **Do the meta-analysis.** Do the meta-analysis, calculating an effect size for each research study used. Summarize the effect sizes for all the research studies used and/or for each classification of participants in the research studies (moderator variables). Some researchers look at the spread in the effect sizes and/or the distribution of effect sizes to determine whether a moderator variable(s) need to be considered. If there is a large spread in the effect sizes and/or the distribution of effect sizes does not resemble a normal (bell-shaped) curve, this may suggest that the influence of a moderator variable(s) should be considered. Probably there should be at least five research studies for each level of a moderator variable. For example, if gender is the moderator variable, at least five research studies with males and five research studies with females

are required. Probably this does not suggest that a meta-analysis study could be conducted using 10 research studies. One of the purposes of meta-analysis is to synthesize the information from a large number of research studies. Often a moderator variable has more than two levels, and there will be considerably more than five research studies for most levels.

6. **Report your results.** Write a report or journal article manuscript based on the meta-analysis. An extensive description of what was done in steps 1 to 5 is vital. The reader of the research report must know exactly what was done in the meta-analysis study in order to interpret and accept the results. In a study by Dishman and Buckworth (1996), the authors listed the 62 sources referenced in the body of their article and the 127 research articles used in the meta-analysis. If this is allowed in a research journal, it is a desirable feature in terms of offering a complete report and a service to future researchers.

COMPUTER PROGRAM

Conducting a meta-analysis becomes more demanding as the number of research studies analyzed increases and as the influence of moderator variables is considered. The use of a computer program to do most of the organizing and computing for the meta-analysis is desirable. Often a computer program is more accurate with computations and provides more information than a person conducting a meta-analysis by hand. The DSTAT program (Johnson 1993) is excellent. It comes with a very comprehensive manual. The program accepts data in a variety of different forms and provides a variety of different values. The sections of the manual are literature review tactics, conducting a meta-analysis review, general program operations and installation, calculation of effect size, management of effect size, analysis of effect sizes, and tutorial. In addition, the manual has an appendix where formulas used in the calculations are presented, as well as a list of references. Schwarzer (1991) has a program called Meta 5.3 which is shareware and follows the Rosenthal (1991) book closely. The program is commonly used. Arthur, Bennett, and Huffcutt (2001) present how to use the SAS statistical package of computer programs to conduct a meta-analysis. Bax, Yu, Ikeda, Tsuruta, and Moons (2006) have a very good program called MIX. The program is well documented and designed to be used by beginners to meta-analysis. The site for MIX is http://www.meta-analysis-made-easy.com.

SELECTED META-ANALYSIS STUDIES

Dishman, R. K., and Buckworth, J. (1996). Increasing physical activity: A quantitative synthesis. *Medicine and Science in Sport and Exercise, 28*(6), 706–719.

Their research intent was to clarify the literature in the area. They conducted a meta-analysis of 127 studies that dealt with the effect of various interventions on increasing physical activity in people. Effects were expressed as correlation coefficients (r) and examined as they varied according to selected moderator variables.

Criteria for including a study and that the studies occurred between 1965 and August 1995 were reported. The authors reported how many studies were excluded. All their methods are well explained. The mean effect was moderately large, r = .34. Effects for each moderator are reported in a table.

The many analyses which can be conducted as part of a meta-analysis are presented in this study. This is an example of using a correlation coefficient as the effect measure. The authors used a computer program called Meta. A bibliography for the 127 research studies used in the meta-analysis is provided. This study is a good example of how to conduct and report a meta-analysis.

Payne, V. G., and Morrow, J. R. (1993). Exercise and VO2max in children: A meta-analysis. *Research Quarterly for Exercise and Sport, 64,* 305–313.

Studies examining the ability of children to improve maximal oxygen uptake (VO2max) have yielded inconsistent findings. The researchers examined the effects of four moderating variables on the VO2max of children. Sixty-nine studies were located, and 28 met the criteria for inclusion.

The authors provided a brief overview of meta-analysis and cited references to studies in human performance where meta-analysis was utilized. They indicated that three computer searches were used to locate research studies. The criteria for including a research study were presented. Effect size (ES) was calculated for each study. Considerable differences in mean ES were found between contrasted groups formed by using the four moderating variables. Effect sizes of .35 to .94 were found. The authors found that the experimental design, cross-sectional or pretest-posttest, for a research study had an influence on the outcome of a study.

This article is easy to read and understand. It is an example of using ES. A bibliography for the 28 studies used in the meta-analysis is provided. This article is a good example and could be read and understood by a person just starting to learn about meta-analysis. Note: Payne, Morrow, Johnson, and Dalton (1997) conducted a meta-analysis of resistance training in children and youth which the interested researcher might read.

Herring, M. P., O'Connor, P. J., and Dishman, R. K. (2010). The effect of exercise training on anxiety symptoms among patients: A systematic review. *Archives of Internal Medicine, 170*(4), 321–331.

Exercise training may help improve anxiety. One hundred seven articles published between 1995 and 2008 were used in the study. All their methods are well explained. The d-formula was used to calculate effect size. The study is a good example of how to conduct and report a meta-analysis. The article is easy to read and understand.

The Cochrane Library (http://www.thecochranelibrary.com) provides systematic reviews for health care decision making. These reviews are basically a meta-analysis.

CRITICISMS OF META-ANALYSIS

Meta-analysis is not the final answer. It only suggests what to do and what to control in a research study. It may be the combining of good and bad studies. It may be the combining of studies with small and large sample sizes. The research participants in the studies combined in the meta-analysis may vary too much in age and gender; or the study may vary too much in research setting, research methods used, and so on, to trust the findings of a meta-analysis. If there is a difference across moderator variables, but the moderator variables were not manipulated in the studies, then an inference concerning cause and effect cannot be made. Thus, a meta-analysis may be an unidentifiable mix applying to nothing specifically. Clearly, without a definition of the research issue and the population of interest before conducting a meta-analysis, this could be a criticism. There were some criticisms of meta-analysis based on methodological/statistical issues but generally these issues are now addressed in the literature in general and in the literature summarized in books like Rosenthal (1991).

Summary of Objectives

1. **Understand why the meta-analysis approach is utilized.**
   Meta-analysis is a means of analyzing the results of many research studies. By reexamining the results of a large number of research studies, researchers are able to draw conclusions that are supported by many studies.

2. **Know how the meta-analysis approach is conducted.**
   Through meta-analysis, the results from available research studies are reanalyzed, and, if necessary, allowances are made for variables that need to be controlled.

12

Historical Research and Action Research

The research approaches discussed in this chapter may not be as commonly used as the approaches discussed in Chapters 8 to 11. These additional approaches are presented for two reasons. One, you need to know the research approaches available to you as a researcher so that you may select the best one for use in your research study. Two, you need to be aware that there are a variety of research approaches and appreciate all of them when reading the research of others. The potential problem is that if all the research you have ever encountered is experimental or is qualitative, you begin to think that it is the only research approach and all other approaches are not research. Often several research approaches are used in a research study. No matter what the research approach, if the research was conducted with good procedures, it is good research.

The two additional research approaches discussed in this chapter are: (1) historical and (2) action. The historical approach is a traditional one although not commonly used in kinesiology research. Research classifications were presented in Chapter 1. Experimental research is conducted to determine what should be done in the *future*. Descriptive research is conducted to describe things in the *present*. And historical research is conducted to describe what happened in the *past*. The action approach is another approach which is not new but not commonly used in kinesiology research.

HISTORICAL RESEARCH

Using the historical approach, the researcher endeavors to record and understand events of the past. In turn, interpretations of recorded history help provide better understanding of the present and suggest possible future directions.

The Nature of Historical Research

Historical researchers, like those conducting experimental and descriptive research, are interested in discovering facts, trying to get at truth. While historians do make observations, they do so through the eyes of other people, those who witnessed a historical event or who wrote about it. Historical studies, like all research studies, involve the collection of data. These data are verified and interpreted following specific standards and then are presented as a report deemed acceptable after critical examination by others.

Historical research is important in kinesiology. Fields within kinesiology have a common past. A thorough study of the past can lead to an understanding of what each field in kinesiology has inherited and what now serves as its roots. Each field has a history and a heritage from which its depth, tradition, and even its present are derived. History repeats itself. Why we do certain things today is based on what has happened to us in the past. What data may exist concerning the origin, growth, and development of the kinesiology disciplines? What problems were present and how were they solved? What societal and cultural pressures have affected kinesiology? What movements have come and gone? Which movements have remained and what form do they now take? Who were the pioneer leaders in each field of kinesiology? What were their contributions? If all of kinesiology was once under the umbrella of physical education, what was the genesis of the separation into what are now many well-defined fields of study? Who were some of the individuals responsible for the separatist movement? What are the historical justifications for changing the name *physical education* to *kinesiology?* What trends, events, and relationships have dictated this name change?

In seeking data to answer these and other critical questions concerning past kinesiology history, we will discover that events occurred, ideas surfaced, and people came and went. More importantly, however, a study of the past can let our professions know how they have been shaped by it. What kinesiology is and what it might become in the future depend largely upon the impressions professionals hold about what kinesiology used to be and how it developed to the point where it is today. The historical approach is oriented to the past and the researcher seeks to cast light on a question of current interest by conducting an intensive study of material that already exists. Historical research can pull all the information in many scattered sources together in one source. Historical research can put on paper what lies in the memories of older people who were present at historical events. If it is not recorded, the information is lost when these people die. Information from individuals who have for many years attended the Masters Golf Tournament in Augusta, Georgia, can shed much light on that historic event and, in fact, the history of golf in the United States.

It frequently is the case in historical research that the collected data cause us to construct new interpretations of an event or person based on the information gained as a result of a study. The assassination of President John F. Kennedy and the origin of the game of baseball are examples of past events whose interpretation has been altered based upon new data. Sometimes historical research is dramatic and gets high visibility when new material not presumed to exist is found. A good example is the discovery of the Dead Sea Scrolls in 1947.

Data Control and Interpretation

Historical research differs from other scholarly work because its subject matter, the past, is difficult to capture. This, in turn, makes interpretation of the past unique and difficult. Historical researchers, like those in experimental and descriptive research, utilize data. However, the researcher of history encounters problems with data that are different than those of the other approaches: (1) These data already exist, and new data cannot be generated, only found, (2) these data cannot be controlled in the same way they are controlled in the other research approaches, and (3) whatever data are found must be analyzed without clarifying the questions being asked.

In experimental research, for example, we often are concerned about the possible effects of extraneous and intervening variables and we try to control them. This is not possible in historical research. Many factors may have affected the historical data, but the historian can exercise no control over these factors. Typical of the factors that might have affected a document or event are memory, politics, censors, greed, jealousy, ulterior motives, ideology, ego, bias, and discrimination. Thus, historical researchers are faced with two problems in the development of their data. The researchers lack the basic elements of control necessary to produce data of the kind and form they wish, and then they must apply some frame of reference to the data if those data are to be meaningful.

The historical researcher cannot interpret words and events by using present-day terminology. All interpretations must be done according to the meanings of that time. The researcher's task is to take information from a given time period and examine and interpret it from within the societal and cultural perspectives of that period. The meaning of words and use of terms change with time. Using the term *sports medicine* in interpreting the meaning of some athletic training event of 50 years ago would be improper because that term, while in vogue now, did not exist in 1942. Even the term *athletic training* would have to be used in the context of that time and not the way we interpret it today. It is important that the researcher become saturated with the educational, political, economic, environmental, and cultural habits of the period being studied. The better the researcher's background knowledge of the time period being studied, the better the interpretation of the facts and the more reliable the final report.

Sources of Historical Data

To provide data about the past, the historian must obtain considerable reliable information. To obtain this information, the researcher will consult two categories of material: *primary sources* and *secondary sources.*

Primary Sources.

Primary source material consists of original documents or remains of documents and physical artifacts, or people who can provide eyewitness evidence where there is no intervening account of an event between its occurrence and its use by the historical researcher. A primary source is connected directly to the event; it is firsthand information. For example, Grosshans (1975) talked to family members and professional colleagues when developing a biography of Delbert Oberteuffer and his professional contributions to the fields of health and physical education.

Primary source material
Original sources in historical research.

Primary sources are of the utmost importance. Historical research should mostly be based on primary sources. The historian always tries to obtain original material. The use of secondary kinds of informational sources when the primary ones are available constitutes a major mistake in this research approach.

Secondary Sources.

Secondhand accounts of historical happenings, hearsay evidence, for example, constitute **secondary source material.** An interpreter is placed between the researcher and the historical event. This person is not tied directly to the event and, consequently, is not an eyewitness. Typical secondary sources are textbooks, newspapers, abstracts, almanacs, encyclopedias, and bibliographies. It should be noted that a source can be primary in one situation and secondary in another. This is particularly true in the case of textbooks and newspapers. Textbooks are normally considered a secondary source. However, if they are used to determine the depth and breadth of the content of such books, they are considered to be primary sources. Stories and written materials change and get taken out of context when repeated or rewritten over time. The good historical researcher has little faith in secondary sources, though they should be studied and checked out for correctness. Sometimes the lack of primary sources will lead the researcher to secondary sources, but this is the exception rather than the rule. In general, a secondary source cannot be depended upon to yield historical truth.

Secondary source material
Secondhand sources in historical research.

Evaluating Historical Data

Historical data, once gathered, must be critically evaluated to determine whether or not it can be considered as fact and, consequently, as historical evidence. This is a difficult and complicated procedure as the researcher attempts to determine such factors as authenticity, genuineness, worth, and accuracy.

External criticism
Method used in historical research to determine the authenticity, genuineness, and validity of the source of data.

External Criticism. The researcher uses **external criticism** to determine the authenticity, genuineness, and validity of the source of the data. Many questions are asked about the author, the time and place in which the document was written, the prevailing conditions of the era in which it appeared, and whether or not the document was a hoax or a forgery. Is the document on the concept of the right-to-life genuine? Did Dr. Jones really write the right-to-life paper? If he did write it, was he competent? Was he a truthful person? What motives did Dr. Jones have when he came out strongly against abortion and birth control devices and substances? Did his religious beliefs influence his stance on the concept? On what scientific studies did he base his stand? Is this Dr. Jones's original piece of work or a duplicated version?

In applying external criticism, researchers use several methods as pointed out by Neutens and Rubinson (2002): (1) Physical and chemical tests of parchment, paper, cloth, wood, ink, paint, or metal are used to determine the age and authorship of a data source, (2) tests of signature, script, handwriting, spelling, and type are used to check authenticity, and (3) consistency in language use, in knowledge and technology of the time period, and documentation are observed closely.

Historians today also enlist the aid of the computer in the authentication of historical data. Such was the case in November 1985 when the manuscript of a poem was discovered. The poem languished unnoticed in the Bodlein Library at Oxford University for 230 years. The poem, a love lyric of nine stanzas, was attributed to William Shakespeare. In an attempt to authenticate the poem as Shakespeare's creation, computer concordance was used. This technique reviewed all of Shakespeare's work and told exactly how often and in what context he used every word he ever wrote. Shakespearean scholars were immediately active with their criticism. Many agreed that the poem was too awful to be genuine and that the quality of lines like "Star-like eyes win love's prize when they twinkle" cast serious doubts about Shakespeare's authorship. They thought the poem was unconventional, that the rhythm was clumsy and the rhymes forced, and the style was utterly unlike Shakespeare's early style.

Internal criticism
Method used in historical research to assess the meaning and accuracy of the source of data.

Internal Criticism. **Internal criticism** assesses the meaning of the content of the document. Interpretations are made to determine the value of the historical data, and the document or event is closely examined to establish its accuracy and worth. Did the event actually occur? If so, did it take place as it was described? How consistent is the writer's account with other reports about the same event? In the right-to-life example, one would seek to determine if Dr. Jones's statements were representative of health, medical, and historical facts. He may have been the true author of the document, but he may have twisted the truth, either accidentally or on purpose. Many of the statements may reflect bias and prejudice, thus negating the accuracy and value of the account. The author's motives for writing a document or describing an event should be carefully examined. It should not be surprising that the writings of medical science researchers and tobacco company researchers differ with regard to the effects of smoking on health. Have the environmentalists taken liberty with the truth when they produce scathing literature concerning the "facts" of human destruction of the environment? Whether the historical event took place is usually quite easily established, but affirming that it happened *as described* is often difficult. In most instances two or more independent sources, preferably primary ones, are needed to verify a historical fact.

Historical researchers, then, use both types of criticism, but especially that of internal criticism. It must be applied to documents, events, and published and unpublished studies in an attempt to avoid conclusions that may end up being quoted and requoted widely, disseminating a great deal of false information over a long period of time.

Oral History

Oral history research is conducted through taped interviews with individuals who are in a position to be able to recall their involvement and perceptions of various events and movements. Much excellent historical data has been obtained by interviewing people who have made contributions to the fields of kinesiology.

There are many ways to handle interviews and the information they provide. For oral history purposes, these seem to be the major considerations:

1. All taped oral history needs to be written down and preferably edited by the person who provided the account.

2. When using the interview technique, the content should be written from the researcher's notes, verbatim as much as is possible.

3. The questions asked and how they are asked are most important. Leading questions should not be asked. The researcher should aim to draw out the individual's personal views and feelings, avoiding any tendency respondents may have to say what they think the interviewer wants to hear.

4. Interviewing can be tiring for the person interviewed. Several sessions with the same person may be necessary, but should last no longer than about one hour.

5. Let the person to be interviewed know in advance what topics will be covered so that some preparation can be made.

6. The person conducting the interview should have read the literature concerning the topic(s) about which questions will be asked.

In analyzing data from oral sources, a strict application of external and internal criticism should be observed. Information provided by the oral source can be very subjective and opinionated. Some people have a tendency to embellish past events to make a better story. With older people, memory can be a problem. The researcher should make every effort to maintain historical standards, at the center of which is objectivity, when evaluating the data and writing the oral history report.

Biographical Research

Biographical historical research presents yet another avenue for the professional in a field of kinesiology to gain further insight into the background of that field. Studying the life, career, and contributions of former leading scholars, teachers, coaches, and administrators can provide a better understanding of the philosophies and movements that are the foundation of current thought and activity in kinesiology. Appropriately, the subjects of biographies have been leaders with outstanding professional credentials, their legacies preserved through careful and objective evaluation of their contributions to their respective fields. At the same time, the heritage of each kinesiology field will be kept and maintained.

Biographical research emphasizes the use of primary source materials and applies external and internal criticism to evaluate the data. Grosshans (1975) completed an excellent biography on Delbert Oberteuffer and his contributions to the fields of health and physical education. Besides extensive personal interviews with Oberteuffer, she talked to his family members, childhood friends, fellow students, professional colleagues, and former employees. In determining the worth of the data obtained from these individuals, Grosshans applied questions, such as:

1. Was the position, location, or association of the contributor favorable for observing the conditions he reported?
2. Did emotional stress, age, or health conditions cause the contributor to make faulty observations or an inaccurate report?
3. Did the contributor report on direct observation, hearsay, or borrowed source material?
4. Did the contributor write the document at the time of the observation, or weeks or years later?
5. Did the contributor have biases concerning any person, professional body, period of history, old or new teaching methods, educational philosophy, or activity that influenced his writing?
6. Did the contributor contradict himself?
7. Are there accounts by other independent, competent observers that agree with the report of the contributor?

The biographer encounters many of the problems typical of most historical research. The following list represents some of the items that can become problematic in a biographical study:

1. Faulty memory of the primary source people.
2. Inability to interview a primary source person of great potential value.
3. Failing to discover a potentially strong primary source person or document.
4. Responses of a living subject of the biography could be biased and could color those of other primary source people.

Hypotheses in Historical Research

Historical studies do not always begin with a hypothesis. If the researcher has no reason or basis for predicting what may or may not be found, then the study will be hypothesis-free. More frequently, however, the researcher develops hypotheses about what the historical data are expected to show. If the gathered evidence supports the predictions, they thus are confirmed. However, they are rejected if the evidence refutes them.

Hence, hypotheses are formulated in an attempt to explain historical phenomena. The goal in testing these hypotheses is to extend our knowledge base concerning historical events, people, and occurrences.

Historical Research in Kinesiology

Interest in historical research in kinesiology has flourished in recent years. In each associated field a group of scholars is devoted to the cultural history of that field of study. Physical education developed a sport history discipline that led to the formation of the North American Society for Sport History (NASSH) in 1973. The publication outlet for sport scholars is the *Journal of Sport History*. Often historical research is published in *Quest*. A little historical research is published in the *Research Quarterly for Exercise and Sport* which has a section editor for history. An increasing number of sport historians are producing a large body of accurate and insightful work. Many of these researchers reside in major universities offering graduate kinesiology programs through which students can pursue advanced degrees in history.

Great strides have been made in recent years by kinesiology educators to increase interest in historical research. Each field maintains archives and holds symposia dealing with historical research. The majority of historical studies conducted by kinesiology graduate students have been sport history reports, biographical sketches of leaders, and treatments of the historical development of agencies, organizations, and athletic conferences. A major and continuing limitation for individuals interested in engaging in historical research has been a lack of sufficient time to complete a historical project. It is difficult to predict in advance just how long the project will take. The search for new data could take years, and the development of concepts and insights in relationship to the data takes additional time. Many individuals do not have the financial resources to permit them to spend an indefinite period completing a historical study. Hence, many individuals in kinesiology, while they may be interested in history, opt to do experimental or descriptive research projects which usually consume less time than historical work. The fields of kinesiology offer a wide range of topics for historical research. Following is a brief list of varied topics that have been studied by professionals, including students, in kinesiology. Some of the journal articles have over 100 references.

1. *A Century of Women's Basketball* (Hult and Trekell 1991).
2. "Prized Performers, but Frequently Overlooked Students: The Involvement of Black Athletes in Intercollegiate Sports in Predominantly White University Campuses, 1890–1972" (Wiggins 1991).
3. *Out of Many, One: A History of the American College of Sports Medicine* (Berryman 1995).
4. "Time Given Freely to Worthwhile Causes: Anna S. Espenschade's Contributions to Physical Education" (Park 2000).
5. "Contesting the Canon: Understanding the History of the Evolving Discipline of Kinesiology" (Wrynn 2003).
6. "Historical Concepts of the Athlete's Heart" (Thompson 2004).
7. "A Fine Balance: Margaret Bell—Physician and Physical Educator" (Wrynn 2005).
8. "The American 'Alliance' of Health and Physical Education: Scholastic Programs and Professional Organizations" (Zieff 2006).

ACTION RESEARCH

What Is Action Research?

Action research is a variation of applied research in which the focus of the project is to meet the immediate, local needs of the research-practitioner. Although counselors, social workers, and nurses, among others, may utilize action research, arguably the most prevalent use of action research over the past decade has been among teachers. Action research enables practicing teachers to conduct research in their own classroom or school in order to bring contextual relevance to research findings. Action research has been carried out in schools around the world in an effort to improve teaching practices and enhance the lives of both children and teachers. Recognizing this growing trend, many colleges and universities have changed the research methods course required in teacher training programs to one that emphasizes action research. Accordingly, the context for action research discussed in this book will be from the perspective of the teacher as the researcher.

Social psychologist Kurt Lewin is often given credit for coining the term action research in the 1940s. Concerned that academic research often yielded findings that had little effect on society or the work of practitioners, he was instrumental in employing a research methodology that was action-oriented and designed to improve conditions and practices in classrooms and other practitioner-based environments. This approach to research was typically conducted in a practicing environment (e.g., individual classroom, a group of grade level classrooms, or the whole school), involved a field-intensive process in which the researcher actively participates in the environment being studied, utilized multiple forms of data, and resulted in the development of an action plan for improving practices, conditions, or the environment. According to Gall, Gall, and Borg (2005), action research was widely used in the 1940s and 1950s, declined in use thereafter, but has recently become more popular, particularly among teacher educators.

Action research draws upon the techniques and methods of scientific inquiry discussed elsewhere in this book, but its purpose is improving local practice rather than producing generalizable knowledge or testing theories. McMillan (2008) defined action research as a systematic investigation conducted by practitioners to provide information to immediately improve teaching and learning. He points out that action research brings together the characteristics of systematic inquiry and professional practice in a teacher's classroom for the purpose of solving a local problem or improving a practice. According to Mills (2011, 6), "action research is any systematic inquiry conducted by teacher researchers, principals, school counselors, or other stakeholders in the teaching/learning environment to gather information about how their particular schools operate, how they teach, and how well their students learn." Mills further proclaims that action research is "done *by* teachers *for* themselves" in an effort to effect positive changes in the school environment and improve student learning. Through action research, teachers engage in a systematic and structured process for obtaining valuable information in order to improve professional practice. Although many benefits of action research have been cited, a key benefit of particular importance in practitioner settings is that it impacts directly on professional practice, thereby reducing the gap between theory and practice.

Characteristics of Action Research

Philosophically, action research is largely founded on *postmodernism* theory, arguing that truth is relative, conditional, situational, and based on previous experience. Thus, action research provides the means for investigating one's own classroom or school (i.e., practicing environment) that is necessarily context-bounded. Although action research may have different purposes and different audiences compared to traditional research, it is our view that action research uses the same basic methods

TABLE 12.1 Characteristics of Action Research Compared to Traditional Research

CHARACTERISTIC	ACTION RESEARCH	TRADITIONAL RESEARCH
Goal/Purpose	Seeks knowledge that may be applied to the local situation with little regard for generalizability	Creation of new, generalizable knowledge; theory testing
Who does the research	Teachers, counselors, principals, practitioners, etc.—insiders	Trained researchers such as scholars and professors—outsiders
Setting	Local settings—classroom, schools, or wherever the practice is implemented	Any setting appropriate for the research question and design
Literature review	Cursory review of literature related to problem being studied	Extensive review of literature with an emphasis on primary sources
Research design	Tends to be nonexperimental or quasi-experimental; simple design; less extensive control	Whatever design is appropriate for the research question; greater emphasis on control
Research participants	Typically students or other individuals with whom the action-practitioner works; purposeful or convenience sampling	Tends to be a representative sample of the population of interest; often selected through systematic sampling
Data collection	Local, convenient measures; often instruments are teacher developed	Standardized measures or techniques with emphasis on reliability and validity of instruments
Data analysis	Primarily descriptive and interpretative; focuses on practical significance	Descriptive and inferential often with complex analyses; focuses on statistical significance
Application of results	Applied directly to local situation and problems; results shared with peers informally; infrequent reporting in professional journals	Emphasis on generalizability and theoretical significance; practical implications may not be important; reported in publications/presentations
Researcher	Considered an insider; personally involved, generally close to the research participants; often the instrument of data collection	Considered an outsider; objective, often unknown to the participants; selects and uses standardized instruments of known value

and procedures of scientific inquiry as seen in other forms of research. Because of its philosophical underpinning, action research is generally more closely associated with qualitative research and, as such, often uses qualitative methods of inquiry. However, the nature of the research question and type of data needed to answer the question should determine whether a qualitative or quantitative approach, or both, should be used. Both qualitative and quantitative approaches may be used in action research. In fact, we believe that mixed methods may be particularly suited for the type of research questions often seen in action research.

Ary, Jacobs, and Sorensen (2010) cite three main characteristics of action research:

1. The research is situated in a local setting and focuses on a local issue.
2. The research is conducted by and for the practitioner.
3. The research results in an action or a change implemented by the practitioner in the local context.

It is also noted that action research is often associated with *reflective practice,* a process in which teachers use a systematic approach for examining their own practice and the impact of their work. In fact, some models of action research include reflection as a specific step in the research process. The distinction between action research and traditional or formal research is not great, most notably in the primary goals of the research. While the goals of traditional research are to test theories and produce generalizable knowledge, action research is focused on obtaining knowledge that is directly applicable to the local situation, with little interest in generalizing the results to other settings. Other differences may exist in the literature review process, the selection of research participants, the type of research design used, the type of measures used, the control of extraneous variables, the type of data analysis used, and the role of the researcher. Table 12.1 summarizes characteristics of action research compared to traditional research discussed elsewhere in this book.

Sample Action Research Study.   Here is an example of action research conducted by an elementary school physical education teacher.

Ms. James is a veteran teacher who recently accepted a new position in an elementary school in a relatively affluent suburb of a large city in the Midwest part of the country. She began to notice that students in her classes seemed bored and unmotivated and generally not engaged in class activities. Furthermore, conversations with parents at various times, including during parent-teacher conferences, revealed a general apathy and, in fact, a negative attitude among parents toward school physical education. Recognizing the increasing rates of obesity among children and the many benefits associated with regular physical activity, Ms. James is concerned that her students are not sufficiently engaged in physical education class and thus are not acquiring the skills and developing the attitudes needed to lead a healthy, active lifestyle. She decides to study the problem to determine why this is occurring and to determine whether she can make changes in the class that will better engage the students and thus improve learning and participation in physical activity.

Ms. James searches the Internet for information concerning student engagement and motivation related to physical activity participation, hoping that some of this information will provide meaningful suggestions that might make a difference in her classes. She even goes to the local college library to continue her literature search and seek more information on the topic. Ms. James has access to extensive student performance information and heart rate data that might provide some insight into students' participation levels during physical education class. In addition, Ms. James decides to keep a personal journal for an entire term to note her reflections on each class period and to record her observations about student behavior. She also conducts a series of interviews with the students, asking them to talk about what they liked and disliked about physical education class and physical activity (exercise) in general. Furthermore, recognizing that parental influence is an important factor affecting children's behavior, Ms. James develops a short questionnaire that is sent to the parents of her students. She is attempting to assess parental satisfaction with the physical education program and to determine parental attitudes toward physical activity participation. By doing these things, Ms. James is engaged in action research. She is utilizing both quantitative and qualitative techniques to gather data that may help to explain why her students seem bored and unmotivated and may help her make meaningful changes in her teaching practice. More information about Ms. James's research will be presented later in this chapter.

The Action Research Process

The action research process follows essentially the same stages as traditional research. We identify five stages in the action research process: (1) identifying the question or problem, (2) developing the research plan, (3) collecting and analyzing the data, (4) interpreting the results and forming conclusions, and (5) developing an action plan. You will note two key differences from the conceptualization of the research process described in Chapters 1 and 2 of this textbook. First, since hypothesis testing is not a fundamental component of action research, we do not include a stage in our description of the action research process in which the researcher formulates a hypothesis. Note, however, that depending upon the nature of the research question, the design of the study, and the type of data collected, hypotheses could be developed and tested in the same manner as in traditional research. Secondly, the action research process includes an additional stage that involves developing an action plan for implementation of the findings in the teaching environment. This stage comes after results have been interpreted and conclusions drawn and represents a unique aspect of action research—acting upon the knowledge gained to improve professional practice. As we previously described in Chapter 2, each stage of the research process involves certain discrete steps that guide the work of the researcher. These same steps apply to the action research process, with only slight adjustments being made to account for the differing nature of action research. Also note that the action research process is cyclical in nature and may be repeated over time as the research-practitioner reflects on the research process and the resulting action plan. In the following we address in more detail the stages of the action research process.

1. Identifying the Question or Problem. The first stage, as is true with all types of research, is to determine what you want to study and then frame this as a research question. Normally, for the teacher-researcher, the question emerges from practices occurring in the teaching and learning environment that raise concerns, issues, or questions. Sometimes the question may simply reflect an interest area or something you feel passionate about. Often the initial question or interest area is rather broad and general, making it unsuitable for scientific investigation. As discussed in Chapter 2, *distillation* is the process of narrowing an initial question to a specific researchable problem. For the teacher-researcher, the distillation process involves gathering more information about the general question—information from self-reflection, information from discussions with colleagues, and information from a review of the professional literature.

As mentioned previously, reflection is an important characteristic of action research as this process enables the teacher-researcher to step back from the world of practice and consider how her or his aims and practices are working. This may facilitate the distillation process and lead to the identification of a research question that is both meaningful and practical. It is also wise to find out what other teachers have done or experienced related to your topic. Their insights, particularly if they have taught the same subject matter, at the same grade level, and in the same setting, may be particularly valuable in zeroing in on a researchable problem and planning the research. Although some authors of action research textbooks downplay the importance of reviewing the literature, most experts agree that it is an invaluable activity. The literature review in action research may not be as extensive as that required for the more traditional types of research, but it is important that teacher-researchers become familiar with and develop a basic understanding of the professional literature related to the question of interest. Moreover, in many cases, reviewing the literature enables the question or research topic to be set in a theoretical context. Being able to relate your question to existing theories adds credibility to your study and provides a framework for interpreting the results. In addition to framing the study and helping to distill the research question, a review of the literature may provide ideas for designing the study and collecting data. And in those rare instances in action research in which hypotheses are needed, the published literature provides a basis for formulating hypotheses. Therefore, the teacher-researcher will want to consult professional journals, books, and Internet sources to search for relevant information related to the question of interest.

2. Developing the Research Plan. The second stage of the action research process is to develop the research plan. Developing the research plan will involve selecting the basic approach to be used to investigate the research question or problem (e.g., quantitative, qualitative, or mixed methods approach) and making decisions about the research participants, experimental protocols, if any, measures to be used, methods of data collection, and analysis techniques. One approach is not better than the other. A review of the action research literature indicates that a qualitative approach may be preferred among educators. We believe that, initially, both quantitative and qualitative approaches should be considered. We also believe that a mixed-methods approach, in which both quantitative and qualitative techniques are used, may be particularly useful for action research studies.

The selection of the participants in action research is often predetermined by the setting and the nature of the research question. Because of the local nature and context-bound setting of the problem being investigated, the selection of appropriate research participants is a critical feature of the action research process. Research participants are generally selected because they are students or other individuals with whom the teacher-researcher usually works. Since generalizability is seldom an aim of action research, rarely would the selection of research participants involve any type of random sampling technique. Sometimes an action researcher wants to actually conduct a study to investigate the effectiveness of some type of treatment intervention or pedagogical technique. When this is the case, the study takes on the basic appearance of experimental research. Yet, because of the limitations imposed by the practicing environment, it is highly improbable that action research can meet all the conditions expected of an experimental study. For instance, in most schools or classrooms, random selection of participants is generally not possible and it is difficult, if not impossible, to randomly assign participants to groups. Moreover, since action research usually takes place in an authentic classroom or school environment, relatively little attention is paid to the control of extraneous variables—variables that could be a source of error in traditional experimental research. These realities mean that experimental studies in action research are more likely to be quasi-experimental research. For example, a study might involve a simple pretest-posttest design in which a group of students (entire class) are given a pretest, participate in some type of intervention, and then take a posttest. The reader is referred to Chapter 8 of this textbook for further discussion of experimental research and various types of experimental designs.

Selecting the appropriate measurement instruments and procedures is a challenge that all researchers face. According to McMillan (2008), a good starting point in determining the data collection procedures is deciding whether quantitative or qualitative measures will be used by themselves or in combination with each other. Researchers conducting formal types of research are particularly concerned that the measures used and the data collection procedures are valid and reliable. Consequently, considerable attention is given to selecting appropriate measures that have established validity and reliability, frequently resulting in the use of standardized instruments or procedures. Where standardized instruments are not available, researchers often conduct pilot studies in order to establish the suitability of the measuring instrument. In action research, on the other hand, the teacher-researcher is more likely to use data-collection methods of convenience. Such methods may include available measures (e.g., test scores, class products, or existing artifacts), interviews, simple questionnaires, and observation. Often the measures are developed by the teacher-researcher rather than being standardized instruments. In such cases, where established validity and reliability likely does not exist, it is important that the measures and procedures be reviewed by others (e.g., teaching colleagues, administrators, university professors, etc.) for clarity and face validity purposes. This helps establish the credibility of the measures and data collection procedures in the absence of extensive testing to determine validity and reliability.

Researchers may choose from a multitude of data collection strategies and measures. We previously identified (see Chapter 4) three methods of data collection applicable to research in kinesiology (and physical education): observation, questioning, and direct measurement. A fourth category of data collection techniques is applicable for action research, *examining,* whereby all sorts of archival and existing documents may be used for gathering data. Clearly, schools and teachers maintain a wide variety of records (e.g., test scores, grade reports, attendance records), student work, minutes of meetings and so forth that may be useful data sources. Note, however, that permission must be obtained for using these data for research purposes. We now recognize there are four basic methods of gathering information having particular application for action research in physical education: *observation, questioning, direct measurement,* and *examining.* In Table 12.2 we identify specific examples of strategies and techniques in each of these categories that may be useful for action researchers in school physical education. In action research, particularly those studies using mixed methods, it is common practice to utilize more than one measure of the phenomenon being studied, thus allowing for *triangulation,* a process in which the researcher uses multiple data sources to facilitate the emerging interpretation. This process brings different perspectives into play and helps foster a more thorough understanding of the phenomenon of interest. Recall in the

TABLE 12.2 Example Methods of Data Collection in Action Research

OBSERVATION	MEASUREMENT	QUESTIONING	EXAMINING
VIEWING THE PARTICIPANTS AND RECORDING DATA IN VARIOUS WAYS	*DIRECT AND INDIRECT MEASUREMENT OF PHYSICAL AND PSYCHOLOGICAL ATTRIBUTES*	*VARIETY OF METHODS OF ASKING THE PARTICIPANTS TO DISCLOSE INFORMATION*	*USING ARCHIVAL DOCUMENTS AND OTHER RECORDS THAT CURRENTLY EXIST*
Field notes	Physiological measures	Formal interviews	Standardized test scores
Checklists	Heart rate data	Informal interviews	Student work/artifacts
Journals	Sport skills tests	Focus group interviews	Heart rate data
Video/audio tapes	Attitudinal scales	Questionnaires	Fitness test scores
Checklists	Physical activity monitoring	Opinion scales	Grade reports
Anecdotal records	Psychological inventories	Checklists	Dietary diaries
Rating scales	Physical fitness tests	Activity self-reports	Lesson plans
	Performance measures		Health records
			Video/audio tapes
			Portfolios

example of Ms. James's study concerning student engagement and motivation, she utilized four sources of data: personal journal entries, student interviews, parental surveys, and student performance records, namely heart rate data. When multiple sources of data show similar results, this strengthens the ability of the researcher to make accurate and meaningful interpretations. We recommend that action researchers use at least two data sources, but probably no more than four, to avoid complicating the interpretation process.

Developing the research plan also involves determining how the collected data will be analyzed. It is one thing to collect data, but now the researcher must make sense out of the information collected, thus the role of data analysis. Data analysis techniques used in action research, just as we see in traditional research, are largely dependent upon the nature of the research question and the type of data collected. Quantitative data may be analyzed using one or more statistical techniques. Most action research in which quantitative data have been collected involves relatively simple statistical procedures, often descriptive statistics used for summarizing data or perhaps correlational statistics for examining relationships. Although more sophisticated statistical analyses may be used in some instances, it is often argued that practical significance is more appropriate than statistical significance in action research studies (Gall, Gall, and Borg 2005). Also note that with the small number of research participants often used in action research, statistical power is low, making it difficult to obtain statistical significance. When qualitative data are collected, which is often the case in action research, analysis is largely inductive in nature. There are three basic approaches to data analysis that are common to action research: reporting, descriptive reality, and grounded theory (Craig 2009). The reporting approach is simply transcribing and summarizing the data (e.g., field notes, recordings, survey responses, student artifacts) with little analysis involved. The descriptive reality approach requires a more systematic analysis of the data, often involving simple coding and integrating (collapsing) data in order to develop a more comprehensive, detailed picture of the situation or phenomenon of interest. The grounded theory approach involves the most in-depth analysis, as the researcher engages in additional coding and examines the data to identify common themes and attributes. Further discussion of both quantitative and qualitative analysis techniques is presented elsewhere in this textbook.

3. Collecting and Analyzing the Data.   The research plan is now put into action and data collected. Leading education experts consider the collection and analysis of research data to be the most important aspects of action research (Gall, Gall, and Borg 2005). We couldn't agree more! In order for action research, often conducted without the control and rigor associated with traditional research, to effect positive change in educational practices and be considered credible within the scientific community, careful attention must be given to the collection of meaningful data and to the thoughtful and considered analysis of the data. This is another reason why the use of more than one data source is advised, so that the results are not entirely dependent on one source of information. In action research, more so than in traditional research, the researcher continuously reviews the data being collected or examined as the research process unfolds. This is part of the reflective process that is an integral component of action research. As the study evolves and data are gathered, action researchers may find it necessary to modify the research plan somewhat to accommodate the serendipitous nature and changing realities of conducting research in an authentic setting. This reflects the basic nature of action research. The process of collecting data for an action research study must follow accepted ethical guidelines applicable to all research involving human participants. This will likely mean obtaining permission from parents to utilize their children or their children's records in the research, and quite possibly assent from the children. A more complete discussion regarding ethics involved in action research is presented later in this chapter.

4. Interpreting the Results and Forming Conclusions.   Once the data have been organized and analyzed in some manner, whether through the use of a statistical procedure or some qualitative strategy, the researcher must now interpret this information in order to make sense of the data collected. Data interpretation is concerned with meanings that emerge from the analysis and leads to the formation of the conclusions. The interpretation stage is a process, which includes ongoing reflection and careful examination of the data in light of existing practices and accepted knowledge in the area of interest. For many teacher-researchers, this is the most challenging aspect of action research. The process of interpretation is significantly aided if the study has been set within a theoretical framework. The use of *concept-mapping* is a strategy seen mostly in qualitative research that may help the action researcher in interpretation. A concept map is essentially a diagram used to help the researcher visualize how different factors (components) relate to the question or problem being investigated. Concept-mapping is particularly beneficial in situations involving multiple data sources, a recommended practice in action research. For example, consider the problem facing Ms. James regarding the lack of motivation and student engagement during physical education class. She collected data from a variety of sources, including student interviews, a parental survey, student heart rate monitoring, as well as her own personal journal. Based on a careful examination of the data collected and the results of the analyses completed, she might create a concept map as shown in Figure 12.1. This may, in turn, help her (1) identify factors that contribute to the problem being investigated, (2) reach a reasonable conclusion, and (3) point to possible solutions.

Action planning
A unique stage within the action research process whereby the researcher identifies local actions that take place based on the findings of the study.

5. Developing an Action Plan.   **Action planning** is the next stage of the action research process. In fact, Ary, Jacobs, and Sorensen (2010) describe action planning as the most important step in action research. Somewhat unique to action research,

FIGURE 12.1
Example Concept Map of Potential Factors Contributing to Lack of Student Engagement in Physical Education Class

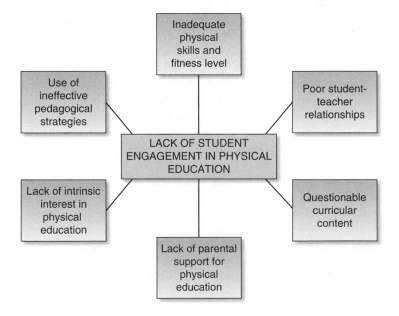

this is the stage in which the teacher-researcher is basically trying to answer the following question: *"Based on what I have learned from this investigation, what should I do now?"* (Mills 2011). Moreover, Mills states that "action planning is also a time for reflection—reflection on where you have been, what you have learned, and where you are going." In the case of Ms. James's study, she would reflect upon her own teaching practices in light of the specific findings from her research and proffer recommended actions that could be implemented which are intended to improve student motivation and engagement during physical education class. Although each action plan is unique, contextually limited, and based on a specific research study, there are several components that are universally applicable. The action plan sets overall goals; establishes specific objectives; describes possible strategies or tasks to be taken; identifies who is responsible; establishes a timeline; and determines resources needed. The action plan resulting from action research may be thought of as an expanded description of recommendations that we normally see in reports of traditional research. But in this case, the action plan describes the actions that the teacher-researcher will take based on the findings of the study. More information about action planning subsequent to action research, including sample templates for developing an action plan, can be found in textbooks by Mills (2011) and Craig (2009).

As previously discussed in this chapter, generalizability is not a goal of action research. Rather, the goal of action research is to better understand and improve local practice. It is not uncommon, however, for teacher-researchers to share the results of their action research with their teaching colleagues, school administrators, parents, students, and others. Usually this is done informally or through online networks or conference/workshop presentations. Although there are a few academic journals that may publish the results of action research studies, writing for publication is seldom a major objective for teachers conducting action research. Many readers of this textbook, however, will find themselves writing not by choice, but in order to complete requirements for an academic degree or professional advancement. Yet, as we discussed in Chapter 1, one of the features that distinguishes scientific inquiry and research from other ways of knowing is the public nature of the activity. Consequently, we believe that "writing-up" and formally publishing action research studies not only provides a permanent record of the study, but also has the potential to help fellow teachers and impact educational policy and practices.

Ethics in Action Research

Action research is bound by the same ethical principles and regulations as other types of research involving human participants. As discussed in Chapter 6, Institutional Review Boards (IRBs) have been created by federal mandate to ensure compliance with governmental regulations pertaining to research involving human research participants. These governmental regulations pertain to research in schools just as they do for research in hospitals and laboratories. Researchers affiliated with universities and colleges, including all faculty, staff, and students conducting research with human participants, will need to obtain IRB approval before initiating any phase of the research. This also applies to teacher-researchers who may be completing a graduate degree as a part-time student. In some cases, the research study may be determined to meet the criteria for an exempt review, but this determination is made by the IRB, not the researcher. Although it is rare that a public or private K-12 school system will have an officially established IRB, most school systems have established procedures in place for conducting research in the classroom setting and for protecting the rights and welfare of human research participants associated with their school. Graduate students conducting research in public or private schools must follow the policies and procedures of both the university IRB and the school district and will likely need approval from the university IRB as well the school district. Because of the variability in guidelines and procedures from one institution to another, you are advised to review the pertinent regulations of both the school district and the university IRB and consult with appropriate officials if you have questions.

It is generally acknowledged by most experts in the field that the researcher must obtain parent or guardian permission in order for their minor children (students) to participate in a research study. Moreover, the assent of the minor to participate in the research is also needed in most cases. Legally effective informed consent is, in fact, a fundamental requirement in the federal regulations. Further discussion of this topic is presented in Chapter 6 and may, of course, be found in the federal regulations (45 C.F.R. 46). In addition, however, action researchers have some unique challenges to address in order to ensure that their research complies with ethical guidelines. Three are discussed here.

Perhaps the most difficult challenge for teacher-researchers to satisfactorily address is actually associated with the very essence of action research—the study is being conducted in a practicing environment in which the researcher (the teacher in this case) is closely associated with the research participants (the students). In fact, teacher-researchers frequently want to use their own students in the research study. Obviously that makes sense for action research. But the problem, from an ethical perspective, is that the teacher is in a position of authority or power over the students (the desired research participants). The ethical principle of autonomy demands that research participants enter the research study voluntarily and with adequate information to make an informed decision. When the researcher is in a position of authority over the participants (or prospective participants) in the study, particularly if they are minor children, it may be impossible for them to decline participation, thus denying the individual the capability of self-determination. Also, the inherent relationship between the teacher and students may foster conditions whereby the students may be subtly coerced or unduly influenced to engage in research activities for which they would not otherwise volunteer. Although teachers do not have direct power or authority over the parents, it is well known that parents often make school-related decisions concerning their children so as to gain favor with the child's teacher or to negate perceived negative consequences. Thus, parents may feel pressured to allow their child to participate in a research study being conducted by their child's teacher. This situation also undermines the principle of autonomy and the capacity to voluntarily choose whether or not to participate in a research study. To avoid the ethical dilemma described above, some IRBs have established policies that prohibit teachers from using their own students as research participants. This is a reason that teacher-researchers need to carefully review pertinent ethical policies and regulations that may affect their planned research and to develop precise and thorough procedures that mitigate the possibility of undue influence affecting the decision regarding research participation of minor students.

A second issue that frequently confronts the teacher-researcher pertains to the use of student records and other materials or data that are routinely collected and maintained in the school setting. Basic student grade reports, standardized test scores, progress reports, activity records, portfolios, heart rate monitor data, and student work samples are examples of such information that are useful data sources for the teacher-researcher. These records or materials are, understandably, individually identifiable. Teachers generally have the ability and license to access such records as the information may be germane to their role as a teacher. Yet, permission from a school administrator may sometimes be required to access certain records. But accessing and using such records and materials for research purposes is quite a different situation. Because the records contain individually identifiable information, permission to access and use the records for research purposes must be obtained not only from an appropriate school authority, but also from the parent or guardian of the minor student. Usually this is addressed through the informed consent document (permission letter) used to obtain parental permission. Although the letters requesting parental permission will be somewhat generic in order to include the required elements of consent as specified by federal regulations, the letters will be unique in that they must specifically identify what will happen to students participating in the research, what records and materials are being requested, and so forth. Check the website of the IRB governing research at your university for a description of the required elements of consent as well as sample documents and guidelines for developing consent documents.

Lastly, protecting the privacy of research participants, particularly when they are students of the teacher-researcher, and maintaining the confidentiality of collected data present unique challenges that must be addressed. A critical factor in conducting research with human research participants is to make sure that their anonymity is protected. Students' identity is obviously known to the teacher. The records maintained by the school contain personally identifiable information. In addition, teacher-researchers wishing to conduct research with students from schools should be aware of federal laws that govern the conduct of these studies and the disclosure of information. Namely, the Family Educational Rights and Privacy Act (FERPA) and the Protection of Pupil Rights Amendment (PPRA) prescribe laws pertaining to research with schoolchildren. FERPA stipulates, among other things, that written permission is required to disclose personally identifiable information from a student's education record. PPRA applies to survey research conducted in schools and stipulates that parents have the right to inspect questionnaires distributed in schools. In addition, PPRA also states that parental permission is required to have minors participate in surveys that ask certain types of sensitive information. As stated above, these permissions are normally sought through a letter sent to parents. It is important that practicing teachers conducting action research studies adhere to applicable federal laws and school policies and carefully develop procedures designed to protect the privacy of student research participants and ensure that private information is kept confidential.

Summary of Objectives

1. **Understand the nature of historical research.** Historical research is used to record and understand the events of the past. Both primary and secondary sources are used as historical data sources.

2. **Explain how action research is used in kinesiology.** Action research is a special type of applied research often conducted by a practicing professional such as a teacher or a nurse for the purpose of meeting the immediate, local needs of the research-practitioner and thus improving professional practice. Although action research employs methods of systematic inquiry seen in other forms of research, action research is ordinarily context-bound, having little generalizability.

3. **Describe characteristics of action research and compare to traditional research.** Action research is usually conducted by and for the practitioner as opposed to a trained researcher or scholar; it is situated in a local setting and focused on a local issue with little regard for generalizability; research participants typically include students or other individuals with whom the research-practitioner works as opposed to a representative sample of a defined population; data collection methods employ locally developed instruments or seek readily available data compared to the use of standardized measures; and results from action research are applied locally with little emphasis given to generalizability or theoretical significance as seen in traditional research.

4. **Identify methods of data collection common to action research.** Data collection in action research utilizes a variety of measures and techniques for gathering information, but generally four basic methods are recognized: observation, questioning, direct measurement, and examining. The action researcher will often use data collection methods of convenience and is less concerned with the validity and reliability of the measures. Existing data, such as test scores or class products, as well as simple surveys or interviews and observational techniques are frequently used in action research.

5. **Understand the ethical challenges of conducting action research in a school setting.** Action research is bound by the same ethical principles and regulations as other types of research involving human participants. In many forms of action research, the research participants are underlings of the researcher (e.g., students or patients). In such situations where the researcher is in a position of authority over the research participant, the researcher must take special care to mitigate the possibility of coercion or undue influence. Moreover, since minor children are often involved in action research in school settings, parental or guardian permission is generally required.

Part Three

Data Analysis

Data are the measures, scores, and other information collected in a research study. Usually, the term *data* is used to refer to the scores of the participants for a variable, although it is not uncommon to have multiple data sets because information was collected on multiple variables. Researchers draw their conclusions based on the data. Presented in Chapters 13 and 14 of Part Three are a variety of commonly used data analysis techniques. It will be useful to be aware of what techniques are available in selecting the most appropriate one for use in your research. Knowledge of these techniques will also make the research literature easier to understand. These techniques typically require some mathematical calculation.

Measurement of research participants with various tests and techniques occurs in a research study in order to collect data. As discussed briefly in Chapter 5, the data must have objectivity and reliability. Further, the interpretations of the data must have validity. Objectivity, reliability, and validity, as well as techniques for estimating them, are discussed in detail in Chapter 15.

13

Descriptive Data Analysis

This chapter presents statistical techniques that can be applied to evaluate a set of scores. You should be familiar with them in order to select the appropriate one for a given situation and to understand the research literature.

After reading Chapter 13, you should be able to

1. Understand several options for organizing and graphing scores.
2. Explain three measures of central tendency.
3. Explain two measures of variability.
4. Explain two measures of group position.
5. Explain how to determine the relationship between scores.
6. Explain measures of association.

This chapter covers techniques and statistics commonly used to describe the characteristics and performance of a group and to interpret the scores of individuals within a group. There are many reasons why we analyze data. For a large group, a simple listing of the scores has no meaning to the researcher or the person reading the research report. Only by applying some analysis to the data can it be condensed to a point where it can be meaningful to all interested people in terms of overall performance or characteristics of the group. Also, to make comparisons between groups, there must be a single score for each group representing the typical score of the group.

    Sometimes it is necessary to describe the performance of an individual within a group. Some data analysis is necessary before the performance of an individual can be compared to the performance of others in the group or to the overall group performance. Before presenting various descriptive data analysis techniques, data analysis basics, types of scores, common units of measure, and computer analysis must be discussed, since these elements influence the data analysis.

DATA ANALYSIS BASICS

There are three distinct steps in data analysis: (1) Select the technique appropriate for the data and the research questions; (2) apply the technique or calculate using the technique; and (3) interpret the result of the technique. Step 2 is often quite difficult when a large amount of data is involved or the analysis technique is complex. Thus, step 2 is best accomplished with the aid of the computer. A computer package will be frequently referenced in Chapters 13 and 14, and no calculational formulas or computational examples will be presented in these chapters unless they help the reader understand the data analysis technique. Using the computer for step 2 takes nothing away from the researcher in terms of decision making but is of great benefit in terms of the time saved and the accuracy of the result. An excellent reference on interpreting statistics is Huck (2008).

In most research studies, a population is identified, a sample is drawn from the population, the research study is conducted on the sample, and the results for the sample are inferred to the population. Thus, sample information **(statistics)** are used to estimate population information **(parameters).** For example, the mean, or arithmetic average, for a sample is a statistic used as an estimate of the mean for a population, which is a parameter. All calculated values in Chapters 13 and 14 will be called statistics. Statistics can be classified in a number of ways. One classification is the descriptive versus inferential statistic. A descriptive statistic is used to describe characteristics of a group, while an inferential statistic is used in the process of making an inference from a sample to a population. Some statistics (the mean is one) can be used in either a descriptive or inferential manner. Chapter 13 focuses on **descriptive statistics.**

Statistics
Values or quantities calculated using information obtained from a sample; used to estimate population information.

Parameters
Values or quantities calculated using information obtained from a population.

Descriptive statistic
Statistic used to describe characteristics of a group.

TYPES OF SCORES

Scores can be classified as either continuous or discrete. **Continuous scores,** as most are in kinesiology, have a potentially infinite number of values allowing variables to be measured with varying degrees of accuracy. Between any two values of a continuous score are countless other values that may be expressed as fractions. For example, 100-yard dash scores are usually recorded to the nearest tenth of a second, but they could be recorded in hundredths or thousandths of a second if timing equipment accurate to that level of precision was available. Body weight accurate to the closest five-pound interval, to the whole pound, or to the half-pound might be recorded depending on how exact the measurement needs to be. **Discrete scores** are limited to a specific number of values and usually are not expressed as fractions. Scores on a throw or shot at a target numbered 5-4-3-2-1-0 are discrete because whole number scores of 5, 4, 3, 2, 1, or 0 are the only ones possible. A score of 4.5 or 1.67 is impossible.

Most continuous scores are rounded off to the nearest unit of measurement when they are recorded. For example, the score of a student who runs the 100-yard

Continuous scores
Scores that have a potentially infinite number of values.

Discrete scores
Scores that are limited to a specific number of values.

dash in 10.57 seconds is recorded as 10.6 because 10.57 is closer to 10.6 than to 10.5. Usually when a number is rounded off to the nearest unit of measurement, it is increased only when the number being dropped is 5 or more. Thus 11.45 is rounded off to 11.5, while 11.44 is recorded as 11.4. A less common method is to round off to the last unit of measure, awarding the next higher score only when that score is actually accomplished. For example, an individual who does eight sit-ups but cannot complete the ninth receives a score of 8.

We can also classify scores as ratio, interval, ordinal, or nominal. How scores are classified influences what calculations may be performed on the data. **Ratio scores** have a common unit of measurement between each score and a true zero point so that statements about equality of ratios can be made. Length and weight are examples, since one measurement may be expressed as two or three times that of another. **Interval scores** have a common unit of measurement between each score but do not have a true zero point. (A score of 0 as a measure of distance is a true zero, indicating no distance. However, a score of 0 on a knowledge test is not a true zero because it does not indicate a total lack of knowledge; it simply means that the respondent answered none of the questions correctly.) Most physical performance scores are either ratio or interval. **Ordinal scores** do not have a common unit of measurement between each score but are ordered in a way that makes it possible to characterize one score as higher than another. Class ranks, for example, are ordinal: If three students receive sit-up scores of 16, 10, and 8, respectively, the first is ranked 1; the next, 2; and the last, 3. Notice that the number of sit-ups necessary to change the class ranks of the second and third students differs. Thus there is not a common unit of measurement between consecutive scores. **Nominal scores** cannot be hierarchically ordered and are mutually exclusive. For example, individuals can be classified by church preference, but we cannot say that one religion is better than another. Gender is another example.

COMMON UNITS OF MEASURE

Many scores are recorded in feet and inches or in minutes and seconds. To analyze scores, they must be recorded in a single unit of measurement, usually the smaller one. Thus distances and heights are recorded in inches rather than feet and inches, and times are recorded in seconds rather than minutes and seconds. Recording scores in the smaller unit of measure as they are collected is less time-consuming than translating them into that form later.

COMPUTER ANALYSIS

Score analysis should be accurate and quick. Particularly when a set of scores is large, say 50 or more, computers should be used to ensure both accuracy and speed. Computers are increasingly available in school districts and universities, agencies,

---

Ratio scores
Scores that have a common unit of measurement between each score and a true zero point.

Interval scores
Scores that have a common unit of measurement between each score, but do not have a true zero point.

Ordinal scores
Scores that do not have a common unit of measurement between each score, but are ordered from high to low.

Nominal scores
Scores that cannot be hierarchically ordered.

and businesses. Each statistical example in this chapter is accompanied by an example of the desktop computer application. Sometimes the output from the desktop computer program will include more information than will have been discussed in the chapter. Do not be concerned if this information is unfamiliar or you do not understand what it means.

Many computer program packages for statistical computations have been developed. Some nationally distributed packages of statistical programs such as SAS and SPSS run on both mainframe and desktop computers. These packages are available on many college campuses. Other packages of statistical programs run on only one type of desktop computer (Windows or Macintosh). Most computer programs provide similar information for any particular statistical technique. The computer examples in Chapters 13 and 14 were generated using a package of statistical programs for a desktop computer because most students, both at present and once they have a job, will have access to desktop computers.

Chapters 13 and 14 will reference computer programs from the SPSS package. If you don't have access to and/or familiarity with any other package of computer programs, you may decide to use this one. SPSS was selected because there is a Windows version of the package and SPSS is commonly used in schools, agencies, labs, and organizations across the country. Also, SPSS is quite complete in meeting the needs of the researcher. There is a small version of SPSS which is called SPSS Student Version. It can be bought in a box containing the program and a manual for approximately $65. One nice feature is that the SPSS and SPSS Student Version operate basically the same, so learning how to use one of them prepares a person to use the other one. Another desirable feature is that data entered with another computer program package can be used by SPSS and data entered using SPSS can be used with another computer program package. A third nice feature of SPSS is that it has graphic capacities. The manuals available with SPSS and SPSS Student Version programs are quite good.

There is a graduate student package of SPSS (GradPack) which can be leased (around $35) for six months (http://www.onthehub.com). Directions for using SPSS and SPSS Student Version are presented in Appendix A. Pavkov and Pierce (2007) is a short, excellent, and inexpensive guide to using SPSS. Many publishers such as Lawrence Erlbaum Associates (2011) and Sage (2011) have SPSS guides. Other references are listed at the back of the SPSS for Windows Basic part of Appendix A.

There is a Macintosh version of SPSS. Also, there are some excellent packages of computer programs for Macintosh. One of these is Statview (SAS 1998) with both a Macintosh and a Windows version. Most packages of computer programs are quite similar in terms of what they can do and how they do it. So there is not much difference among packages of computer programs. Once you learn one package of computer programs, you can easily use another package. Larose (1998) is a short and inexpensive guide to using SAS for Windows.

The SPSS package of programs requires that the data be entered and then an analysis program selected. Normally after the data are entered they will be saved before any analysis is undertaken. If the data are not saved, when the computer is turned off the data are lost. If the data ever need to be reanalyzed because of a mistake in the original analysis, or if a different analysis becomes necessary, the data must be entered again. Doing additional analysis on the data happens quite often. If there are large amounts of data, reentering the data represents a considerable inconvenience. Thus, when using SPSS or some other computer program package, it is a good idea to enter and save the data prior to analyzing the data.

All instructions in Chapters 13 and 14 and Appendix A concerning how to use the computer assume that the Windows version of SPSS is being used. The instructions for SPSS and for Student SPSS 11.0 are quite similar. The example computer printouts in the book are based on SPSS output.

The steps to follow in getting into SPSS, entering the data, saving the data, and editing the data are presented in sections 1 through 4 of the SPSS for Windows Basics part of Appendix A. The steps used to analyze the data and print the output of the analysis are presented in sections 5 and 6 of the document. Sections 7 through 9 of this part of Appendix A have additional useful information. Note that in the SPSS for Windows Statistical Procedures part of Appendix A there are directions for using the analysis procedure selected in section 5 of the SPSS for Windows Basics part of Appendix A.

ORGANIZING AND GRAPHING SCORES

Simple Frequency Distributions

The 50 scores in Table 13.1 are not very useful in their present form. They become more meaningful if we order the scores to find out how many participants received each score. To do this, we first find the lowest and highest scores in the table. Now

TABLE 13.1 Knowledge Test Scores for 50 Participants				
66*	67	54	63	90
56	56	65	71	82
68	68	76	55	78
47	58	68	78	76
46	68	68	90	62
58	49	62	84	75
75	65	66	72	73
71	75	83	83	64
60	76	65	79	56
68	70	48	77	59

* Number Correct

we find the number of participants who received each score between the lowest (46) and the highest (90).

Once the scores are ordered, it is easy to make up a simple frequency distribution of the results (see columns 1 and 2 of Table 13.2). We used to make the simple frequency distribution by hand listing the scores in descending order with the best

TABLE 13.2 Simple Frequency Distribution of Knowledge Test Scores of 50 Participants in Table 13.1

SCORE	FREQUENCY	PERCENT	VALID PERCENT	CUMULATIVE PERCENT
46.00	1	2.0	2.0	2.0
47.00	1	2.0	2.0	4.0
48.00	1	2.0	2.0	6.0
49.00	1	2.0	2.0	8.0
54.00	1	2.0	2.0	10.0
55.00	1	2.0	2.0	12.0
56.00	3	6.0	6.0	18.0
58.00	2	4.0	4.0	22.0
59.00	1	2.0	2.0	24.0
60.00	1	2.0	2.0	26.0
62.00	2	4.0	4.0	30.0
63.00	1	2.0	2.0	32.0
64.00	1	2.0	2.0	34.0
65.00	3	6.0	6.0	40.0
66.00	2	4.0	4.0	44.0
67.00	1	2.0	2.0	46.0
68.00	6	12.0	12.0	58.0
70.00	1	2.0	2.0	60.0
71.00	2	4.0	4.0	64.0
72.00	1	2.0	2.0	66.0
73.00	1	2.0	2.0	68.0
75.00	3	6.0	6.0	74.0
76.00	3	6.0	6.0	80.0
77.00	1	2.0	2.0	82.0
78.00	2	4.0	4.0	86.0
79.00	1	2.0	2.0	88.0
82.00	1	2.0	2.0	90.0
83.00	2	4.0	4.0	94.0
84.00	1	2.0	2.0	96.0
90.00	2	4.0	4.0	100.0
Total	50	100.0	100.0	

score first. Now we use the computer and the SPSS Frequencies program by default (automatic setting) lists scores in ascending order with the smallest score first. This assumes that the smallest score is the worst score. We might as well start following what is done by SPSS if we make a simple frequency distribution by hand. In most cases, the higher scores are better scores, but this is not true when, for example, distance running event times, number of accidents, or number of errors are being measured. A **simple frequency distribution** of times from a distance running event should list the higher scores first. We always want to list the scores from worst to best with the worst score first. In SPSS, if the smallest score is the worst score, nothing has to be done. However, if the smallest score is the *best* score, the SPSS program must be told to list the scores in descending order (largest score first and best score last). How to do this is explained in the Frequencies program directions.

From a simple frequency distribution we can determine the range of scores at a glance, as well as the most frequently received score and the number of participants who received each score. For example, from Table 13.2 we can see that the scores ranged from 46 down to 90, that the most frequently received score was 68, and that scores had a frequency of 3 or less in all cases but one.

Where the number of scores is large, forming a simple frequency distribution is time consuming without a computer. Using a computer, scores can be entered and analyzed with any one of a number of programs. Most statistical packages for mainframe and desktop computers include a frequency count program.

The Frequencies program in SPSS is one such program. The directions for using the Frequencies program are presented in section 1 of the SPSS for Windows Statistical Procedures part of Appendix A.

The output from SPSS for the data in Table 13.1 is presented in Table 13.2. From Table 13.2 it can be seen that test scores ranged from 46 to 90, and six participants scored 68.

Some researchers use a frequency count program to screen their data for extreme scores or incorrect scores before conducting any more complex analysis. It is a wise thing to do because scores do get incorrectly recorded and entered into the computer.

Grouping Scores for Graphing

The scores and their frequencies in Table 13.2 could be presented in the form of a graph that shows the general shape of a score distribution. Based on the shape of a score distribution, decisions are made about how to interpret the performance of the group measured. If there are many different scores, the graph is usually formed by grouping like scores together. In grouping a set of scores, we try to form about 15 (10–20) groupings by dividing the difference between the largest and smallest scores by 15, and rounding off the result to the nearest whole number if necessary.

$$\text{Interval size} = \frac{\text{largest score} - \text{smallest score}}{15}$$

The interval size tells us how many scores to group together. Design the first grouping to contain the worst score. Table 13.3 is a grouping of the data in Table 13.2 using an interval size of three.

Figure 13.1 is a graph of the data in Table 13.1 using SPSS. SPSS used different intervals from those in Table 13.3. Test scores (sometimes midpoints of

TABLE 13.3 Grouping of the Knowledge Test Scores in Table 13.2

GROUPING	FREQUENCY
44–46	1
47–49	3
50–52	0
53–55	2
56–58	5
59–61	2
62–64	4
65–67	6
68–70	7
71–73	4
74–76	6
77–79	4
80–82	1
83–85	3
86–88	0
89–91	2

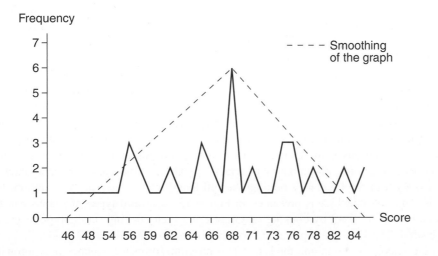

FIGURE 13.1
Graph of the knowledge test scores in Table 13.1.

FIGURE 13.2
A normal curve.

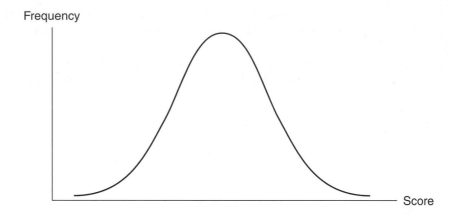

Frequency

Score

Frequency polygon
A line graph of scores
and their frequencies.

Normal curve
A symmetrical curve
centered around a point
with a defined base to
height ratio, indicating
a balanced (or normal)
distribution; also called
a bell-shaped curve.

Skewed curve
An asymmetrical curve,
indicating an unbalanced
distribution.

Leptokurtic curve
A curve that is more
sharply peaked than a
normal curve, indicating
an extremely homogeneous
group.

Platykurtic curve
A curve that is less sharply
peaked than a normal
curve, indicating an
extremely heterogeneous
group.

Histogram
A bar graph of scores and
their frequencies.

intervals) are listed along the horizontal axis with low scores on the left to high scores on the right. The frequency is listed on the vertical axis starting with 0 and increasing upward. Going up from a score until the graph line is hit and then going to the left until the vertical axis is hit, the frequency for a score can be obtained. For example, the frequency for the score 56 is 3. This graph was formed by connecting the plotted frequencies for the scores. The graph is called a **frequency polygon.**

Smoothing out the frequency polygon creates a curve that, by its shape, tells us the nature of the distribution. In Figure 13.1, the smoothing out is indicated by the broken line. If that line resembles the curve in Figure 13.2, the graph is called a **normal curve** or *bell-shaped curve.* The normal curve is often used as a model. If the graph of the data resembles the normal curve (data are normally distributed) one decision is made, but if the graph does not resemble the normal curve a different decision is made.

The graph of the data may not resemble the normal curve. When a smoothed graph has a long, low tail on the left, indicating that few participants received low scores, it is called a *negatively skewed curve.* When the tail of the curve is on the right, the curve is called *positively skewed.* A curve is called **leptokurtic** when it is more sharply peaked than a normal curve and **platykurtic** when it is less sharply peaked (Figure 13.3). Leptokurtic curves are characteristic of extremely homogeneous groups. Platykurtic curves are characteristic of heterogeneous groups.

A computer can be utilized to form a graph. An option of most computer programs is any number of groupings and several different types of graphs. Another type of graph that is quite common is a **histogram.** Again, the frequencies for the scores (sometimes midpoints of intervals) are plotted, and bars are constructed at the height of the frequency running the full length of the interval. A histogram for the data in Table 13.1 is presented in Figure 13.4. Several types of graphs can be obtained with SPSS by clicking on Graphs and then clicking on the type of graph desired. The Histogram program forms a histogram with about 10 scores (interval midpoints) by default, and the Line Chart program forms a frequency polygon with

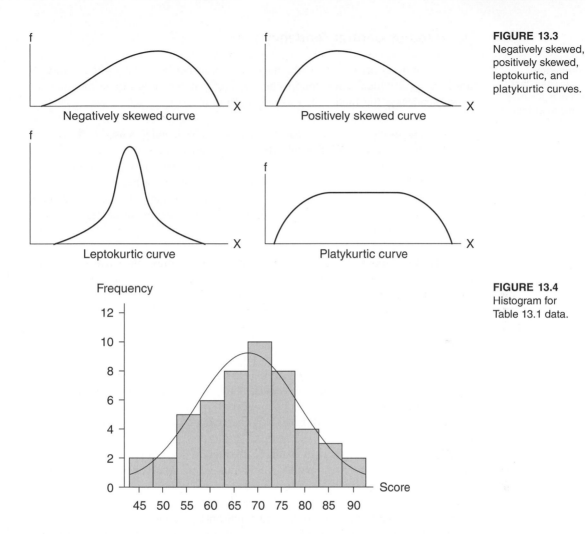

FIGURE 13.3
Negatively skewed, positively skewed, leptokurtic, and platykurtic curves.

FIGURE 13.4
Histogram for Table 13.1 data.

about 15 to 20 scores (interval midpoints) by default. An option with the Histogram program is to have a normal curve superimposed on the histogram as was done in Figure 13.4. Directions for these programs are in sections 17 and 18 of the Statistical Procedures part of Appendix A. Other types of graphs and how to construct graphs are presented in most basic statistics books, such as Moore (2010).

DESCRIPTIVE VALUES

Once a large set of scores has been collected, certain descriptive values can be calculated; these values will summarize or condense the set of scores and give it meaning. Descriptive values are used by researchers primarily to describe the performance of a group or compare its performance with that of another group.

Measures of Central Tendency

Central tendency
A descriptive value that indicates those points at which scores tend to be concentrated.

Mode
A measure of central tendency used with nominal data that indicates the score most frequently received.

Median
A measure of central tendency used with ordinal data that indicates the middle score.

Mean
A measure of central tendency, used with interval or ratio data, that is the sum of the scores divided by the number of scores.

One type of descriptive value is the measure of **central tendency,** which indicates those points at which scores tend to be concentrated. There are three measures of central tendency: the mode, the median, and the mean.

Mode.   The **mode** is the score most frequently received, and it is used with nominal data. In Table 13.2 the mode is 68: More participants received a score of 68 than any other one score in the set. It is possible to have several modes if a number of scores tie for most frequent. The mode is not a stable measure because the addition or deletion of a single score can change its value considerably. Unless the data are nominal or the most frequent score is desired, other measures of central tendency are more appropriate.

Median.   The **median** is the middle score; half the scores fall above the median and half below. It requires data that are at least ordinal. It cannot be calculated unless the scores are listed in order from best to worst. For example, the median score for the nine numbers 4, 3, 1, 4, 10, 7, 7, 8, and 6 is 6 since it is the middle score.

$$10, \ 8, \ 7, \ 7, \ 6, \ 4, \ 4, \ 3, \ 1$$

$$\uparrow \text{Median}$$

Notice that the value of the median is affected only by the position, not the value, of each score. If, in the example above, the scores were 10, 8, 7, 7, 6, 3, 2, 1, and 0, the median would still be 6. This characteristic of the median is sometimes a limitation.

When scores are listed in a simple frequency distribution, we can obtain a value of the median by a computational formula. This value of the median is usually a fractional number.

Mean.   The **mean** is ordinarily the most appropriate measure of central tendency for interval or ratio data. It is affected by both the value and the position of each score. The mean ($\bar{x}$) is the sum of the scores divided by the number of scores. Notice that the scores need not be ordered hierarchically to calculate the mean. For example, the mean for the scores in Table 13.1 is 67.78, the sum of the randomly ordered scores divided by 50.

When the graph of the scores is a normal curve, the mode, median, and mean are equal. When the graph is positively skewed, the mean is larger than the median; when it is negatively skewed, the mean is less than the median. For example, the graph for the scores 2, 3, 1, 4, 1, 8, and 10 is positively skewed with a mean of 4.14 and a median of 3.

The mean is the most common measure of central tendency. But when scores are quite skewed or lack a common interval between consecutive scores (e.g., with ordinal scores), the median is the best measure of central tendency. The mode is used only when the mean and median cannot be calculated (e.g., with nominal scores) or when the only information wanted is the most frequent score (e.g., most common uniform size, most frequent error).

Measures of Variability

A second type of descriptive value is the measure of **variability,** which describes the data in terms of their spread or heterogeneity. For example, consider these scores for two groups:

GROUP 1	GROUP 2
9	5
1	6
5	4

Variability
A descriptive value that describes the data in terms of their spread or heterogeneity.

For both groups, the mean and median are 5. If you simply report that the mean and median for both groups are identical without showing the data, another person could conclude that the two groups have equal or similar ability. This is not true: Group 2 is more homogeneous in performance than is group 1. A measure of variability is the descriptive term that indicates this difference in the spread, or heterogeneity, of the data. There are two such measures: the range and the standard deviation.

Range.   The **range** is the easiest measure of variability to obtain and is the one used when the measure of central tendency is the mode or median. The range is the difference between the highest and lowest score. For example, the range for the data in Table 13.2 is 44 (90 − 46). The range is neither a precise nor stable measure because it depends on only two scores and is affected by a change in either of them. For example, the range for the data in Table 13.2 would have been 38 (84 − 46) if the participants who scored 90 had instead scored 84 or less.

Range
A measure of variability that is the difference between the highest and lowest score.

Standard Deviation.   The **standard deviation** is the measure of variability used with the mean. It indicates the amount that all the scores differ from the mean. The more the scores differ from the mean, the larger the standard deviation. The minimum value of the standard deviation is 0, indicating that all scores were the same value. Presented below is a formula illustrating how the standard deviation is defined.

Standard deviation
A measure of variability that indicates the amount that all the scores differ from the mean.

$$s = \sqrt{\frac{\Sigma(x - \bar{x})^2}{n - 1}}$$

In the formula, s is the standard deviation, x is a score, $\bar{x}$ is the mean, n is the number of scores, and Σ is a summation sign. There is a much easier formula than this one for calculating s.

If the data are normally distributed, few if any scores will be more than three standard deviations away from the mean. For example, if the mean is 60 and the standard deviation 10, the lowest score might be around 30 ($\bar{x} - 3s = 60 - 30$) and the highest score might be around 90. Often, when a score is more than three standard deviations from the mean, it is called an **outlier** and may be removed from the data. The researcher is concerned that the outlier score is not correct or the participant did not belong in the group.

Outlier
An extremely high or low score that does not seem typical for the group tested.

The mean, standard deviation, and other useful statistics can be obtained with SPSS using either the Descriptives program or the statistics option in the Frequencies program. Because the median is provided with the Frequencies program but not with the Descriptives program, many researchers use the Frequencies program. Directions for these programs are presented in sections 1 and 2 of the Statistical Procedures part of Appendix A. Read the directions for both programs before selecting one. If the Frequencies program is selected, pay attention in the directions to selecting and turning off options in the program. The output from the Frequencies program for the data in Table 13.1 is presented in Table 13.4.

Variance
A measure of variability that is the square of the standard deviation.

Variance. A third measure of variability is the **variance.** It is not a descriptive statistic like the range or standard deviation, but rather, a useful statistic in certain

TABLE 13.4 All the Statistics Output from SPSS for the Data in Table 13.1

N	Valid	50
	Missing	0
Mean		67.7800
Std. Error of Mean		1.5184
Median		68.0000
Mode		68.00
Std. Deviation		10.7367
Variance		115.2771
Skewness		−.058
Std. Error of Skewness		.337
Kurtosis		−.392
Std. Error of Kurtosis		.662
Range		44.00
Minimum		46.00
Maximum		90.00
Sum		3389.00

other statistical procedures and interpretations of statistics that will be discussed later. The variance is the square of the standard deviation. If, for example, the standard deviation is 4, the variance is 16.

MEASURING GROUP POSITION

Percentile Ranks and Percentiles

Sometimes a researcher needs to indicate the position or rank of participants within a group based on their test scores. This can be accomplished by the use of **percentile ranks** and **percentiles.** Although their calculations differ, their interpretations are basically the same, so the two terms are used interchangeably in the literature. Both statistics indicate the percentage of participants below a particular score. Thus, if a researcher reports that the percentile rank (PR) for a score of 28 is 60, this indicates that 60 percent of the participants scored below the score of 28. However, the researcher might report that a participant with a score of 28 scored at the 60th percentile (P). Percentile ranks and percentiles are often calculated when developing norms.

> **Percentiles or percentile ranks**
> A descriptive value that indicates the percentage of participants below a designated score.

One disadvantage of percentile ranks is that they are ordinal scores. There is no common unit of measure between consecutive percentile rank values because they are position measures. Thus, it is inappropriate to add, subtract, multiply, or divide percentile rank values. Another disadvantage of percentile ranks is that small changes in score values near the mean result in large changes in percentile ranks. Baumgartner, Jackson, Mahar, and Rowe (2007) present a detailed coverage of percentile ranks and percentiles.

Percentiles and percentile ranks computer programs are available, but they are not common in packages of statistical programs like SPSS. Some researchers use the cumulative percent values presented in Table 13.2 as an estimate of percentile ranks. Computer programs usually assume that a large score is good. When this is not true (score is number of auto accidents), subtract the percentile rank of each participant from 100 to get the correct value. How to obtain percentiles and percentile ranks using SPSS are presented in sections 14 and 15 of the Statistical Procedures part of Appendix A. Percentiles for the data in Table 13.1 are presented in Table 13.5.

Standard Scores

Researchers use **standard scores** when they have data on participants from several different tests, and they want all the data in the same unit of measurement. An example of this is the sit-up, mile-run, skin-fold, and sit-and-reach tests common to many fitness batteries. Test scores for a test are converted to standard scores by the formula

> **Standard scores**
> Scores that are used to change scores from different tests to a common unit of measurement.

$$z = \frac{x - \bar{x}}{s}$$

TABLE 13.5 Percentiles for the Data in Table 13.1	
PERCENTILE	**SCORE**
5	47.5500
10	54.1000
15	56.0000
20	58.0000
25	59.7500
30	62.3000
35	64.8500
40	65.4000
45	66.9500
50	68.0000
55	68.0000
60	70.6000
65	72.1500
70	75.0000
75	76.0000
80	76.8000
85	78.3500
90	82.9000
95	86.7000
100	90.0000

z score
A standard score with mean 0 and standard deviation 1.0.

where z is a standard score, x is a test score, $\bar{x}$ is the mean for the test, and s is the standard deviation for the test. Thus, for each test, test scores are converted to z **scores** by using the formula. Once all test scores are converted to z scores, the researcher can obtain the sum of the z scores for each participant or determine on which test the participant scored best.

A z score indicates how many standard deviations a test score is from the mean. Thus, a z score of 1.5 indicates the test score was 1.5 standard deviations above the mean. Typically z scores are between -3.0 and 3.0 and are fractional. The mean z score is 0, and the standard deviation for a distribution of z scores is 1.0.

Computer programs to obtain z scores are usually available. Most packages of statistical programs have a transformation feature that could be used to calculate new scores (like z scores) using scores already entered into the computer. To accomplish this, first enter the scores into the computer, then obtain the mean and standard deviation for the scores using the computer, and finally, using the transformation feature, calculate z scores. With SPSS, z scores can be obtained using an option in the Descriptives program. In sections 16 and 17 of the Statistical Procedures part of Appendix A, there is a description of how to get z scores and the sum of z scores. The z scores for the data in Table 13.1 are presented in Table 13.6.

There is another standard score called a T score, which physical education teachers often use in preference to z scores. Baumgartner, Jackson, Mahar, and Rowe (2007) discuss T scores in detail.

TABLE 13.6 z Scores for the Data in Table 13.1

CASE	SCORE	z SCORE	CASE	SCORE	z SCORE
1	66	−0.166	26	62	−0.538
2	56	−1.097	27	66	−0.166
3	68	0.020	28	83	1.418
4	47	−1.935	29	65	−0.259
5	46	−2.029	30	48	−1.842
6	58	−0.911	31	63	−0.445
7	75	0.672	32	71	0.300
8	71	0.300	33	55	−1.190
9	60	−0.725	34	78	0.952
10	68	0.020	35	90	2.070
11	67	−0.073	36	84	1.511
12	56	−1.097	37	72	0.393
13	68	0.020	38	83	1.418
14	58	−0.911	39	79	1.045
15	68	0.020	40	77	0.859
16	49	−1.749	41	90	2.070
17	65	−0.259	42	82	1.324
18	75	0.672	43	78	0.952
19	76	0.766	44	76	0.766
20	70	0.207	45	62	−0.538
21	54	−1.283	46	75	0.672
22	65	−0.259	47	73	0.486
23	76	0.766	48	64	−0.352
24	68	0.020	49	56	−1.097
25	68	0.020	50	59	−0.818

Mean   = 67.78
Std Dev = 10.74

DETERMINING RELATIONSHIPS BETWEEN SCORES

There are many situations in which researchers would like to know the relationship between scores on two different tests (e.g., the relationship between beliefs about the importance of leisure time pursuits and leisure time practices). Sometimes the major objective of the research is to determine relationships, but in other studies it may be a minor objective. To determine if there is a relationship between two variables, every participant must be measured on each variable. There are two different techniques to determine score relationships: a graphing technique and a mathematical technique called correlation.

The graphing technique is not as precise as the mathematical technique, but prior to computers it was easier and quicker. Many of the terms used in the mathematical technique come from the graphing technique. Presently, with the availability of computers, many researchers are using the graphing technique initially to check some of the assumptions underlying the mathematical technique and as a way to graphically show the relationship. They then use the mathematical technique to obtain a value that precisely indicates the amount of relationship between the two variables.

The Graphing Technique

To graph a relationship, the computer develops a coordinate system with values of one variable listed along the horizontal axis and values of the other variable listed along the vertical axis. It plots a point for each participant above his/her score on the horizontal axis and opposite his/her score on the vertical axis, as shown in Figure 13.5. The graph that results is called a **scattergram.**

Scattergram
A graph that shows the relationship between two variables.

FIGURE 13.5
Graph of a positive relationship between scores.

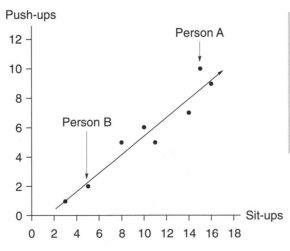

Person	Sit-ups	Push-ups
A	15	10
B	5	2
C	11	5
D	10	6
E	14	7
F	3	1
G	16	9
H	8	5

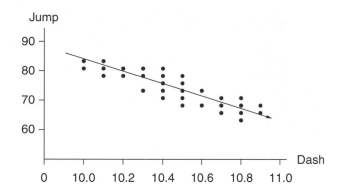

FIGURE 13.6
Graph of a negative relationship between scores.

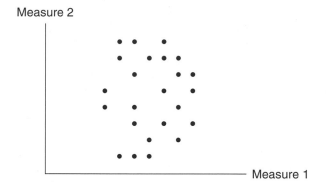

FIGURE 13.7
Graph of no relationship between scores.

The point plotted for participant A is at the intersection of sit-up score 15 and push-up score 10, the scores the participant received on the two tests. The straight line—the **line of best fit** or the *regression line*—represents the trend in the data, in this case that participants with large sit-up scores have large push-up scores, and vice versa. When large scores on one measure are associated with large scores on the other measure, the relationship is positive. When large scores on one measure are associated with small scores on the other measure, the relationship is negative (Figure 13.6).

The closer the plotted points to the trend line, the higher or larger the relationship. The maximum relationship occurs when all plotted points are on the trend line. When the plotted points resemble a circle, making it impossible to draw a trend line, no linear relationship exists between the two measures being graphed (Figure 13.7).

Computer programs contain scattergram graphic programs that facilitate plotting data. An example of a computer-generated graph using SPSS and the data in Figure 13.5 is presented in Figure 13.8. To obtain a scattergram using SPSS, follow the directions in section 20 of the Statistical Procedures part of Appendix A.

Line of best fit
A straight line that represents the trend or relationship in the data; also known as the *regression line*.

FIGURE 13.8
Computer-generated
scattergram of the data
in Figure 13.5.

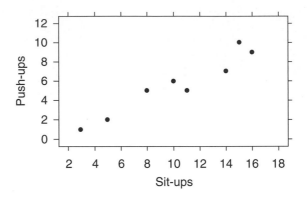

The Correlation Technique

Correlation
A mathematical technique
for determining the
relationship between
two sets of scores.

Correlation coefficient
A value indicating the
degree of relationship
between two sets of
scores.

Correlation is a mathematical technique for determining the relationship between two sets of scores. The formula was developed by Karl Pearson to determine the degree of relationship between two sets of measures (called X measures and Y measures).

A **correlation coefficient** (r) has two characteristics, direction and strength. Direction of the relationship is indicated by whether the correlation coefficient is positive or negative, as indicated under the graphing technique. Strength of the relationship is indicated by how close the r is to 1, the maximum value possible. A correlation of 1 ($r = 1$) shows a perfect positive relationship, indicating that an increase in scores on one measure is accompanied by an increase in scores on the second measure. A perfect negative relationship ($r = -1$) indicates that an increase in scores on one measure is accompanied by a decrease in scores on the second. (Notice that a correlation of -1 is just as strong as a correlation of 1.) Perfect relationships are rare, but if one exists, it is exactly described by a mathematical formula. An example of a perfect positive and a perfect negative relationship is shown in Table 13.7. When the correlation coefficient is 0 ($r = 0$), there is no linear relationship between the two sets of scores.

Because the relationship between two sets of scores is seldom perfect, the majority of correlation coefficients are fractions (e.g., .93, $-.85$). The closer the correlation coefficient is to 1 or -1, the stronger the relationship. When the relationship is not perfect, the scores on one measure only tend to change with a change in the scores on the other measure. Look, for example, at Table 13.8. The correlation between height and weight is not perfect: Participant C, whose height is 75 inches, is not heavier than Participant E, whose height is only 70 inches.

Rho
A value indicating the
degree of relationship
between two sets of
ranks; also known as
Spearman's rho and
*rank order correlation
coefficient*.

When the scores for the two sets of scores are ranks, a correlation coefficient called **rho** or *Spearman's rho* or the *rank order correlation coefficient* may be

TABLE 13.7 Examples of Perfect Relationships

PARTICIPANT	HEIGHT	WEIGHT	PARTICIPANT	100-YARD DASH	PULL-UPS
A	60	130	A	10.6	14
B	52	122	B	10.6	14
C	75	145	C	11.2	8
D	66	136	D	11.7	3
E	70	140	E	10.5	15
	$r = 1$			$r = -1$	
Exact formula: weight = height + 70			Exact formula: dash = 12 − .1 (pull-ups)		

TABLE 13.8 Example of an Imperfect Correlation

PARTICIPANT	HEIGHT	WEIGHT
A	60	130
B	52	125
C	75	145
D	66	136
E	70	150
	$r = .91$	

calculated. The formula is just a simplification of the Pearson correlation formula and will produce the same result when applied to the two sets of ranks, provided that no tied ranks exist. Rho is commonly included in computer statistical programs.

Interpreting the Correlation Coefficient. A high correlation between two measures does not usually indicate a cause-and-effect-relationship. The perfect height and weight relationship in Table 13.7, for example, does not indicate that an increase in weight *causes* an increase in height. Also, the degree of relationship between two sets of measures does not increase at the same rate as does the correlation coefficient. The true indicator of the degree of relationship is the **coefficient of determination**—the amount of variability (variance) in one measure that is explained by the other measure. The coefficient of determination is the square of the correlation coefficient (r^2). For example, the square of the correlation coefficient

Coefficient of determination
A value that indicates the amount of variability in one measure that is explained by the other measure.

in Table 13.8 is .83 ($.91^2$), meaning that 83 percent of the variability in height scores is due to the individuals having different weight scores.

Thus, when one correlation coefficient is twice as large as another, the larger coefficient really explains four times the amount of variation that the smaller coefficient explains. For example, when the r between height and weight is .80 and the r between strength and athletic ability is .40, the r^2 for height and weight is $.80^2$, or 64 percent, and the r^2 for strength and athletic ability is $.40^2$, or 16 percent.

Remember: When you interpret a correlation coefficient, there are no absolute standards for labeling a given r as "good" or "poor"; only the relationship you want or expect determines the quality of a given r. For example, a correlation coefficient of .67 between leg strength and distance run scores for males might lead you to expect a similar correlation coefficient in comparing leg strength and distance run scores for females. If the relationship between the females' scores was only .45, you might label that correlation coefficient "poor" because you expected it to be as high as that of the males.

There are two reasons why correlation coefficients can be negative: (1) opposite scoring scales and (2) true negative relationships. When a measure on which a small score is a better score is correlated with a measure on which a larger score is a better score, the correlation coefficient probably will be negative. Consider, for example, the relationship between scores on a speed event like the 50-yard dash and a nonspeed event like the high jump. Usually, the best jumpers are the best runners, but the correlation is negative because the scoring scales are reversed. Two measures can be negatively related as well. We would expect, for example, a negative correlation between body weight and measures involving support or motion of the body (e.g., pull-ups).

Linear relationship
A relationship between two variables best represented graphically by a straight line.

Curvilinear relationship
A relationship between two variables best represented graphically by a curved line.

The Question of Accuracy. In calculating r, we assume that the relationship between the two sets of scores is basically linear. A **linear relationship** is best shown graphically by a straight line, as is the trend line in Figure 13.5. However, a relationship between two sets of scores may be best represented by a curved line, indicating a **curvilinear relationship.** If a relationship is truly curvilinear, the correlation coefficient will underestimate the relationship. For example, r could equal 0 even when a definite curvilinear relationship exists. Learning curves and fatigue curves are typically curvilinear. The correlation between age and most physical performance measures (e.g., strength) is curvilinear. An example of a curvilinear relationship is presented in Figure 13.9.

Although we need not assume when calculating r that the graph of each of the two sets of scores is a normal curve, we do assume that the two graphs resemble each other. If they are dissimilar, the correlation coefficient will underestimate the relationship between the scores. Considerable differences in the two graphs are occasionally found, usually when the number of people tested is small. For this

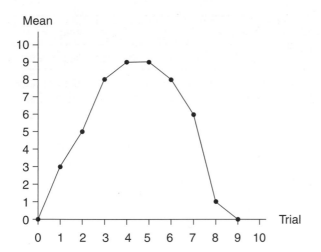

Practice trial	Group mean
1	3
2	5
3	8
4	9
5	9
6	8
7	6
8	1

FIGURE 13.9
Example of a curvilinear relationship between group performance and practice trials within a day when learning a new skill.

reason, the correlation coefficient ideally should be calculated using the scores of several hundred people.

Other factors also affect the correlation coefficient. One is the reliability of the scores; low reliability reduces the correlation coefficient. Another factor is the range in the scores; the correlation coefficient will be smaller for a homogeneous group than for a heterogeneous group. Generally, the range in scores increases as the size of the group tested increases. Certainly, the measurements or test scores for small groups exhibit a greater tendency than those of large groups to be either more homogeneous or more heterogeneous than is typical for the group measured and the test administered. This is another reason to calculate the correlation coefficient for only large groups. Moore (2010) covers this subject in greater detail.

When the group tested is large or when the researcher wants the correlation between all possible pairings of more than two variables (sex, age, height, weight, etc.), a computer is the most efficient way to generate the correlation coefficients. Programs for calculating correlation coefficients are commonly found in statistical packages for computers. In SPSS, correlations are obtained by following the directions presented in section 11 of the Statistical Procedures part of Appendix A. Before clicking on OK to do the analysis, click on a score deletion option. (Listwise deletion is not using the scores of a subject who has any missing scores. Pairwise deletion is not using the scores of a subject who has missing scores on the two variables being correlated.)

The correlations for the data in Table 13.9 are presented in Table 13.10 using SPSS. The correlations between any two variables are found by finding the value listed in the cell formed by the row and column of the two variables. For example, the correlation between height and weight is .91.

TABLE 13.9 Individual Physical Characteristic Data of 40 Participants

PARTICIPANT	SEX	AGE	HEIGHT	WEIGHT	PARTICIPANT	SEX	AGE	HEIGHT	WEIGHT
1	0	6	123.0	22.5	21	1	7	122.7	23.8
2	0	6	115.0	24.9	22	1	7	132.9	33.9
3	0	6	115.0	22.7	23	1	7	128.8	28.3
4	0	6	121.5	24.3	24	1	7	133.6	30.2
5	0	6	116.5	19.7	25	0	8	136.0	31.8
6	1	6	119.6	21.9	26	0	8	129.0	26.8
7	0	7	124.6	24.5	27	1	8	128.2	27.6
8	0	7	111.8	19.3	28	1	8	131.1	28.8
9	0	7	120.3	19.8	29	1	8	139.1	31.1
10	0	7	119.0	21.3	30	1	8	124.1	25.4
11	0	7	119.5	21.3	31	1	9	137.1	34.8
12	0	7	132.0	26.9	32	1	9	134.6	31.9
13	0	7	122.5	22.7	33	1	9	137.6	29.8
14	0	7	128.5	31.6	34	1	9	140.1	34.4
15	0	7	119.5	21.3	35	1	9	140.2	32.3
16	1	7	126.0	24.3	36	1	9	149.9	36.6
17	1	7	132.2	29.3	37	0	10	140.5	29.0
18	1	7	136.8	28.9	38	0	10	131.5	29.6
19	1	7	125.8	25.5	39	0	10	146.4	35.5
20	1	7	116.9	22.6	40	0	10	136.5	28.1

Sex: 0 = female, 1 = male
Age: In years
Height: In centimeters
Weight: In kilograms

TABLE 13.10 Correlations among All Variables for the Data in Table 13.9

	SEX	AGE	HEIGHT	WEIGHT
SEX	1.00			
AGE	0.13	1.00		
HEIGHT	0.36	0.77	1.00	
WEIGHT	0.41	0.67	0.91	1.00

MEASURES OF ASSOCIATION

Epidemiological research is conducted in many disciplines. In kinesiology, researchers in public health and physical activity commonly conduct epidemiological research. Dishman, Washburn, and Heath (2004) in their book, *Physical Activity Epidemiology,* address the topic. Neutens and Rubinson (2002) have a chapter on analytical epidemiological studies. Dishman, Washburn, and Heath (2004) state that a research design is the way research participants are grouped according to some variable like physical activity or fitness, or other factors that might explain the occurrence of health-related events like injury, disease, or death. The intent of the research design is to allow the researcher to conclude that the independent variable (e.g., physical activity or fitness) explains changes in the dependent variables (e.g., disease, injury, or death). So, the purpose is to determine if there is a cause-and-effect relationship between an independent variable and a dependent variable. Dishman, Washburn, and Heath (2004) indicate that studies must show a statistically meaningful association between physical activity, or fitness, and health (disease, injury, or death). The most common statistics used to measure the size of an association are relative risk, odds ratio, and attributable risk. These statistics are not presented in all statistics books. They are commonly presented in research and statistics books in health and epidemiology (Sullivan 2008). In addition to Dishman, Washburn, and Heath (2004), Kuzma and Bohnenblust (2005), *Basic Statistics for the Health Sciences,* and Neutens and Rubinson (2002), *Research Techniques for the Health Sciences,* present the formulas for these statistics. An overview of these three measures of association is presented below.

Data in an epidemiological study are typically organized and analyzed in a two rows and two columns table (2 × 2 table). The rows correspond to the levels of the independent variable (risk factor) and the columns correspond to the levels of the dependent variable (health characteristic). In a 2 × 2 table, the value in each of the four cells (squares) is the number of people with the row and column classification. For example, in Table 13.11 the rows are inactivity (no exercise) and the columns are a health problem (a disease). In Table 13.11, 200 people were inactive and 60 of them had health problems. **Relative risk** (RR) is the percent of incidence (health problem) rate for inactive people divided by the percent of incidence rate for active people:

$$\text{Inactive percent rate} = 60/200 = 30, \quad \text{Active percent rate} = 40/400 = 10$$

$$\text{RR} = 30/10 = 3.0$$

RR is interpreted as the health problem and is three times more likely to occur in the inactive group than in the active group.

Relative risk
Likelihood that a group with a risk factor will have a health characteristic in comparison to a group without a risk factor; see also *odds ratio.*

TABLE 13.11 Example of a Two-by-Two (2 × 2) Table

		HEALTH PROBLEM		
		Yes	No	Total
INACTIVITY	Yes	60	140	200
	No	40	360	400
	Total	100	500	600

Odds ratio
An estimate of relative risk.

Odds ratio (OR) is a common measure of association. It is an estimate of relative risk. It is the ratio or odds of health problems in inactive people relative to the odds of health problems in active people. In Table 13.11, OR = (60)(360)/(140)(40) = 3.8. The interpretation of the odds ratio is similar to relative risk. Inactive people have 3.8 times the odds of having health problems as compared to active people.

Attributable risk
Percentage of cases in the total group that occur in the group with a risk factor.

Attributable risk (AR) is an index of the percent of cases in the total group that occur in the inactive group, so it is calculated as the difference in the percent of cases for the total group and the inactive group divided by the percent of cases for the total group. In Table 13.11,

Total group percent = 100/600 = 16.7   Inactive group percent = 60/200 = 30.0

$$AR = (30 - 16.7)/16.7 = 80\%$$

Summary of Objectives

1. **Understand several options for organizing and graphing scores.** Researchers use frequency distributions and graphing techniques such as scattergrams, histograms, and curves, to show relationships and trends in data.

2. **Explain three measures of central tendency.** Central tendency is a descriptive value indicating the points at which scores tend to be concentrated. The mode is the most frequently received score; it can only be used with nominal data. The median represents the middle score—the point at which, when scores are listed in order, half the scores fall above and half fall below. The mean is the average score—the sum of all the scores divided by the total number of scores. The mean is most useful for interval or ratio data.

3. **Explain two measures of variability.** A measure of variability is a descriptive value indicating the amount of variability or spread in the set of scores. The range is used when the data are not interval or ratio. It is the difference between the largest and smallest score. The standard deviation is used when the data are interval or ratio. It indicates the variability or spread of the scores around the mean.

4. **Explain two measures of group position.** Percentile ranks and percentiles are calculated to indicate the position or rank of participants within a group.

5. **Explain how to determine the relationship between scores.** The relationship between scores on two different tests can be determined by using a graph, but the common method is to calculate a correlation coefficient. A correlation coefficient of 1.0 or −1.0 indicates a perfect relationship.

6. **Explain measures of association.** A measure of association is a value indicating the relationship between an independent variable and a dependent variable.

14

Inferential Data Analysis

OBJECTIVES

This chapter presents statistical tests that researchers commonly use in analyzing their data. You should be familiar with them in order to select the appropriate one(s) in your research and to understand the research of others as reported in research journals.

After reading Chapter 14, you should be able to

1. Identify the different research designs and statistical tests commonly used.
2. Understand the five-step hypothesis-testing procedure and how it is reported in research journals.
3. Understand and evaluate common statistical tests when they are used in the research literature.

The data analysis techniques discussed in this chapter are those most commonly used by researchers to analyze their data. These are the techniques you are most likely to use as a researcher and to see in the research literature as a consumer of research. Not all data analysis techniques available can be discussed in this chapter. On occasion you will need to use techniques or will see techniques in the literature that have not been discussed in this chapter. It is hoped that what you learn here will provide you with the foundation to understand these additional techniques.

No statistical training is assumed in order to understand the material in this chapter. The material presented should prepare you to understand the statistical information presented in the research literature. This chapter is not a comprehensive coverage of each statistical technique as would be found in a statistics book, so some of you may want to consult a statistics book. Others may want to skip some of the more advanced topics (e.g., two-way ANOVA). Moore (2010) and Kuzma and Bohnenblust (2005) are excellent statistics books covering most of the statistical techniques presented. Green and Salkind (2005) have a comprehensive explanation of many statistical techniques based on using SPSS to analyze the data.

Ways of obtaining copies of SPSS were presented in Chapter 13. Selected statistics books are referenced throughout the chapter.

INFERENCE

This chapter focuses on **inferential statistics.** A researcher typically identifies or defines a population to which the findings of the research are to apply; states a research hypothesis about the population; selects a sample(s) from the population using random sampling procedures; conducts the research study on the sample(s); and, finally, infers the results of the study to the population (see steps in research, Chapter 2).

Inferential statistics
Statistics used in the process of making inference from a sample to a population.

> *Example:* The researcher wants to determine which of three teaching methods (A, B, or C) is the best way to teach rope skipping to third-grade boys. The researcher defines the population as third-grade boys in Georgia. The research hypothesis is that teaching method A is superior to the other two methods. Using random sampling procedures, the researcher selects three samples of 50 participants each from the population. The study is conducted by teaching a different method of skipping rope to each sample and administering a rope-skipping test to all participants at the end of the study. After analyzing the rope-skipping data, the researcher finds that method B is the superior teaching method. The researcher infers this finding to the population by stating that the research hypothesis is false and method B is the superior method for teaching third-grade boys in Georgia.

Let us examine this example further. The rope-skipping test has 20 points possible. The mean rope-skipping test scores for groups A, B, and C are 10.5, 15.9, and 12.1, respectively. In regard to the differences in the means, one position the researcher could take is that any difference indicates that the teaching methods are not equally effective and that teaching method B is the superior method. This position however, ignores the possibility of **sampling error** which may have partially or totally caused the differences among the groups in mean score. Sampling error occurs when a sample is not 100 percent representative of the population. Sampling error is the difference between the value of a population parameter (e.g., population mean) and that of the corresponding sample statistic (e.g., sample mean). Therefore, the differences among groups A, B, and C in mean score could be due to sampling error. Essentially, all samples should have started the experiment with the same mean, but due to sampling error the sample means differed. This could be what caused the differences at the end of the experiment, rather than any differences in the effectiveness of the three treatments. As a result, the differences among the sample means may be a **real difference** due to the treatments not being equally effective, or the differences may be due to sampling error.

Sampling error
Difference among group means because the samples are not 100 percent representative of a population; the extent to which sample values (statistics) deviate from those that would be obtained from the entire population (parameter).

Real difference
Difference among group means because the groups are different and not due to sampling error.

If the differences among the means in the rope-skipping example are large, it is reasonable to conclude the differences are real and the treatments are not equally effective. However, if the differences among the means are small, they may well be due to sampling error. The question becomes, Are the differences among the sample means (10.5, 15.9, 12.1) large enough to indicate a real difference? Posing this question to a group of people, some would say yes and some would say no, but many would say they could not tell. The researcher needs a standard procedure to follow in reaching such a decision. Standardization increases the likelihood that researchers following the procedure will reach the same conclusion. Agreement among researchers in this situation is desirable.

HYPOTHESIS-TESTING PROCEDURE

Hypothesis testing involves a five-step procedure that researchers use to decide whether to accept or reject the research hypothesis based on the information collected on the sample(s) in the research study. Though they may execute these steps, researchers may not report all five in their written report or journal article. This five-step procedure, which can be used in a variety of situations, is explained below. Following this explanation, a number of different research designs are presented showing how the hypothesis-testing procedure is used.

Step 1: State the Hypotheses

Statistical hypothesis
Hypothesis tested with a statistical test.

Research hypothesis
A tentative explanation or prediction of the eventual outcome of a research problem; normally this is the outcome expected by the investigator.

A researcher starts out with a statement concerning what may be the situation at the population level. If the research involves multiple groups, the statement is that the groups are equal in terms of the measure of interest in the research. Since this is a statement of no or null difference, this statement is called the *null hypothesis* (described in Chapter 5) and is indicated using the symbol H_0. This is the **statistical hypothesis,** and it does not have to agree with the **research hypothesis.** In the rope-skipping example, the research hypothesis is that method A is superior, but the null hypothesis is that all three methods are equally good. At least one, and often two, alternate hypotheses symbolized by H_1 and H_2 must be stated to provide a hypothesis to accept if H_0 is rejected.

Step 2: Select the Probability Level

Alpha level
Probability level selected that warrants rejection of the null hypothesis.

The difference between the population statement in the null hypothesis and what is found in the sample(s) in the research studies is due either to the null hypothesis being false or to sampling error. To make an objective decision, the researcher will conduct a statistical test at the fourth step of the five-step hypothesis-testing procedure. The results of the statistical test provide the probability of the sample finding occurring if the null hypothesis is true. If the probability is small, the null hypothesis is rejected and the difference is considered to be real. Otherwise, the null hypothesis is accepted and the difference is considered to be due to sampling error. In step 2 the researcher selects some probability level that warrants rejection of the null hypothesis. This probability level is called the **alpha level** (α) and is usually specified as .05 or .01.

Step 3: Consult the Statistical Table

Most researchers examine the appropriate statistical table to find the value that the statistical test of the sample would need to equal or exceed in order to reject the null hypothesis at the chosen alpha level. Many computer programs provide a probability value (p) for the value of the statistical test selected in step 4. In this case, the researcher rejects the null hypothesis if the p value is less than or equal to the alpha level.

Step 4: Conduct the Statistical Test

In this step the statistical test is calculated. The statistical test may be calculated by hand or by using a computer.

Step 5: Accept or Reject the Null Hypothesis

In the final step, the decision is made either to accept or to reject the null hypothesis. If the value of the statistical test is greater than the table value or if the p value for the value of the statistical test is less than the alpha level, the null hypothesis is rejected. If the opposite is true, the null hypothesis is accepted.

Accepting the null hypothesis does not prove it is true, only that it is plausible. The null hypothesis could be false by such a small amount that the statistical test did not detect it (e.g., H_0: $\mu = 10$ when really $\mu = 10.03$). So some researchers use the terms *fail to reject* and *reject* rather than *accept* and *reject*. A statement in the research literature that the statistical test was **significant** indicates that the value of the statistical test warranted rejection of the null hypothesis. More specifically, it indicates that the difference between the null hypothesis population statement and what was found in the sample(s) in the research seems to be a real difference and not due to sampling error. Therefore, a statement that the statistical test was **nonsignificant** indicates that the null hypothesis was retained, and any differences were attributed to sampling error.

The five-step hypothesis-testing procedure is applied in the examples that follow. Each uses a different research design and statistical test. Some additional explanation of the steps in the research process is provided along with the examples. The most extensive explanation of the steps occurs in the first example. The presentation of the five-step hypothesis-testing procedure in subsequent examples is abbreviated to save space. Since the same five-step procedure is followed in each example, make sure you understand the one-group t test example well before venturing on to other examples. The t test and analysis of variance (ANOVA) examples generally apply to situations in experimental research (Chapter 8) while chi-square test examples usually apply to situations in descriptive research (Chapter 9).

Significant
Value of the statistical test that warrants rejection of the null hypothesis; differences among groups are real differences.

Nonsignificant
Value of the statistical test does not warrant rejection of the null hypothesis; differences among groups are sampling error.

ONE-GROUP *t* TEST

A researcher believes the mean percentage of body fat for a population of male workers is 18 percent. To test this hypothesis, the researcher randomly selects a sample of 41 men from the population and measures their percentage of body fat.

Step 1: The researcher's hypothesis is that the mean percentage of body fat is 18, so the null hypothesis is that the population mean (μ) is 18 (H_0: $\mu = 18$). As alternatives to this hypothesis, the researcher thought it possible that the mean could be less than 18 (H_1: $\mu < 18$) or greater than 18 (H_2: $\mu > 18$).

Step 2: An alpha level of .05 is selected.

One-group *t* test
A statistical test used with one sample.

Step 3: A **one-group *t* test** will be the statistical test, and the sample size is 41. The researcher uses the *t* tables to find that in order to reject the null hypothesis at an alpha level of .05, the value of the *t* test has to be at least ±2.021. Step 3 is not needed if a computer program is used because a *p* value is calculated and can be compared to the selected alpha level in step 2 (.05 in this case).

Step 4: The researcher calculates the mean for the body fat measurements and calculates the *t* test.

$$\bar{x} = 16.50, s = 2.50$$

$$t = \frac{\bar{x} - \mu}{SE} = \frac{16.50 - 18}{SE} = -3.85$$

where SE is the standard error (calculated by using a formula presented in a statistics book or by the computer program). In this case because the formula is simple, $SE = \dfrac{s}{\sqrt{n}} = \dfrac{2.50}{\sqrt{41}}$.

Step 5: Since the calculated value of *t* (-3.85) at step 4 is less than the tabled value of *t* (-2.021) at step 3, the researcher concludes that the difference between the null hypothesis value (18 percent) at step 1 and the sample value (16.50 percent) at step 4 is real and not due to sampling error. The researcher rejects the null hypothesis and accepts the most likely alternate hypothesis, which in this case is H_1. The population mean is less than 18 percent, since the sample mean is less than 18 percent.

Degrees of freedom
A value associated with a statistical test which is used when finding a table value of the statistical test.

At step 3 when the researcher used the *t* tables (see Appendix B) to identify the *t* value needed for rejecting the null hypothesis, the **degrees of freedom** and the alpha level had to be lined up to find the *t* value. The degrees of freedom for this *t* test was *(n − 1)* where *n* is the sample size. Because there are two alternate hypotheses, the researcher uses the alpha level under a two-tailed test. For a two-tailed test this value is always interpreted as both plus and minus. If there is only the one alternate hypothesis, the alpha level under the one-tailed test is used; the value read from the table is interpreted as plus if the alternate hypothesis is greater than (H_1: μ >) and minus if the alternate hypothesis is less than (H_1: μ <). The tabled value is sometimes called the **critical value.** All values at or beyond the critical value are in the **critical region.** If the value of the statistical test used at step 4 is equal to or greater than the tabled value found at step 3 (in the critical region), the difference and the statistical test are called significant (the difference is considered to be real), and the null hypothesis is rejected at step 5. If the value of the statistical test is not equal to or greater than the table value, the difference and statistical test are called nonsignificant (the difference is considered to be due to sampling error), and the null hypothesis is accepted.

At step 4, the larger the difference between the hypothesized population mean (18) and the sample mean (16.50), the larger the value of *t*. Also, the standard error (*SE*) is an indication of the amount of sampling error.

This one-group *t* test just studied is one of three *t* tests available. Fortunately, most computer packages of statistical programs contain all three *t* tests. In SPSS, the *t* test for one group is called One-Sample *T* Test. Directions for its use are presented in section 3 of the Statistical Procedures part of Appendix A.

The scores of three groups on a first aid test are presented in Table 14.1. The scores of group A are analyzed using SPSS to test the null hypothesis that the population mean equals 10 (H_0: μ = 10). The alternative hypotheses are H_1: μ > 10 and H_2: μ < 10. The alpha level is set at .05. The *t* test output is presented in Table 14.2. The sample mean is 12.0. Notice that the computer provides a probability value (*p* value—.025, in our example) (SPSS calls it sig.) so that it is not necessary

Critical value
The tabled value of the statistical test needed to reject the null hypothesis.

Critical region
The region at which all values of the statistical test are at or beyond the critical value.

TABLE 14.1 Scores for Three Groups on a First Aid Test

GROUP A	GROUP B	GROUP C
12	7	13
15	10	14
10	11	10
11	8	9
9	9	12
14	10	11
12	12	11
13	9	15

TABLE 14.2 Output for the One-Group t Test of Group A in Table 14.1

N	8
Mean	12.00
Std. Deviation	2.00
Mean Difference	2.00
t	2.83
df	7
Sig. (2-tailed)	.025

to look up the table value. Since the p value is less than the alpha level, H_0 is rejected and H_1 is accepted.

TWO INDEPENDENT GROUPS t TEST

Two independent groups t test
A statistical test used with two independent samples.

The **two independent groups t test** is used either when two samples are drawn from the same population and each is administered a different treatment or when a sample is drawn from each of two populations. In the first case, two samples of 75 each are drawn from a population of female college freshmen, and each sample is taught by a different method. After the treatments (methods) are administered, each sample represents a different population: a population of freshmen who have received or will in the future receive the particular treatment. In the second case, two samples of 40 are drawn, one from a population of athletes and one from a population of nonathletes. Both samples represent different populations; the question is whether there is a difference between the two samples in mean performance as an indication of a difference at the population level.

The t test for two independent groups can be obtained with SPSS. The data of groups A and B in Table 14.1 are used to demonstrate this analysis and the five-step hypothesis-testing procedure. When entering the data into the computer each participant must have two scores: one identifying group membership and the other being the score of the participant. An example of this for the first two scores in group A and then group B in Table 14.1 is shown below.

CASE	ID	SCORE	
1	1	12	ID was the name the researcher used to identify
2	1	15	group membership (1 = A group, 2 = B group),
3	2	7	and SCORE was the name the researcher used
4	2	10	for the score of a subject.

To conduct the t test using SPSS, refer to section 4 of the Statistical Procedures part of Appendix A.

Step 1: H_0: $\mu_A - \mu_B = 0$ (hypothesis that population means are equal)

H_1: $\mu_A - \mu_B > 0$ (hypothesis that A population mean is greater)

H_2: $\mu_A - \mu_B < 0$ (hypothesis that B population mean is greater)

Step 2: Alpha $= .05$

Step 3: The t test table critical value is based on degrees of freedom equal to $(n_1 + n_2 - 2)$ where n_1 is the sample size for group A and n_2 is for group B. The degrees of freedom is 14 (or $8 + 8 - 2$). The table value for an alpha of .05 under a two-tailed test and degrees of freedom 14 is ± 2.145.

Step 4: The scores of each group are analyzed and the t test calculated.

$$t = \frac{\bar{x}_A - \bar{x}_B}{SE}$$

where SE is based on the two sample variances and is an estimate of the amount of sampling error.

The results of the computer analysis are presented in Table 14.3.

Step 5: The calculated t value from step 4 is compared with the table t value at step 3 or the computer p value with the alpha level at step 2.

The computer provided a p value (sig.) of .015. No matter whether the calculated t value of 2.76 is compared with the table t value of ± 2.145, or the p value of .015 is compared with the alpha level (.05) in step 2, the difference between the means for A and B groups is significant, and the null hypothesis (H_0) is rejected in favor of H_1 because the t value is positive and group A has the larger mean.

TABLE 14.3 Output for the Two Independent Groups t Test for Groups A and B in Table 14.1

ITEM	GROUP A	GROUP B
N	8	8
Mean	12.00	9.50
Std. Deviation	2.00	1.60
t	2.76	
df	14	
Sig. (2-tailed)	.015	

TWO DEPENDENT GROUPS *t* TEST

Two dependent groups *t* test
A statistical test used with two dependent groups or columns of scores.

Repeated measures
A two dependent groups *t*-test design where participants are tested before and after a treatment.

One example of the **two dependent groups *t* test** is a **repeated measures** design, and the other example is a *matched pairs* design (discussed in Chapter 8). In either case there are two columns of scores and some degree of correlation or dependency between them. With the repeated measures design, a population is defined from which a sample is drawn using random sampling procedures. Participants are tested initially, an experimental treatment is administered, and the participants finally retested. Usually, the same test is administered both before and after the treatment so the research situation is called a test-retest design or pretest-posttest design. With paper-and-pencil tests, one form of the test (form A) could be administered at pretest and form B of the test could be administered at posttest. The purpose of this research design is to determine if an experimental treatment is effective.

The research question could also be investigated using two independent groups, with one group receiving the experimental treatment (experimental group) and the other receiving no treatment (control group). The repeated measures design is more efficient and precise than the two independent groups design because all participants receive the treatment and act as their own control. In Chapter 8 the repeated measures design is described as having numerous internal and external validity problems; however, this design is commonly used.

With the matched pairs design, a population is defined and some measure(s) is collected on each member of the population that the researcher feels must be controlled in the research study. The researcher wants the two groups involved in this design to start the experiment basically equal in terms of the measure(s) collected. Participants are paired on this measure(s), with one participant from each pair randomly assigned to each of the two groups. Each group receives a different treatment, so there may be one experimental group and one control group, or there may be two experimental groups. After the groups receive the treatments, they are measured and the data are analyzed to determine if the groups seem equal in mean performance.

> *Example:* The population is college freshmen at a large university. Two different methods of teaching a large lecture class are going to be compared. A gender score and IQ score are obtained for each of the 600 members of the population. For two students to be paired, they have to be of the same gender and have IQ scores that differ by no more than 5. One hundred pairs are formed. One participant from each pair is randomly assigned to each teaching method. Participants are taught by their assigned teaching method for 15 weeks. After that, all participants take a knowledge test. The data are analyzed to determine if the two teaching methods seem to be equally effective.

The matched pairs design is an alternative to the two independent groups design but is more precise in that the two groups start the experiment equal on at least the measure(s) used for forming pairs. Loss of participants can be a problem with the matched pairs design because some members of the population cannot be paired, and during the experiment, if one member of a pair is lost from the experiment, the other member of the pair must be removed from the study.

The t test is the same for the repeated measures design and matched pairs design.

$$t = \frac{\bar{x}_I - \bar{x}_F}{SE}$$ for repeated measures where $\bar{x}_F$ is the mean for the final scores

or

$$t = \frac{\bar{x}_1 - \bar{x}_2}{SE}$$ for matched pairs where $\bar{x}_2$ is the mean for group 2

with degrees of freedom equal to $n - 1$, where n is the number of participants for a repeated measures design or the number of pairs for a matched pairs design. An example of the five-step hypothesis-testing procedure with a repeated measures design is presented below.

Suppose eight participants are selected and initially (I) measured for number of mistakes made when juggling a ball. The participants are then taught to juggle and finally (F) measured. Let us say that, in Table 14.1, the group A scores are the initial scores and the group B scores are the final scores. To determine if the participants improved in juggling ability as a result of the juggling instruction, a t test for dependent groups is conducted.

Step 1: H_0: $\mu_I - \mu_F = 0$ (Hypothesis that final and initial means are equal at the population level.)

H_1: $\mu_I - \mu_F < 0$

Step 2: Alpha $= .05$

Step 3: Find the t test table value with degrees of freedom equal to $n - 1$, where n is the number of participants. In this example, the degrees of freedom is 7 (8 − 1) and the tabled t value is −1.895 for an alpha of .05 in a one-tailed test.

Step 4: Analyze the initial and final data, and calculate the t test.

$$t = \frac{\bar{x}_I - \bar{x}_F}{SE}$$

The repeated measures t test can be obtained with SPSS. The data are entered in pairs by participant with the initial and final score for participant 1 (12, 7) entered first, followed by the initial and final score for participant 2 (15, 10), and each of the remaining participants

TABLE 14.4 Output for the Repeated Measures *t* Test Treating the A and B Group Data in Table 14.1 as Repeated Measures

ITEM	SCORE 1	SCORE 2
N	8	8
Mean	12.00	9.50
Std. Deviation	2.00	1.60
Mean Difference	2.50	
t	2.89	
df	7	
Sig. (2-tailed)	.023	

(see Table 14.1). To conduct the *t* test using SPSS, follow the procedures presented in section 5 of the Statistical Procedures part of Appendix A. The printout of this analysis is presented in Table 14.4.

Step 5: Because the *p* value in Table 14.4 is less than the .05 alpha level selected at step 2, the difference between the initial and final means is significant and the null hypothesis is rejected. Notice that the calculated *t* exceeds the tabled *t,* and the same conclusion is drawn. Also notice that because the measured variable is number of mistakes, the final mean of 9.50 is superior to the initial mean of 12.00. Therefore, the researcher concludes that the treatment is effective.

DECISION ON ALTERNATE HYPOTHESES AND ALPHA LEVEL

Before considering other research designs and statistical tests, selection of alternate hypotheses and the alpha level must be explained in greater detail. With the five-step hypothesis-testing procedure at least one, and often two, alternate hypotheses are stated. Usually two alternate hypotheses are stated because the null hypothesis and the two alternate hypotheses cover all possibilities. The researcher believes that if the null hypothesis is false it could be in either direction, and the researcher is interested in both alternatives. For example, all possibilities are covered in the situation where H_0: mean IQ is 100; H_1: mean IQ is less than 100; and H_2: mean IQ is greater than 100. The researcher may have decided that the teaching method to be used will depend on which hypothesis is accepted. However, in situations where the researcher knows there is only one alternative to the null hypothesis or only one alternative is of interest to the researcher, only one alternative hypothesis is stated. For example, in a repeated measures design the researcher usually knows that the treatment will either have no effect or a positive effect; the treatment will not make the participants worse. Another example is situations where a traditional method is being compared with a new method. Only if the new method is superior to the traditional method will the researcher recommend a change in method.

It is important to remember that the number of alternate hypotheses determines whether the statistical test is one-tailed or two-tailed. If there are two alternate hypotheses, the statistical test is two-tailed. Notice in the t tables that for any degrees of freedom and alpha level, the value for a one-tailed test is smaller than for a two-tailed test. The smaller the table value, the easier it is to reject the null hypothesis. Thus, acceptance or rejection of the null hypothesis may be dependent on the number of alternate hypotheses.

While examining the t table, notice that for any degrees of freedom, the smaller the alpha level, the larger the table value. Selection of the alpha level also influences the acceptance or rejection of the null hypothesis. Traditionally researchers have used an alpha level of .05 unless there were reasons for selecting a different value. The second most commonly used alpha level is .01. Using an alpha level of .01 rather than .05 makes it more difficult to reject the null hypothesis, meaning the smaller the alpha level, the larger the difference must be between what is hypothesized at the population level and what is found at the sample level. In situations where rejecting the null hypothesis has major implications, researchers tend to use alpha levels of .01 or even .001. For example, if rejecting the null hypothesis means that an effective traditional drug is going to be replaced by a new drug, the researcher might use an alpha level of .01 or .001 because the researcher wants to be particularly confident that the new drug is superior to the effective traditional drug.

A diagram of the four possible outcomes of a research study is presented in Figure 14.1. In any research study, the null hypothesis is either true or false, but the researcher never knows for sure which is correct. Based on the statistical test, the researcher either accepts or rejects the null hypothesis. If the null hypothesis really is true, and based on the statistical test the researcher accepts it, this is a good decision. However, if the researcher rejects a null hypothesis that is really true, this is called a **type I error.** A type I error is defined as rejecting a true null hypothesis. The probability of making a type I error is equal to the alpha level. Therefore, the researcher usually selects the alpha level based on the seriousness of a type I error. Researchers always use small alpha levels as a way of protecting themselves against making a type I error.

Type I error
Rejection of a true null hypothesis.

	Decision	
	Accept	**Reject**
H_0 **True**	Good decision	Type I error
False	Type II error	Good decision

FIGURE 14.1
Four possible outcomes in a research study.

Type II error
Acceptance or non-rejection of a false null hypothesis.

If the null hypothesis really is false, and based on the statistical test the researcher rejects it, this is also a good decision. But if the researcher did not reject a false null hypothesis, this is called a **type II error.** The probability of making a type II error is symbolized by *beta* (β). A type II error is defined either as accepting a false null hypothesis or not rejecting a false null hypothesis. Many things can influence the probability of making a type II error. The larger the alpha level, the smaller the probability of making a type II error. Since the alpha level also affects the probability of a type I error, most researchers do not try to influence the probability of a type II error with the alpha selection. The larger the sample size, the smaller the probability of a type II error, and sample size is often something the researcher can control. The more false the null hypothesis, the less likely a type II error will occur. This is not something the researcher controls, but it should be kept in mind when small differences are found in a research study.

Statistical power
Probability of not making a type II error.

The term **statistical power** is commonly found in the research literature. Statistical power is the probability of not making a type II error, so power is the probability of rejecting a false null hypothesis. Power equals one minus beta ($1 - \beta$). One-tailed tests have more statistical power than two-tailed tests, and a two dependent groups design has more statistical power than a two independent groups design. Everything that decreases the probability of making a type II error, increases statistical power.

ANALYSIS OF VARIANCE

Analysis of variance (ANOVA)
A statistical test with two or more groups.

Many research problems or questions involve more than two treatment groups. In these situations, **analysis of variance (ANOVA)** is used to analyze the data. Actually, ANOVA can also be used when there are just two treatment groups, so in this situation it could be used rather than a *t* test. There are many different ANOVA designs. An overview of the technique should help in understanding each design.

Sums of squares (SS)
Variability values in ANOVA.

Mean square (MS) value
Values used in ANOVA to calculate an F statistic.

Using the ANOVA technique, the total variability in a set of scores is divided into two or more components. These variability values are called **sums of squares (SS).** A degrees of freedom value (df) is obtained for both the total variability value and each of the component values. The sum of squares value for each component is divided by its degrees of freedom value to obtain a **mean square (MS) value.** The ratio of two mean square values is an *F* statistic, which is used to test the null hypothesis. The *F* test is conducted at step 4 of the five-step hypothesis-testing procedure.

One-Way ANOVA

One-way ANOVA
A statistical analysis used with two, or more, independent groups.

One-way ANOVA is an extension of the two independent groups design already discussed, but typically involves statistical analysis of three or more independent groups. Some statistics books refer to this test as a one-way ANOVA because each score only has one classification (group membership). The placement of the score in the group has no effect on the data analysis. Actually, a one-way ANOVA can be used with two or more independent groups, so it could be used in place of the t test for two independent groups. The null hypothesis being tested is that the populations represented by the groups (samples) are equal in mean performance. The one alternate hypothesis is that the population means are not equal.

Some explanation of the one-way ANOVA is necessary to understand how the technique is used and how to interpret the output from the computer analysis. Also, a few symbols are necessary in order to develop formulas for determining degrees of freedom.

Two or more independent groups each receive a different treatment. The number of groups will be represented symbolically by K, and the total number of scores by N. For the data in Table 14.1, $K = 3$ and $N = 24$. All the scores in all the groups are combined into one set of scores, and the mean is calculated. The variability of the scores from this mean is the total variability for the set of scores and is called the sum of squares total (SS_T). The sum of squares total is divided into sum of squares among groups (SS_A) and sum of squares within groups (SS_W).

$$SS_T = SS_A + SS_W$$

Group means are calculated; if these group means are not equal, the sum of squares among groups is greater than zero. Thus, SS_A is an indication of differences among the groups. The sum of squares within groups is an indication of how much the scores in the groups differ from their group mean. Thus, if in any groups all scores are not the same value, SS_W will be greater than zero.

Each sum of squares has a degrees of freedom value. The degrees of freedom for total (df_T) is divided into a degrees of freedom among (df_A) and within (df_W) groups.

$$df_T = df_A + df_W,$$

where $df_T = N - 1$, $df_A = K - 1$, $df_W = N - K$.

Applied to the data in Table 14.1,

$$df_T = 24 - 1 = 23, \ df_A = 3 - 1 = 2, \ df_W = 24 - 3 = 21$$

The sums of squares values for among and within groups are divided by their degrees of freedom to provide mean square (MS) values, and an F statistic is calculated from the two mean square values:

$$MS_A = \frac{SS_A}{df_A}, \ MS_W = \frac{SS_W}{df_W}, \ F = \frac{MS_A}{MS_W}$$

Any F statistic is represented by two degrees of freedom values in the F table. The first degrees of freedom value is for the numerator and the second degrees of freedom value is for the denominator of the F statistic. The numerator degrees of freedom is df_A and the denominator degrees of freedom is df_W. So,

$$F = \frac{MS_A}{MS_W}$$

has degrees of freedom equal to $(K - 1)$ and $(N - K)$.

The F table is presented in Appendix C. The first degrees of freedom value is read across the top of the table, and the second degrees of freedom value is read down the left side of the table. Two table values appear where the line down from the first degrees of freedom value and across from the second degrees of freedom value intersect. The larger value is the F value needed for significance at the .01 alpha level, and the other level is for the .05 alpha level. If the degrees of freedom is 2 and 21, the table values are 3.47 for alpha equals .05 and 5.78 for alpha equals .01.

An example of the five-step hypothesis-testing procedure using the data in Table 14.1 follows:

Step 1: H_0: $\mu_A = \mu_B = \mu_C$ (The three population means are equal.)

H_1: $\mu_A \neq \mu_B \neq \mu_C$ (The three population means are not equal.)

Step 2: Alpha = .05

Step 3: Find the critical value in the F test table with degrees of freedom $(K - 1)$ and $(N - K)$ at the alpha level selected. In this example, the degrees of freedom are 2 and 21 so the table value is 3.47 for alpha equals .05.

Step 4: Analyze the data using a one-way ANOVA. In SPSS, one-way ANOVA is conducted by following the directions in section 6 of the Statistical Procedures part of Appendix A. As in the t test for two independent groups, when the data are entered, there must be a variable identifying group membership and a score for each participant. In SPSS, the dependent variable is the data variable and the factor variable is the variable identifying group membership. Applied to the data from Table 14.1, the one-way ANOVA output is presented in Table 14.5. The group means are 12.00, 9.50, and 11.88. The statistical test is the F ratio, and it can be seen that the F ratio is 4.45 and the p value of the F ratio is .024.

Step 5: Since the p value of .024 is less than the alpha level of .05, a researcher concludes that there is a significant difference among the group means and accepts the alternate hypothesis. The same decision is made if the F ratio of 4.45 is compared with the table value of 3.47 in step 3.

SOURCE	SS	DF	MS	F	SIG.
TABLE 14.5 Output for the One-Way ANOVA for the Data in Table 14.1					
Among	31.75	2	15.88	4.45	.024
Within	74.88	21	3.57		
Total	106.63	23			
GROUP	**N**	**MEAN**			
A	8	12.00			
B	8	9.50			
C	8	11.88			

Repeated Measures ANOVA

The **repeated measures ANOVA** design is an extension of the t test for two dependent groups design, using repeated measurement of participants. Each participant is measured on two or more occasions. If there are only two measures for each participant, the repeated measures ANOVA design is an alternative to the t test for dependent groups design. However, if there are more than two measures for each participant, the repeated measures ANOVA design must be used. The repeated measures ANOVA design is also referred to as a one-way ANOVA with repeated measures. The null hypothesis being tested is that, at the population level, the means for the repeated measures are equal. The alternate hypothesis is that the means are not equal.

> **Repeated measures ANOVA**
> A statistical analysis where each participant is measured on two or more occasions.

Suppose a group of participants is drawn from a population using random sampling procedures. Before the experimental treatment is administered the participants are initially tested. The experimental treatment is then administered for nine weeks, and every three weeks the participants are tested. The data layout for this study is presented in Table 14.6.

The data layout is two-dimensional since each score has two classifiers—a row designation (participant) and a column designation (repeated measure). The score of 10 for participant A must be placed in the Initial Test column of the row for participant A (each row-column intersection is called a **cell**), or it is in the wrong cell. Notice in the one-way ANOVA previously discussed, that each score had only the single classification of group membership.

> **Cell**
> A row-column intersection in a two-dimensional data layout.

Again, some symbolism is needed to develop degrees of freedom formulas. The total number of scores is N, the number of repeated measures is K, and the number of participants is n. In Table 14.6, $N = 32$, $K = 4$, and $n = 8$. In this ANOVA design, sum of squares total (SS_T) is partitioned into the following

	INITIAL	3-WEEK	6-WEEK	9-WEEK
TABLE 14.6 Repeated Measures ANOVA Example Data				
PARTICIPANTS	**TEST**	**TEST**	**TEST**	**TEST**
A	10	13	15	16
B	5	9	10	13
C	11	12	12	13
D	6	9	12	14
E	6	8	10	12
F	5	6	10	13
G	8	10	11	13
H	9	11	13	14

components: sum of squares participants (SS_P); sum of squares repeated measures (SS_M); and sum of squares interaction (SS_I).

$$SS_T = SS_P + SS_M + SS_I$$

The minimum value for each of the sum of squares values is zero. The SS_T is greater than zero if all N scores are not the same. The SS_P is greater than zero if participants differ in mean score across repeated measures. The SS_M is greater than zero if the means for repeated measures are not equal. The SS_I is greater than zero if all participants did not follow the same scoring pattern across the repeated measures. In Table 14.6, SS_I is greater than zero because the scores for participant A increased by three, then by two, then by one from test to test, but the other participants demonstrated different patterns. Each of these terms has a degrees of freedom (df) value.

$$df_T = df_P + df_M + df_I$$

The formulas for the degrees of freedom are as follows:

$$df_T = N - 1 \qquad df_P = n - 1 \qquad df_M = K - 1 \qquad df_I = (n - 1)(K - 1)$$

In Table 14.6, $df_T = 32 - 1 = 31$, $df_P = 8 - 1 = 7$, $df_M = 4 - 1 = 3$, and $df_I = (8 - 1)(4 - 1) = 21$.

Mean square values are obtained for participants, for repeated measures, and for interaction components. The statistical hypothesis being tested is that the means for the repeated measures are equal. To form the F statistic the mean square value indicating the differences among the means for the repeated measures (MS_M)

becomes the numerator, and the mean square value indicating sampling error (MS_I) becomes the denominator. The F test takes this form:

$$F = \frac{MS_M}{MS_I}$$

with $K - 1$ degrees of freedom and $(n - 1)(K - 1)$ degrees of freedom.

An example of the five-step hypothesis-testing procedure is presented using the data in Table 14.6.

Step 1: H_0: $\mu_{initial} = \mu_3 = \mu_6 = \mu_9$

   H_1: $\mu_{initial} \neq \mu_3 \neq \mu_6 \neq \mu_9$

Step 2: Alpha $= .05$

Step 3: Find the table value of F with degrees of freedom $K - 1$ and $(n - 1)$ $(K - 1)$ at the .05 alpha level. The value of F with degrees of freedom 3 and 21 at the .05 alpha level is 3.07.

Step 4: The easiest way to conduct a repeated measures ANOVA with SPSS is to use the Reliability program. In this program the columns are called items, so for the repeated measures ANOVA the repeated measures are the items. To get the column (repeated measure) means and the ANOVA summary table, the Statistics option in the Reliability program must be selected as described in the directions for the Reliability program (see section 13 of the Statistical Procedures part of Appendix A). The Reliability program was used to analyze the data in Table 14.6. The output from the computer is presented in Table 14.7. The repeated measures

TABLE 14.7 Output for the Repeated Measures ANOVA for the Data in Table 14.6 Using the Reliability Program

SOURCE	SS	DF	MS	F	SIG.
Between People	82.47	7	11.78		
Between Measures	158.34	3	52.78	48.39	.000
Residual	22.91	21	1.09		
Total	263.72	31	8.51		

	Measure	Mean	Std. Deviation
	Initial	7.50	2.33
	3-week	9.75	2.25
	6-week	11.63	1.77
	9-week	13.50	1.20

means vary from 7.50 to 13.50. The repeated measures F value is 48.39, which is greater than the table value of F at step 3. The p value of .000 for repeated measures is less than the alpha level at step 2. Using either indicator, the calculated F value for repeated measures is significant, so H_1 is accepted. The F value for participants is not of interest in this analysis.

Labels for the sources or components in the ANOVA vary among statistics books and computer programs. Knowing what to expect in the ANOVA summary table helps the reader interpret the labels. In Table 14.7 the residual source is the interaction source. Other computer programs may label the interaction source as error, or as PT to suggest a participant (P) by treatment (T) interaction.

Step 5: Based on step 4, conclude that H_0 is false; accept H_1 that the treatment means are not equal.

Another way to conduct a repeated measures ANOVA using SPSS is using the General Linear Model with Repeated Measures program. (This program is not on Student SPSS.) The General Linear Model with Repeated Measures program can analyze data from a variety of designs with one or more groups. The analysis for one group with repeated measures is easier to interpret than a design with multiple groups. However, the output from this SPSS program is more complicated than the output for the ANOVA examples discussed up to this point. Pavkov and Pierce (2007) have a very good presentation on how to interpret the printout from the General Linear Model with Repeated Measures program. Undoubtedly other books have a good presentation and discussion of the program. Liu (2002) has an excellent tutorial on analyzing repeated measures data and interpreting the SPSS output in which he discusses several repeated measures designs. See section 7 of the Statistical Procedures part of Appendix A for directions on how to conduct a repeated measures ANOVA.

The General Linear Model with Repeated Measures program was used to analyze the data in Table 14.6. With this program the repeated measures were labeled Initial, Week3, Week6, and Week9. The output for the analysis of the data in Table 14.6 is presented in Table 14.8. Much of the information in Table 14.8 has not been presented and explained up to this point. So the discussion of the information in Table 14.8 is as simplified as possible. First, look at the Tests of Between-Subjects Effects information. In the example data analysis of this test is probably not important, and the F value should be significant. The F value is 304.83 which is significant at the .000 level. The next thing to look at in Table 14.8 is Mauchly's Test of Sphericity. The result of the Mauchly test determines whether a univariate test or multivariate test should be used for the repeated-measures ANOVA. If the approximate chi-square value is not significant, then the univariate test should be used. If the chi-square value is significant, then use a multivariate test. The approximate chi-square value is 9.994 with significance at .079. So the

TABLE 14.8 Output for the General Linear Model with Repeated Measures for the Data in Table 14.6

WITHIN-SUBJECTS FACTORS
Measure: MEASURE_1

FACTOR1	DEPENDENT VARIABLE
1	INITIAL
2	DAY3
3	DAY6
4	DAY9

DESCRIPTIVE STATISTICS

	MEAN	STD. DEVIATION	N
INITIAL	7.5000	2.32993	8
DAY3	9.7500	2.25198	8
DAY6	11.6250	1.76777	8
DAY9	13.5000	1.19523	8

MULTIVARIATE TESTS*

EFFECT		VALUE	F†	HYPOTHESIS DF	ERROR DF	SIG.
FACTOR1	Pillai's Trace	.912	17.367	3.000	5.000	.004
	Wilks' Lambda	.088	17.367	3.000	5.000	.004
	Hotelling's Trace	10.420	17.367	3.000	5.000	.004
	Roy's Largest Root	10.420	17.367	3.000	5.000	.004

* Design: Intercept; Within Subjects Design: FACTOR1
† Exact statistic.

MAUCHLY'S TEST OF SPHERICITY*

Measure: MEASURE_1

WITHIN SUBJECTS EFFECT	MAUCHLY'S W	APPROX. CHI-SQUARE	DF	SIG.	EPSILON‡		
					GREENHOUSE-GEISSER	HUYNH-FELDT	LOWER-BOUND
FACTOR1	.174	9.994	5	.079	.502	.609	.333

Tests the null hypothesis that the error covariance matrix of the orthonormalized transformed dependent variables is proportional to an identity matrix.
* Design: Intercept; Within Subjects Design: FACTOR1
‡ May be used to adjust the degrees of freedom for the averaged tests of significance. Corrected tests are displayed in the Tests of Within-Subjects Effects section.

TESTS OF WITHIN-SUBJECTS EFFECTS

Measure: MEASURE_1

SOURCE		TYPE III SUM OF SQUARES	DF	MEAN SQUARE	F	SIG.
FACTOR1	Sphericity Assumed	158.344	3	52.781	48.389	.000
	Greenhouse-Geisser	158.344	1.505	105.230	48.389	.000
	Huynh-Feldt	158.344	1.827	86.686	48.389	.000
	Lower-bound	158.344	1.000	158.344	48.389	.000
Error(FACTOR1)	Sphericity Assumed	22.906	21	1.091		
	Greenhouse-Geisser	22.906	10.533	2.175		
	Huynh-Feldt	22.906	12.787	1.791		
	Lower-bound	22.906	7.000	3.272		

(Continued)

TABLE 14.8 *Concluded*

TESTS OF WITHIN-SUBJECTS CONTRASTS

Measure: MEASURE_1

SOURCE	FACTOR1	TYPE III SUM OF SQUARES	DF	MEAN SQUARE	F	SIG.
FACTOR1	Linear	158.006	1	158.006	61.639	.000
	Quadratic	.281	1	.281	.797	.402
	Cubic	.056	1	.056	.158	.703
Error(FACTOR1)	Linear	17.944	7	2.563		
	Quadratic	2.469	7	.353		
	Cubic	2.494	7	.356		

TESTS OF BETWEEN-SUBJECTS EFFECTS

Measure: MEASURE_1

Transformed Variable: Average

SOURCE	TYPE III SUM OF SQUARES	DF	MEAN SQUARE	F	SIG.
Intercept	3591.281	1	3591.281	304.830	.000
Error	82.469	7	11.781		

approximate chi-square value is not significant at the .05 level, and the univariate test should be used. Look at the Tests of Within-Subject Effects in Table 14.8. The values for sphericity assumed are the values of interest, and note they are the same as the values in Table 14.7. The F value of 48.39 is significant at .000, so H_0 is rejected and H_1 is accepted. Note: If the Mauchly test had been significant, the multivariate test most frequently used is Wilks' lambda which is found under Multivariate Tests in Table 14.8. The Wilks' lambda is 17.367 with significance .004.

Random Blocks ANOVA

Random blocks ANOVA
A statistical analysis where participants similar in terms of a variable are placed together in a block and then randomly assigned to treatment groups.

Earlier in this chapter, a matched pairs *t* test design was presented. In this design pairs are formed by pairing two participants. Then, using random procedures, one participant from each pair is assigned to one group, and the other participant is assigned to a second group. The **random blocks ANOVA** design is an extension of the matched pairs *t* test when there are three or more groups, and is the same as the matched pairs *t* test when there are two groups. In the random blocks design, participants similar in terms of a variable(s) are placed together in what is called a *block,* rather than a *pair* as in the *t* test. The number of participants in each block is equal to the number of treatment groups in the research study.

TABLE 14.9 Example Data Layout for a Random Blocks ANOVA Design

BLOCK	GROUP 1	GROUP 2	GROUP 3	• • •	GROUP K
1	X	X	X	• • •	X
2	X	X	X	• • •	X
3	X	X	X	• • •	X
•	•	•	•		•
•	•	•	•		•
•	•	•	•		•
n	X	X	X	• • •	X

Note: X = a test score

The procedures used in the matched pairs *t* test might serve as a helpful reference for this design.

After participants are assigned to groups, each group receives a different treatment, and at the end of the study the data are collected. The random block design has all the advantages and disadvantages of the matched pairs *t* test.

Table 14.9 is an example data layout for a random blocks design. Notice that the same notation is used in this design as is used for the repeated measures ANOVA design. In fact, blocks are like participants, treatment groups are like repeated measures, and the hypothesis tested is that the group means are equal. Thus, the analysis for the random blocks design is the same as the analysis for the repeated measures ANOVA design.

Two-Way ANOVA, Multiple Scores per Cell

Two-way ANOVA is a term used by most authors of statistics books and computer programs. A variety of other terms referring to the same design are commonly found in statistics books and the research literature as well. In a two-way ANOVA design, each score has a row and a column classifier.

The two ANOVA designs previously discussed involved just one score per cell. Three examples of two-way ANOVA designs with multiple scores in each cell are presented next. The data analysis is the same in all three examples. In each example, it is possible to test several statistical hypotheses that require different *F* tests. An explanation of the data analysis follows each example.

The first example is a random blocks design with more than one score per cell. This is the same as the previous random blocks design except that enough participants are placed in each block to have multiple scores per cell. For example, if there are 5 treatment groups, the number of participants in each block has to be 10, 15, or some other multiple of 5. The statistical hypothesis is always that the

Two-way ANOVA
An ANOVA design with rows and columns. Also called *two-dimensional ANOVA*.

TABLE 14.10 Example Data Layout for a Factorial ANOVA (Gender × Treatment)

	TREATMENT GROUP		
GENDER	**A**	**B**	**C**
Female	2, 1, 3, 2, 3	6, 3, 4, 5, 6	5, 4, 7, 6, 8
Male	4, 3, 2, 3, 1	4, 5, 7, 6, 8	10, 9, 10, 8, 11

treatment groups are equal in mean score; additional statistical hypotheses of interest are tested in certain situations.

Factorial design
A two-way ANOVA design with rows representing a classification or treatment and columns representing a treatment.

The second example is referred to as **factorial design.** In this two-way data layout, the rows represent some classification of the participants (e.g., gender, age, school grade), the columns identify the treatment group, and there are multiple participants in each cell. In Table 14.10, participants are classified by gender with five females and five males randomly assigned to each treatment group. Data are collected at the end of the research study after the groups experienced the treatments. The analysis for this example design could be referred to as a *two-dimensional ANOVA* or a 2 × 3 (gender × treatment) ANOVA. Gender has two levels and treatment has three levels because there are two classifications of gender and three treatment groups.

In this example, the researcher is interested in testing the statistical hypothesis that the treatment group (column) means are equal. The row variable may be a dimension if the researcher wants to test a second statistical hypothesis that the row means are equal. Or it is possible that this hypothesis is not of interest to the researcher, so the row variable is a dimension used to gain experimental control as discussed in the experimental research chapter. In the Table 14.10 example, gender as a dimension will be a source in the ANOVA summary table. If gender is not a dimension, the design is a one-way ANOVA with three treatment groups, gender is not a source in the ANOVA summary table, and any differences between the genders in mean score are put into the "within" component of the one-way ANOVA. Since in the one-way ANOVA, $F = MS_{among}/MS_{within}$, putting the gender difference into the within component will decrease the value of the F test and increase the chances of making a type II error.

A third statistical hypothesis can be tested in this example: no interaction between the row variable and the column variable. In terms of Table 14.10, this hypothesis is that any differences in the effectiveness of the treatments are the same for both genders. The no interaction hypothesis will be discussed later in the chapter.

The third example is also a factorial design, but rows are levels of one treatment, columns are levels of a second treatment, and there are multiple participants in each cell. It is commonly used because it is a combination of two treatments. For example, in Table 14.11 treatment A is the number of days per week people

TABLE 14.11 Example Data Layout for a Factorial ANOVA (Days × Minutes)			
TREATMENT	**B1**	**B2**	**B3**
A1	12, 10, 9, 11, 10	10, 11, 9, 10, 11	10, 9, 8, 7, 8
A2	14, 12, 13, 15, 12	8, 9, 10, 9, 11	6, 7, 5, 6, 4

Note: A1 = 1 day/week; A2 = 3 days/week; B1 = 15 minutes/day; B2 = 30 minutes/day; B3 = 45 minutes/day.

participated in an adult fitness program (A1 = 1 day, A2 = 3 days); treatment B is how many minutes per participation day people participated (B1 = 15 minutes, B2 = 30 minutes, B3 = 45 minutes). Five participants are randomly assigned to receive each treatment combination. For example, the A1B1 group participated 1 day a week, 15 minutes a day. The experimental period is six months. At the end of that period, all participants are tested on a fitness test where a low score reflects high fitness.

Three null hypotheses are usually tested in this ANOVA design. The first hypothesis is that there is no interaction between the row and column variables. If there is no interaction, the difference between any two column means is the same for each row, and vice versa. If there is no interaction effect, the difference between the A1B1 and A1B2 cell means is the same as the difference between the A2B1 and A2B2 cell means. The second hypothesis is that the row means are equal. If the hypothesis is true, the A1 and A2 row means are equal. The third hypothesis is that the column means are equal. If the hypothesis is true, the B1, B2, and B3 column means are equal.

The particular symbols used to represent two-way ANOVA designs with multiple scores per cell apply to all three of the example designs that have been presented. The symbol C represents the number of columns in the design; the number of rows in the design is R. The number of scores in each cell is represented by n; the total number of scores in the whole design is represented by N, which is equal to CRn (columns × rows × cell size). In Table 14.11, $C = 3$, $R = 2$, $n = 5$, and $N = 30$.

In the two-way ANOVA design with multiple scores per cell, the sum of squares total (SS_T) is partitioned into a sum of squares columns (SS_C), a sum of squares rows (SS_R), a sum of squares interaction (SS_I), and a sum of squares within (SS_W):

$$SS_T = SS_C + SS_R + SS_I + SS_W$$

The minimum value for each of these sum of squares is zero. The SS_T is greater than zero if all N scores are not equal. The SS_C is greater than zero if the means for the columns are unequal. The greater the inequality among the columns, the larger SS_C. Likewise, the more the row means differ, the larger is SS_R. There will be no interaction ($SS_I = 0$) if the pattern of differences among column means is the same for each row, and vice versa. Finally, SS_W will equal zero if for each cell all scores in the cell are the same value.

Each of these sum of squares values has an associated degrees of freedom value. So

$$df_T = df_C + df_R + df_I + df_W,$$

$$\text{where } df_T = N - 1, \quad df_C = C - 1,$$

$$df_R = R - 1, \quad df_I = (C - 1)(R - 1),$$

$$df_W = (C)(R)(n - 1).$$

As always, each of the parts of SS_T is divided by its degrees of freedom (df) to produce a mean square (MS) value. So

$$MS_C = SS_C/df_C, \quad MS_R = SS_R/df_R, \quad MS_I = SS_I/df_I, \quad MS_W = SS_W/df_W.$$

These mean square values are used to form the F tests for the various statistical hypotheses. All three potential hypotheses are presented below, although a researcher might not test a hypothesis if it is not of interest.

Typically the first hypothesis tested is one of no interaction. The alternate hypothesis (H_1) is one of interaction. The hypothesis is tested with $F = MS_I/MS_W$ with degrees of freedom $(C - 1)(R - 1)$ and $(C)(R)(n - 1)$. A significant F value could affect how subsequent F tests are calculated and/or how the overall data analysis is conducted. Discussion of this issue is left to books such as Winer, Brown, and Michels (1991), Maxwell and Delaney (2004), Keppel and Wickens (2004), and other experimental design books.

A second hypothesis tested is that the column means are equal. The alternate hypothesis is that the column means are not equal. This test is usually with $F = MS_C/MS_W$ and degrees of freedom $(C - 1)$ and $(C)(R)(n - 1)$. Occasionally, the denominator is not MS_W; this will alter the second degrees of freedom value. Remember, for any F test the first degrees of freedom value is for the numerator and the second degrees of freedom value is for the denominator. In the F test just presented, the numerator will always be MS_C. Notice that the numerator of any F test corresponds to the hypothesis being tested. The hypothesis in the last example dealt with the column means, so the numerator of the F test was MS_C.

A third hypothesis tested is that the row means are equal. The alternate hypothesis is the row means are not equal. This hypothesis is seldom tested in a random blocks design. The F test is normally $F = MS_R/MS_W$ with degrees of freedom $(R - 1)$ and $(C)(R)(n - 1)$.

The following is an example of the data analysis for a factorial design using the data in Table 14.11. Remember, these data are fitness test scores, so small scores are better than large scores.

Step 1:   A. First hypothesis tested is that there is no interaction between rows and columns.

H_0: $\mu_I = 0$ (mean interaction [μ_I] = 0)

H_1: $\mu_I \neq 0$ (mean interaction > 0)

B. Second hypothesis tested is that the row means are equal.

H_0: $\mu_1 = \mu_2$ (row means are equal)

H_1: $\mu_1 \neq \mu_2$

C. Third hypothesis tested is that the column means are equal.

H_0: $\mu_1 = \mu_2 = \mu_3$ (column means are equal)

H_1: $\mu_1 \neq \mu_2 \neq \mu_3$

Step 2:   Alpha = .05

Step 3:   Find the table value for each of the three hypotheses stated in step 1 for the alpha level stated in step 2.

A. $F(2,24) = 3.40$ (for testing interaction) (F with 2 and 24 degrees of freedom = 3.40)

B. $F(1,24) = 4.26$ (for testing row means)

C. $F(2,24) = 3.40$ (for testing column means)

Step 4:   A factorial ANOVA is conducted on the data in Table 14.11 using SPSS. In entering the data there is a variable for treatment A, treatment B, and the score of a participant. For example, if the variable names used are Row, Column, and Score, the data entered for the first person in cell A1B1 are 1, 1, 12 (Row = 1, Column = 1, Score = 12). See the "Two Independent Groups t Test" for more on data coding of groups. The directions for using SPSS to conduct a factorial ANOVA are presented in section 8 of the Statistical Procedures part of Appendix A. The dependent variable is the data variable and the factors variable is the variable used to form the rows and columns in the factorial ANOVA. Select the Means option. The output of the data analysis is presented in Table 14.12. Notice that a summary of the ANOVA, row means, column means, and cell means is provided in this output.

    Based on Table 14.12, there is a significant interaction effect. This is determined either by noting that the F ratio for the interaction effect from the computer (15.89) exceeds the tabled F (3.40) or noting that the significance value (p value) for the interaction effect from the computer (.000) is less than the alpha level (.05) specified in step 2. Figure 14.2 is a plot of the means that illustrates the significant interaction. The significant interaction can be easily seen in the graph because the lines formed by the cell means are not parallel. For those

TABLE 14.12 Output for the Two-Way ANOVA for the Data in Table 14.11

SOURCE	SS	DF	MS	F	SIG.
Rows	0.53	1	0.53	0.42	.523
Columns	116.27	2	58.13	45.89	.000
Rows × Columns	40.27	2	20.13	15.89	.000
Error	30.40	24	1.27		
Total	187.47	29	6.46		

Row	N	Mean
1:	15	9.67
2:	15	9.40

Column	N	Mean
1:	10	11.80
2:	10	9.80
3:	10	7.00

Row/Column	N	Mean
1 and 1	5	10.40
1 and 2	5	10.20
1 and 3	5	8.40
2 and 1	5	13.20
2 and 2	5	9.40
2 and 3	5	5.60

FIGURE 14.2
A plot of the cell means for the data in Table 14.11.

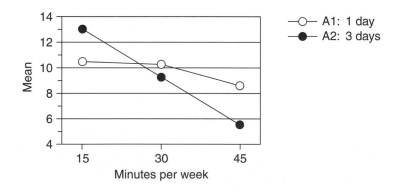

who exercised only one day per week (A1), 45 minutes of exercise per week is better than 15 or 30 minutes; however, the group that exercised three days per week (A2) improved its fitness by exercising more minutes per day.

Significant interactions are reacted to in many different ways depending on the research situation and the type of interaction that the graph of the means appears to show. A discussion of how to interpret significant interactions is beyond the scope of this book. However, in the factorial design example discussed, the significant interaction might invalidate the F tests on row means and on column means. In this case, **simple effects tests** are conducted. Simple effects tests could be comparing the column means for each row or the row means for each column. For example, the test could check for differences among the three column means for row 1 and then for row 2.

Simple effects tests
Tests to compare the column means for each row or the row means for each column in a two-way ANOVA design.

As presented in Table 14.12, there is not a significant difference between the row means ($F = .42$, $p = .523$). For the difference to be significant, the F value would have to be at least 4.26, or the p value would have to be .05 or smaller.

There is, however, a significant difference among the column means. In Table 14.12 the F value for columns is 45.89, which exceeds the table value of 3.40; the p value is .000, which is less than the alpha level of .05. An inspection of the column means shows that the means get progressively smaller as the participants exercise longer per day.

Step 5: The researcher concludes, based on the findings at step 4, that there is an interaction between number of days per week of exercise (rows) and length of each exercise session (columns). Also, the researcher concludes that the three lengths of an exercise session (columns) are not equally effective. However, the researcher concludes that the number of days per week of exercise (rows) are equally effective.

Other ANOVA Designs

The ANOVA designs presented are those most often found in the research literature. Many more ANOVA designs are possible and can be found in the research literature. Whole statistics courses are taught on ANOVA designs from texts like Keppel and Wickens (2004), Maxwell and Delaney (2004), and Winer, Brown, and Michels (1991). One- and two-way ANOVA designs have been discussed, but three- and four-way ANOVA designs are not uncommon in the research literature. Many computer programs will analyze up to an eight-way ANOVA. However, researchers should be cautious when designing studies that require an ANOVA design larger than a three way because they are usually complex and the many interaction terms are difficult to interpret.

ASSUMPTIONS UNDERLYING STATISTICAL TESTS

The statisticians who developed the t and F statistical tests based these tests on certain assumptions. Researchers should be aware of these assumptions and try to satisfy them. Failure to at least partially satisfy the assumptions underlying a statistical test invalidates the test. The assumptions underlying statistical tests sometimes vary from test to test. Assumptions underlying each of the statistical tests discussed up to this point are presented in most statistics books. Presented below is a discussion of assumptions common to most of these statistical tests.

First, it is assumed scores are at least interval (see Chapter 13). In some situations, and with some data, it may be acceptable to use the statistical tests with ordinal scores.

Random sampling of participants is assumed when using the statistical tests. In theory, the researcher has access to all members of the population, and from this population one or more samples is randomly selected. Sample size should be a small percentage of population size. However, in many studies the researcher does not have access to all members of the population, and almost all of the accessible members of the population are included in the sample. If random sampling is used for sample selection in such cases, most researchers accept that the random sampling assumption is met.

With the t test for two independent groups, one-way ANOVA, and factorial ANOVA, it is assumed that the groups are independent of each other. Groups are independent if the selection and placement of any individual into a particular group has no bearing on what other participants are selected or placed into that group. The assumption of independence is not totally met in some studies where volunteer participants are used. For example, a researcher wants to have an experimental group and a control group. If potential participants are volunteers, ideally some are randomly selected and assigned to the experimental group, some are randomly selected and assigned to the control group, and some are not selected as participants. However, only 60 people volunteer and 5 people say they will not participate in the study unless they are in the experimental group. So the researcher puts the 5 people in the experimental group, randomly selects 25 other people for the experimental group, and places the remaining 30 volunteers in the control group. Basically, the assumption of independence is met.

It is also assumed that scores are normally distributed at the population level (i.e., the graph resembles a normal curve; see Chapter 13). The best evidence that this assumption is true is that sample scores are normally distributed. With small sample sizes, scores are often not normally distributed even if scores at the population level are normally distributed. For this reason, a group size of 30 is considered the minimum sample size, and larger sample sizes are recommended. Often researchers have fewer than 30 available participants for each group, so the groups are smaller. Fortunately, as long as the assumption of normal distribution is basically met, the statistical tests are justified.

In studies using multiple samples, the populations they represent are assumed to be equally variable. The assumption is checked by comparing the samples. If the variance (see Chapter 13) for any group equals the variance for the other groups, the assumption is met. As long as the assumption of equal variability is basically met, the application of the statistical test is appropriate.

A researcher can do several things to improve the probability that the assumptions underlying a statistical test are basically met. Be sure that the members of the population available for selection as participants are truly representative of the population; in most studies this means having a large number of people from which to sample. Large sample sizes are definitely advantageous. With multiple groups, it is recommended that approximately the same number of participants be included in each group.

EFFECT SIZE

Statistically significant differences among groups in mean score are not necessarily practically significant differences. For example, if there was a statistically significant difference between two groups in mean IQ with the means 101.55 and 102.49, this is really not enough difference to have any practical significance in that both groups are basically average in mean IQ. Although not very obvious from what has been presented concerning t tests and F tests in ANOVA, the larger the sample size, the larger the statistical power to reject the false null hypothesis—even when it is false by a very small and practically unimportant amount. Thus, in the IQ example above, since the sample size was very large, the difference between 101.55 and 102.49 was statistically significant. If the sample size had been smaller, probably the difference would not have been significant. You can see an example of the influence of sample size (n) on the statistical test by looking at the formula for a single group t test which was presented earlier in this chapter: $t = (\bar{x} - \mu)/(s/\sqrt{n})$. Notice as n gets larger, the denominator gets smaller and the t test value gets larger. If the t test value is large enough, the null hypothesis can be rejected.

A way to decide whether the statistically significant difference is a practically significant difference is to calculate an *effect size* (ES). We studied effect size in Chapter 11, "Meta-analysis."

$$ES = \frac{\text{mean score of Group A} - \text{mean score of Group B}}{\text{standard deviation for one group or the standard deviation for the combined (pooled) groups}}$$

Cohen (1988) states that an effect size less than .20 is small, around .50 is medium, and greater than .80 is large. In most cases, if the effect size is large, the difference between the two means has practical implications, whereas a small-effect size is less likely to have practical significance. Statistics books like Winer, Brown, and

Michels (1991) and Murphy and Myars (2003) have an excellent discussion of statistical power and effect size. Lipsey (1990) is totally devoted to the topic.

OVERVIEW OF TWO-GROUP COMPARISONS

Two-group comparisons
Statistical techniques to compare groups two at a time following a significant *F* in ANOVA. Also called *multiple comparisons* and *a posteriori comparisons*.

Two-group comparisons are sometimes referred to as *multiple comparisons* or *a posteriori comparisons*. These techniques are used to compare groups two at a time following a significant *F* test in ANOVA. Having rejected H_0 that the group means are equal and accepted H_1 that the group means are not equal, the researcher wants to compare pairs of means to determine if they differ significantly. For example, if there are three groups (A, B, and C), this involves comparing A to B, A to C, and B to C.

There are several techniques developed specially for two-group comparisons. It is important for beginning researchers to know something of these techniques in case there is need to use them and in order to have some understanding of their application in the research literature. Some of the techniques commonly used are by Scheffe, Tukey, Duncan, Newman-Keuls, and Bonferroni. Discussion of the techniques can be found in statistics books like Keppel and Wickens (2004) and Winer, Brown, and Michels (1991). Which technique to use is influenced partly by personal preference and partly by the research situation.

Two-group comparison techniques may differ in terms of three important attributes: per-comparison error rate, experiment-wise error rate, and statistical power. Each of these attributes should be considered when selecting a technique for a particular research situation. **Per-comparison error rate** is the probability of making a type I error in a single two-group comparison. **Experiment-wise error rate** is the probability of making a type I error somewhere in all of the two-group comparisons conducted. Statistical power is the probability of not making a type II error in a two-group comparison.

Per-comparison error rate
Probability of making a type I error in a single two-group comparison.

Experiment-wise error rate
Probability of making a type I error somewhere in all the two-group comparisons conducted.

Scheffe's technique, for example, controls type I errors very well, but is lacking in statistical power unless sample sizes are large. Tukey's technique does not control type I errors as well, but has better statistical power than Scheffe.

Two-group comparisons are conducted after a significant *F* test in any ANOVA design, provided there are three or more levels or groups associated with the *F* test. For example, if for the data in Table 14.11 there is a significant *F* test for columns, then two-group comparisons are conducted; but a significant *F* test for rows indicates that the two row means are not equal, making two-group comparison unnecessary.

In statistics books, two-group comparisons are very often discussed after one-way ANOVA, and in packages of statistical computer programs two-group comparisons are often part of the one way ANOVA program. Further, computer programs may not contain all of the two-group comparison techniques. Thus, using a particular two-group comparison with ANOVA designs other than a one way may require hand calculation of the two-group comparison. A hand calculation is not difficult with the information provided in the computer printout for the ANOVA conducted to justify the two-group comparisons. SPSS provides many two-group comparison techniques with both the one-way and two-way programs. Within these programs, click on Post Hoc Tests to select the desired two-group comparison. With a two-way ANOVA, you must specify if two-group comparisons are for rows or columns or both.

REVIEW OF ANALYSIS OF COVARIANCE

Analysis of covariance (ANCOVA) was discussed briefly in Chapter 8; it would be helpful to review that material before proceeding. ANCOVA is an alternative to most ANOVA designs, and it is commonly found in the research literature. Basically, ANCOVA statistically adjusts the difference among the group means on the criterion (data) variable to allow for the fact that the groups differ in mean score on some other variable(s) and then applies ANOVA to the adjusted criterion variable. A variable used for adjusting the data is called the *covariate,* and the data variable is called the *variate*. If there is no adjustment in the variate, ANOVA and ANCOVA yield the same results.

One reason for using ANCOVA is to reduce error variance (reflected in the denominator of the F test) in a design. Another reason is to adjust for the inequality of groups at the start of the research study in terms of one or more variables that need to be controlled in the research study.

ANCOVA is more complex than ANOVA in terms of the assumptions underlying its use, data collection, and analysis. Prior to using ANCOVA, the researcher should become familiar with the technique by consulting statistics books like Huck (2008), Keppel and Wickens (2004), and Winer, Brown, and Michels (1991). Manuals for packages of statistical computer programs often include good explanations of statistical techniques. In SPSS, ANCOVA is in the two-way ANOVA program referenced earlier.

OVERVIEW OF NONPARAMETRIC TESTS

Another way in which a statistic can be classified is by whether it is a **parametric statistic** or a **nonparametric statistic.** All of the statistical tests discussed so far have been **parametric tests** in that interval data and normal distribution of the scores for each population are assumed. This section discusses statistical tests that do not require that these two assumptions be met. **Nonparametric** statistical tests are used when the data are not interval or the data are interval but not normally distributed. For example, small sample sizes per group ($n < 10$) seldom yield data that are normally distributed. An overview of nonparametric statistical tests is presented, and then one commonly used test, chi-square, is discussed in detail.

Parametric statistic
Statistic that requires interval data and a normal distribution.

Nonparametric statistic
Statistic that has no requirement of interval data and normal distribution.

Parametric tests
Statistical tests that assume interval data and normal distribution of scores.

Nonparametric tests
Statistical tests that do not assume interval data and normal distribution of the scores.

Books devoted entirely to nonparametric statistical tests include Siegel (1956), which is a classic but is out of print; and Siegel and Castellan (1988), which is a revision of Siegel. Nonparametric statistics courses are available at most universities. Many statistics books have a chapter devoted to the common nonparametric statistical tests. For each of the common parametric statistical tests discussed in this chapter, there is an alternative nonparametric statistical test. Where parametric statistical tests deal with the mean, nonparametric statistical tests deal with the median, ranks, and frequencies. Note that the second-best measure of central tendency is the median, and the mode is based on frequencies. Often, nonparametric statistical tests do not have as much statistical power as parametric statistical tests. However, random sampling is still assumed with nonparametric statistical tests.

The Kruskal-Wallis one-way ANOVA by ranks and the Friedman two-way ANOVA by ranks are two nonparametric statistical tests commonly found in the research literature. Both of these statistical tests can be found in statistical packages for the computer. SPSS has a Nonparametric Tests program.

The chi-square (χ^2) statistical test is a nonparametric test often used by researchers conducting descriptive research. Most general statistics books discuss the chi-square test. The *one-way (goodness of fit)* and *two-way (contingency table) chi-square tests* are discussed in detail in subsequent paragraphs because of their many uses in research studies.

One-Way Chi-Square

One-way (goodness of fit) chi-square tests
A nonparametric statistical test using frequencies arranged in columns.

In a research study where a **one-way or goodness of fit chi-square test** is used to analyze the data, the researcher hypothesizes some distribution for the data of a population. Based on the distribution of sample data, the researcher either accepts or rejects the hypothesis. Again, the five-step hypothesis-testing procedure is used. An example will help to clarify this test.

Suppose a researcher is interested in determining whether freshmen at a university are satisfied with living in a dorm. The population of university freshmen is 6,000. A sample of 1,000 students is selected using random procedures. A four-item questionnaire with five possible answers (strongly agree, agree, neutral, disagree, strongly disagree) per item is sent to the sample. Eight hundred students return the questionnaire. Prior to mailing the questionnaires to the sample, the researcher hypothesizes that the population distribution on items is 10 percent strongly agree, 10 percent strongly disagree, 20 percent agree, 20 percent disagree, and 40 percent neutral. These hypothesized percentages generate the **expected frequency** for each answer, whereas the number of participants in the sample selecting each answer generates the **observed frequency** for each answer. Presented in Table 14.13 are the frequencies of response (observed frequencies) for the sample to each item of the questionnaire. Presented in Table 14.14 are the expected frequencies for each answer to the questionnaire in Table 14.13. Are the observed

Expected frequency
The frequency hypothesized or expected for an answer in a chi-square test.

Observed frequency
The frequency in the sample for an answer in a chi-square test.

TABLE 14.13 Frequency of Responses of a Sample ($n = 800$) to a Four-Item Questionnaire about Dorm Conditions

ITEM	STRONGLY AGREE	AGREE	NEUTRAL	DISAGREE	STRONGLY DISAGREE	N
1. Food is great.	50	135	400	200	15	800
2. Roommate is terrible.	70	150	350	170	60	800
3. Public dorm area is a mess.	100	200	325	145	30	800
4. Own room is nice.	20	100	200	300	180	800

TABLE 14.14 Expected Frequencies for Questionnaire Items in Table 14.13 ($n = 800$)

ANSWER	HYPOTHESIZED %	EXPECTED FREQUENCY
Strongly Agree	10	80
Agree	20	160
Neutral	40	320
Disagree	20	160
Strongly Disagree	10	80
Total	100	800

frequencies and expected frequencies for a questionnaire item in close enough agreement to accept the hypothesized distribution of responses?

The one-way or goodness of fit chi-square test is used with the five-step hypothesis-testing procedure to determine whether the observed and expected frequencies are in agreement with each other. This chi-square test is called *one way* because the response of each subject to an item has only one classification— which answer was selected. The *goodness of fit* name comes from the chi-square test as a test of the extent to which the expected and observed frequencies were in agreement. The less the agreement between the expected and observed frequencies for the answers to an item, the larger the chi-square value. If there were perfect agreement, the chi-square value would be zero. The one-way chi-square test has degrees of freedom equal to the number of different responses to an item or number of different observed values of a variable (K) minus one (df $= K - 1$). The tabled values of chi-square are provided in Appendix D. Tabled values are positioned where the degrees of freedom row and alpha-level column intersect.

TABLE 14.15 Output for the One-Way Chi-Square for Item 1 in Table 14.13 and the Expected Values in Table 14.14

		N		800	
		Chi-Square		97.97	
		df		4	
		Sig.		.000	
Observed N					
50	135	400	200	15	
Expected N					
80.00	160.00	320.00	160.00	80.00	

The five-step hypothesis-testing procedure is presented using the responses to item 1 in Table 14.13.

Step 1: H_0: Model or distribution of responses is 10%-20%-40%-20%-10%

H_1: Model is not correct

Step 2: Alpha = .05

Step 3: Since there are five different answers to the item, the degrees of freedom is 4 (5 − 1). With df = 4 and alpha = .05, the tabled chi-square value is 9.49.

Step 4: Analyze the data item by item. The data for item 1 in Table 14.13 is analyzed. Using the one-way Chi-Square program in SPSS, the output presented in Table 14.15 was obtained. Both the chi-square value and p value indicate significance. The directions for using this program are presented in section 9 of the Statistical Procedures part of Appendix A.

Step 5: The researcher concludes that the hypothesized model is not correct.

Two-Way Chi-Square

Two-way (contingency table) chi-square tests Nonparametric statistical test using frequencies arranged in rows and columns.

In a research study where a **two-way** or **contingency table chi-square test** is used to analyze the data, the researcher has hypothesized that, for a population, two variables are independent of each other or uncorrelated. Based on the data of a sample from the population, the researcher accepts or rejects the hypothesis. As always, the five-step hypothesis-testing procedure is followed. The following example is an easy way to present this chi-square test.

A questionnaire is sent to a sample of 100 former participants in an industrial fitness program, and 30 of them return it. Participants are asked to indicate their gender, age, and response to each of three items about the fitness program. The data from the questionnaire is presented in Table 14.16. The researcher

TABLE 14.16 Data from a Questionnaire Completed by Former Participants in an Industrial Fitness Program					
PARTICIPANT	**GENDER**	**AGE**	**I-1**	**I-2**	**I-3**
1	1	2	2	3	2
2	1	3	2	4	2
3	2	2	1	3	2
4	1	1	2	3	1
5	2	3	3	2	3
6	2	1	2	4	3
7	2	2	3	2	1
8	1	2	2	2	2
9	1	1	3	3	3
10	2	2	3	4	3
11	1	3	2	3	3
12	1	2	1	2	1
13	1	1	1	2	3
14	1	2	2	2	3
15	2	3	2	3	2
16	2	2	1	2	2
17	1	3	2	3	3
18	2	3	3	3	2
19	2	3	1	2	2
20	1	1	2	2	3
21	1	2	3	3	3
22	1	3	2	2	1
23	2	1	1	2	1
24	2	1	3	2	1
25	1	3	3	4	3
26	1	1	2	2	2
27	2	3	3	4	3
28	1	2	1	2	1
29	2	3	2	3	1
30	1	3	1	4	1

Gender: 1 = Female, 2 = Male
Age: 1 = 18–25, 2 = 26–39, 3 = 40–60
Item: 1 = Strongly Agree, 2 = Agree, 3 = Disagree, 4 = Strongly Disagree

hypothesizes that males and females respond in a similar manner to item 1. This is equivalent to believing that gender and response to item 1 are independent of each other.

The two-way or contingency chi-square test is applied to the data following the five-step hypothesis-testing procedure to determine whether the researcher's belief seems to be true. This chi-square test is called *two way* because the response of each participant to an item has two classifications on it. In this example, the two classifications are answer selected and gender. If the percent of males and females selecting an answer to an item is the same and this prevails for each answer choice within an item, the chi-square value of the item is zero (e.g., if 15 percent of the males and 15 percent of the females selected strongly disagree, 40 percent of each gender selected disagree, and so forth). In this example, response to the item is independent of gender since both genders responded in the same manner.

With a two-way chi-square test, a two-dimensional table is developed with the rows identifying the levels or values of one variable and the columns identifying the levels of the other variable. The number of participants in each cell of the two-dimensional table is then determined. The degrees of freedom for the two-way chi-square test is $(n - 1)(K - 1)$ where n = number of rows and K = number of columns in the two-dimensional table. Tabled values of chi-square are provided in Appendix D.

The five-step hypothesis-testing procedure is presented using the gender and item 1 (I-1) data from Table 14.16.

Step 1: H_0: Gender and I-1 are independent of each other

H_1: Gender and I-1 are dependent

Step 2: Alpha = .05

Step 3: Since gender has two levels or values (1 and 2) and I-1 has three levels (1, 2, and 3), the degrees of freedom is $2(2 - 1)(3 - 1)$. With df = 2 and alpha = .05, the tabled chi-square value is 5.99.

Step 4: Analyze the data item by item. The data for gender and I-1 in Table 14.16 are analyzed using the Two-Way Chi Square program in SPSS. The directions for using this program are presented in section 10 of the Statistical Procedures part of Appendix A. Note: In the directions a number of statistics and options should be selected to obtain a complete printout. Computer output for this analysis is presented in Table 14.17.

First cell frequencies and total frequencies for each row and column are provided in Table 14.17. Seventeen females (row code 1) and 13 males answered item 1. Eight participants strongly agreed (column code 1), 13 participants agreed, and 9 participants disagreed with item 1. Ten females agreed (row code 1 and column code 2) with item 1. Then percents of total, row percents, and column percents are provided for each cell. The females who strongly agreed (row code 1 and column code 1) are 13.33 percent of all 30 participants (percent of total), 23.53 percent of all 17 females (row percents), and 50 percent of all 8 participants who strongly agreed (column percents). Finally test statistics and coefficients (not introduced in this chapter) are provided. The Pearson chi-square is the statistic to use. Neither the chi-square value (4.313) nor p value (.116) indicate significance.

Step 5: Accept H_0 that males and females responded in a similar manner to I-1.

OVERVIEW OF MULTIVARIATE TESTS

A third classification of statistics is the **univariate statistic** versus the **multivariate statistic.** The statistical tests discussed to this point have been **univariate tests** in that each participant contributed one score to the data analysis, or in the case of repeated measures contributed one score per cell. With **multivariate tests,** each participant contributes multiple scores. So, for example, in the case of a multivariate one-way ANOVA, each participant contributes a knowledge test score, a physical performance score, and an attitude test score. The purpose of the data analysis is to determine if there is a difference among the groups in terms of a composite score composed of the three test scores.

Books devoted entirely to multivariate statistical tests are available, such as Huberty and Olejnik (2006). Multivariate statistics courses are offered at most universities. Usually these courses are the third to fourth course in a sequence of statistics courses. For each of the common univariate statistical tests discussed in this chapter there is usually a parallel multivariate statistical test. Multivariate statistical tests that parallel the t test and ANOVA procedures are common in the research literature. Other multivariate techniques often used by researchers are canonical correlation, discriminant analysis, and factor analysis. Discussion of these techniques is beyond the scope of this book.

Multivariate statistical tests can be found in statistical packages for the computer such as SPSS. In SPSS multivariate ANOVA tests are under General Linear Model, discriminant analysis is under Classify, and factor analysis is under Dimension Reduction. Use of multivariate statistical tests is common in the research literature.

As a word of caution, multivariate statistical tests are fairly complex, and so some formal training and experience are recommended before using them in a research study. The use and understanding of multivariate statistical tests are usually too much to expect of the typical master's student or doctoral student who has had only minimal statistical training. Just because a researcher collects some data

Univariate statistic
Statistic for which each participant contributes one score to the data analysis.

Multivariate statistic
Statistic for which each participant contributes multiple scores to the data analysis.

Univariate tests
Tests for which each participant contributes one score to the data analysis.

Multivariate tests
Tests for which each participant contributes multiple scores to the data analysis.

TABLE 14.17 Output of the Two-Way Chi-Square for Gender and I-1 in Table 14.16

GENDER * I1 CROSSTABULATION

			| 1.00	| 2.00	| 3.00	TOTAL
GENDER	1.00	Count	4	10	3	17
		Expected Count	4.5	7.4	5.1	17.0
		% within GENDER	23.5%	58.8%	17.6%	100.0%
		% within I1	50.0%	76.9%	33.3%	56.7%
		% of Total	13.3%	33.3%	10.0%	56.7%
	2.00	Count	4	3	6	13
		Expected Count	3.5	5.6	3.9	13.0
		% within GENDER	30.8%	23.1%	46.2%	100.0%
		% within I1	50.0%	23.1%	66.7%	43.3%
		% of Total	13.3%	10.0%	20.0%	43.3%
TOTAL		Count	8	13	9	30
		Expected Count	8.0	13.0	9.0	30.0
		% within GENDER	26.7%	43.3%	30.0%	100.0%
		% within I1	100.0%	100.0%	100.0%	100.0%
		% of Total	26.7%	43.3%	30.0%	100.0%

CHI-SQUARE TESTS

	VALUE	DF	ASYMP. SIG. (2-SIDED)
Pearson Chi-Square	4.313	2	.116
Likelihood Ratio	4.461	2	.107
Linear-by-Linear Association	.569	1	.450
N of Valid Cases	30		

and analyzes it by using a multivariate statistical test on the computer is no guarantee that the output from the computer is good or that the interpretation of the output is correct. There is a saying among computer users that applies here: Garbage in, garbage out. Bad data going into the computer results in bad information coming out of the computer.

OVERVIEW OF PREDICTION-REGRESSION ANALYSIS

The terms *correlation, regression,* and *prediction* are so closely related in statistics that they are often used interchangeably. **Correlation** refers to the relationship between two variables. When two variables are correlated, it becomes possible to make a prediction. **Regression** is the statistical model used to predict performance on one variable from another. An example is the prediction of percent body fat from skinfold measurements.

> **Correlation**
> A mathematical technique for determining the relationship between two sets of scores.

Practitioners and researchers are interested in predicting scores that are either difficult or impossible to obtain at a given moment. **Prediction** is estimating a person's score on one measure based on the individual's score on one or more other measures. Although prediction is often imprecise, it is occasionally useful to develop a prediction formula.

> **Regression**
> The statistical model used to predict performance on one variable from another.

> **Prediction**
> Estimation of a person's score on one measure based on the individual's score on one or more other measures.

Simple Prediction

Simple prediction involves predicting an unknown score (Y) for an individual by using that person's performance (X) on a known measure. To develop a simple prediction, or regression formula, a large number of participants must be measured, and a score on the independent or predictor variable X and the dependent or predicted variable Y must be obtained for each. Once the formula is developed for any given relationship, only the predictor variable X is needed to predict the performance of an individual on measure Y. An example of simple prediction is predicting college grade point average (Y) with high school grade point average (X). One index of the accuracy of a simple prediction equation is the correlation coefficient (r).

> **Simple prediction**
> Prediction of an individual's score on a measure based on the individual's score on another measure.

Prediction being a correlational technique, there is a line of best fit or regression line that can be generated (see graphing technique, Chapter 13). In the case of simple prediction, this is the regression line for the graph of the X variable on the horizontal axis and the Y variable on the vertical axis.

The general form of the simple prediction equation is

$$Y' = bX + c.$$

> **Slope**
> Angle of the graphed prediction line; rate of change in the predicted score with a change in the predictor score.

The, Y' is a predicted Y score. The b is a constant multiplying X and represents the slope of the regression line. The **slope** is the rate at which Y' changes with change on X and X is the score of a person. The constant is called the **Y-intercept** and is the point at which the line crosses the vertical axis. It is the value of Y' that corresponds to an X of 0. Sometimes computer programs report the simple prediction equation in terms of slope and Y-intercept.

> **Y-intercept**
> The point where the graphed prediction line crosses the Y-axis; the value of the predicted score when the predictor score is zero.

An individual's predicted score Y' does not equal the actual score Y unless the correlation coefficient used in the formula is perfect—a rare event. Thus, for each individual there is an error of prediction. The standard deviation of this error is called the **standard error of prediction.** The standard error of prediction is another index of the accuracy of a simple prediction equation.

If the prediction formula and standard error seem acceptable, the researcher should check the accuracy of the prediction formula on a second group of individuals similar to the first. This process is called **cross-validation.** If the formula works satisfactorily for the second group, it can be used with confidence to predict score Y for any individual who resembles the individuals used to form and cross-validate the equation. If the formula does not work well for the second group, it is considered to be unique to the group used to form the equation and has little value in predicting performance in other groups.

Standard error of prediction
The standard deviation for the errors of prediction; an index of the accuracy of a prediction equation.

Cross-validation
Method for checking the accuracy of a prediction equation on a second group of individuals similar to the first group.

Multiple Prediction

Multiple prediction
Prediction of an individual's score on a measure based on the individual's scores on several other measures.

A prediction formula using a single measure X is usually not very accurate for predicting a person's score on measure Y. **Multiple prediction** (or regression) techniques allow Y scores to be predicted using several X scores (e.g., the prediction of college grade point average based on high school grade point average and SAT scores).

A multiple regression equation has one intercept and one b value for each independent variable. The general form of two- and three-predictor multiple regression equations are

$$Y' = b_1X_1 + b_2X_2 + c \text{ (two-predictor)}$$

$$Y' = b_1X_1 + b_2X_2 + b_3X_3 + c \text{ (three-predictor)}$$

The multiple correlation coefficient R is one index of the accuracy of a multiple prediction equation. The minimum and maximum values of R are 0 and 1, respectively. A second index, percentage of variance in the Y scores explained by the multiple prediction equation, is R^2. A third index of the accuracy of a multiple prediction equation is the standard error of prediction. Whole books have been written on multiple regression by Cohen, Cohen, West, and Aiken (2003) and Pedhazur (1997).

Simple prediction can be accomplished by using a multiple prediction computer program since, if only one X score is entered as data, it is simple prediction. In SPSS, Linear Regression is the program which does multiple prediction. The directions for using this program are presented in section 12 of the Statistical Procedures part of Appendix A. There are many options in this program which are not discussed in this book.

Nonlinear Regression

The regression models discussed to this point assume a linear relationship, but this assumption is not the case for all data. For example, when relating age and strength, the relation is linear for the ages of 10 through 17 because the person is growing and gaining muscle mass; for ages 18 through 65, however, the relationship is nonlinear (or is curvilinear) because increasing age through this period is usually accompanied by a loss of strength. As explained earlier, if the relationship is curvilinear, the linear correlation will be lower than the true correlation. Computer programs have what is termed a **polynomial regression** program to compute the curvilinear correlation. Polynomial regression analysis is beyond the scope of this book.

Polynomial regression
A regression model which does not assume a linear relationship; a curvilinear correlation coefficient is computed.

OVERVIEW OF TESTING CORRELATION COEFFICIENTS

Correlation was introduced as a descriptive statistical technique in the previous chapter. As such, the correlation coefficient is usually viewed as an indication of the relationship between two variables for a group. However, it is not uncommon for a researcher to state a hypothesis about the correlation in a population, randomly select a sample from a population, calculate a correlation coefficient for the sample, and based on the sample correlation coefficient, accept or reject the hypothesis. It is common for a researcher to apply the five-step hypothesis-testing procedure to correlation coefficients. The commonly applied statistical tests on correlation coefficients are usually presented in general purpose statistics books. Less commonly applied statistical tests on correlation coefficients and statistical tests involving multiple prediction or regression are presented in books like Pedhazur (1997). A brief overview of two statistical tests on correlation coefficients is presented because these tests are common in the research literature and will provide a basic understanding of their application.

> *Situation 1:* H_0: The correlation coefficient at the population level is zero. H_1: The correlation coefficient is greater than zero. If the correlation coefficient for the sample is considerably larger than zero, H_0 is rejected. The researcher states that the correlation coefficient is significant, which indicates that the coefficient is significantly greater than zero and did not happen by chance.

> *Situation 2:* H_0: The correlation between two variables is the same for each of two populations. H_1: The correlation coefficients are not equal. If the correlation coefficients for each of the two independent samples differ considerably in value, H_0 is rejected and the researcher concludes that there is a difference between the two correlation coefficients.

SELECTING THE STATISTICAL TEST

Selecting the appropriate statistical test for a given research situation is sometimes difficult for the inexperienced researcher. In terms of the statistical tests discussed in detail in this chapter, Figure 14.3 may be helpful in selecting the appropriate statistical test. Starting at the top of the figure, move down the figure selecting options until a statistical test is selected at the bottom of a path of lines. For

FIGURE 14.3
A chart for selecting the appropriate statistical test.

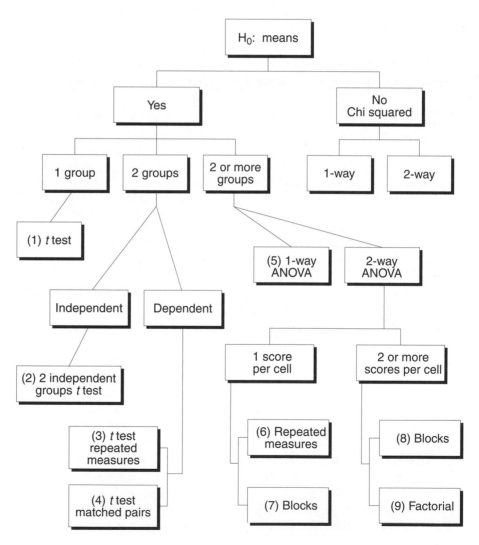

example, the null hypothesis concerns means (move to YES), there are three independent groups (move to 2 or more groups and then one-way ANOVA), and so the statistical test is a one-way ANOVA.

Summary of Objectives

1. **Identify the different research designs and statistical tests commonly used.** Among the research designs and statistical tests most commonly used are the *t* test and analysis of variance (ANOVA), both generally used in experimental research, and chi-square tests, usually used in descriptive research situations.

2. **Understand the five-step hypothesis-testing procedure and how it is reported in research journals.** The five steps involved in testing a hypothesis are (1) stating the hypothesis; (2) selecting the probability level; (3) consulting the statistical table; (4) conducting the statistical test; and (5) accepting or rejecting the null hypothesis. All five steps will not be reported in a journal article.

3. **Understand and evaluate common statistical tests when they are used in research literature.** The reader of a research article must be able to basically understand the statistical tests reported. Also, the reader must be able to determine if the statistical tests are appropriate and correctly interpreted for the research situation.

15

Measurement in Research

OBJECTIVES

In this chapter, we present measurement concepts and techniques commonly used in research. You should be familiar with these concepts and techniques in order to select the appropriate techniques in your research and to understand the research reported in research journals.

After reading Chapter 15, you should be able to

1. Discuss objectivity in terms of what it is, why it is important, and how it is estimated.
2. Discuss reliability in terms of what it is, why it is important, and how it is estimated.
3. Discuss validity in terms of what it is, why it is important, and how it is estimated.
4. Identify things to consider both when preparing to test participants in a research study and when testing them.

Measurement of the participants in a research study in regard to physical ability, physical characteristics, knowledge, attitudes, beliefs, practices, and so on, is part of conducting experimental research and most descriptive research studies. The data collected must have certain essential characteristics in order for them to be considered acceptable evidence upon which research conclusions are based. These essential characteristics are discussed, and then a few other measurement considerations are presented. These measurement considerations contribute to the characteristics of acceptable data.

ESSENTIAL CHARACTERISTICS OF DATA

Data as used here means a set of scores. Data may be obtained by using a variety of techniques or instruments, such as knowledge tests, paper-and-pencil instruments, physical performance tests, testing equipment, and so on. From here on, a data-gathering technique will be called a **test,** and the scores obtained by using a

Test
A data-gathering technique to obtain a set of scores.

technique will be called *data* or *test scores*. Often people will say a **good test** must have objectivity, reliability, and validity, but it is actually the data that must be good because important decisions are made based on the data. From here on, the terms *good test* and *test is good* will be used as often as possible to mean a test for which acceptable objectivity, reliability, and validity of the data have been determined. That a test is good must be documented before data collection begins in the research study, no matter whether the test was developed by another person or by the researcher. Thus, documentation that a test is good almost always occurs in a pilot study with individuals who are similar to the participants in the research study. The age, sex, experience, and such characteristics of the individuals used in the pilot study, as well as the test itself, may influence whether the test is good. So a good test for one group may not be a good test for another group. Further, all tests do not have the same potential to yield data with objectivity, reliability, and validity. Some tests are better than others.

Objectivity, reliability, and validity were briefly discussed in Chapter 5 as a step in the research process. Discussed in this chapter are methods used to document the objectivity, reliability, and validity of data and terms which are used in research articles to describe these methods. Thus, after studying this material, researchers will know what methods exist and readers of research will recognize the methods and terms. Usually, the computations involved with these methods are not shown, but if you are interested in the computations, consult measurement books like Baumgartner, Jackson, Mahar, and Rowe (2007), Crocker and Algina (2008), and Nunnally and Bernstein (1994). In some situations, a formula must be presented for the reader to understand a method or see the difference between methods. In these cases, computations with these formulas may be presented in order for the reader to understand the formula. However, in these situations, computations are kept to a minimum and as simple as possible.

The three essential characteristics of data will be defined and briefly discussed in the order they should be determined. First is **objectivity.** If objectivity exists, two or more people could administer a test to a group and obtain the same or very similar data. If objectivity does not exist, the data of a group are unique to whoever administered and scored the test. Objectivity is important because the data obtained should not be dependent on who administered the test. If the data have objectivity, it is possible for them to have reliability. In fact, objectivity is sometimes called *rater reliability.*

Reliability is defined as consistency of test scores. If reliability exists, people's test scores are not changing over a short period of time. This could be from trial to trial if a test is administered multiple times within a day (like multiple trials one after another or multiple administrations with some short time elapsing between administrations). Or this could be from day to day if a test is administered on two different days. This could be from item to item of a knowledge test. Reliability is important because the researcher wants to be sure that the data collected are a true indication of the ability of the people tested. Without reliability, the data

Good test
A test for which acceptable objectivity, reliability, and validity of the data have been determined; also described by the *test is good.*

Objectivity
The degree to which multiple scorers agree on the values of collected measures or scores; also called *rater reliability.*

Reliability
Degree to which a measure is consistent and unchanged over a short period of time.

Validity
The degree to which
interpretations of test
scores or measures
derived from a measuring
instrument lead to correct
conclusions.

are unique to the testing session and would be entirely different if collected at some other time. If the data have reliability, it is possible for them to have validity.

If **validity** exists, interpretations based on the data are correct. For validity to exist, the data must be measures of what they are supposed to measure and the interpretations based on the data are correct. In other words, the reason all people don't have the same test score is that they differ in terms of the attribute the test measures. To the extent that other things influence the data, the data are not perfectly valid. Validity is vital and the most important characteristic of data. It allows the researcher to make important decisions based on the data, with confidence that the decisions are based on correct information.

The essential characteristics of data (objectivity, reliability, and validity) must be established before collecting research data so the researcher is assured that conclusions are based on correct information. Occasionally, researchers estimate the objectivity, reliability, and validity of the data as part of the data collection procedure for the research study. This is taking a big risk—because if the data are not valid, they should be discarded. They are not good enough to use when drawing conclusions.

If it has been documented by another person that the test is good for the type of people to be tested in the research study, then it is quite acceptable for the researcher to use the test without documenting it himself/herself. However, it would be a good research practice if the researcher checked the objectivity and reliability himself/herself to get a better understanding of the test and the data the test provides. That another person has documented that the test is good indicates only that the test has the potential to be a good test. If the test is administered improperly, it will not be a good test.

If it has not been documented that the test is good for the type of people to be tested in the research study, then the researcher must take the time to develop this documentation. This could be necessary because the test is a new one the researcher developed, a major modification of a documented test, or documented for a different type of people than the researcher will be testing in the research study. The age, sex, experience, and such characteristics of the people tested may influence the reliability and validity of the data. Documenting that the test is good does not have to be done with a large number of people, at least initially. If, for example, the test does not yield reliable data, this might as well be established using 30 rather than 300 people. If the test yields reliable data for 30 people, it would be wise to check that this is true for a larger group. However, much of the documentation of tests found in the literature is based on the test scores of 30 to 50 people. Documenting that a test is good must be conducted in a systematic manner, starting with objectivity and ending with validity. An example of this is the study by Baumgartner, Oh, Chung, and Hales (2002). If any of the three essential characteristics of data is not present, try to improve the test, and then check the characteristic again. There is no use in finding that a test does not yield data which allows valid interpretations and not knowing whether that is due to lack of reliability, the test not measuring what it is supposed to measure, or the interpretations of the data are not correct.

Thus, when the researcher must document that a test is good, the documentation is done in a pilot study before conducting the actual research study. A small group, maybe 30 to 50 people, is used in the pilot study. After the test is found to yield good data, it is used with confidence in the research study. As will be found later in this chapter, usually more test scores per person must be collected in the pilot study than in the research study because it takes more test scores per person to determine objectivity, reliability, and validity of the data.

Many different techniques are used to document the objectivity, reliability, and validity of the data. The technique used may be dependent on what is to be documented. Whether the test is a paper-and-pencil test or a physical performance test may influence the technique used. The type of paper-and-pencil test or physical performance test may even influence the technique used. Finally, when several techniques are available, the technique used may be personal choice. Certainly one technique does not fit all situations, so the selection of a technique must be a knowledgeable one.

Before discussing techniques used to estimate objectivity, reliability, and validity, it must be recognized that the discussion is a brief overview of techniques which are available. The discussion should be enough that a researcher knows what techniques are available and can select the appropriate technique, or a reader of research articles can recognize and understand the techniques used. The techniques discussed are taught in measurement courses at the undergraduate and graduate level.

Objectivity, reliability, and validity are commonly determined by calculating a correlation coefficient. Correlation was discussed in Chapter 13; you might review it before continuing. A **correlation coefficient** indicates the degree of relationship between two sets of scores collected on a group of people. Typically, correlation coefficients between zero and one (positive or negative) are obtained. The closer the correlation coefficient is to one, the higher the degree of relationship between the two sets of scores. There are a number of different types of correlation coefficients used to indicate the objectivity, reliability, and/or validity of the data. Most of the correlation coefficients can vary from -1.00 to 1.00, so the interpretation of the correlation coefficient is usually the same no matter the type of correlation coefficient.

Correlation coefficient
A value indicating the degree of relationship between two sets of scores.

Objectivity

To determine objectivity, at least two scorers, raters, or judges (usually two) must independently score a group of people on the test. With physical performance tests, this would be each scorer independently scoring each person as he/she performed the test. For example, two individuals independently time each person as he/she runs the mile for time. For paper-and-pencil tests or instruments like a questionnaire, this would be each scorer independently scoring the test or instrument. For example, two individuals independently grade a knowledge test. No matter what the situation, for each person tested there will be a score from each scorer. The score organization will be as presented in Table 15.1.

TABLE 15.1 Data for Two Scorers to Determine Objectivity

PERSON	SCORER-1	SCORER-2
A	4*	4
B	4	3
C	3	3
D	2	3
E	3	2
F	3	3
G	5	4
H	4	3
I	1	2
J	3	2

* Scores are ratings on a 5-point scale with 5 = excellent and 1 = terrible.

Objectivity coefficient
A correlation coefficient indicating the relationship between the scores of the scorers.

Intraclass correlation coefficient
A correlation coefficient calculated as an estimate of objectivity and reliability.

The correlation coefficient indicating the relationship between the scores of the scorers is called the **objectivity coefficient.** The **intraclass correlation coefficient** (R) is the coefficient calculated as the objectivity coefficient. The R can vary from 0.00 to 1.00. It is calculated using values which come from a statistical technique called analysis of variance (ANOVA). The ANOVA technique was discussed in Chapter 14. There are many different ANOVA designs; the design used is dependent on how the data are organized. We will always organize our data so the rows are people and the columns are a repeated measure, as in Table 15.1. In Table 15.1, scorers are the repeated measure because each person was scored by each scorer (each person has two scores on the measure). The ANOVA design we use to calculate R is called a two-way or repeated measures ANOVA with one score per cell. A cell in an ANOVA design is identified by a row and a column. For example, in Table 15.1 the intersection of a row (Person A) and a column (Scorer-1) is a cell with the score four (4) in it. With the ANOVA technique a summary table is used to present the results of the ANOVA. The ANOVA is usually done using the computer, which provides the ANOVA summary table. Several different components are identified under a heading called "sources of variation" in the ANOVA summary table. For each of these sources, values called "sum of squares" (SS), "degrees of freedom" (DF), and "mean square" (MS) are presented in the ANOVA summary table. The data in Table 15.1 were analyzed using a computer program called Reliability Analysis, in the SPSS package of statistical programs. The ANOVA summary table and other information for the analysis are presented in Table 15.2. In terms of calculating an intraclass correlation coefficient (R), we are interested in the mean square (MS) value for the sources People and Interaction. The mean square for

TABLE 15.2 Means and ANOVA Summary Table for the Data in Table 15.1

	MEAN	STD. DEVIATION	CASES
Scorer 1	3.20	1.14	10
Scorer 2	2.90	.74	10

ANALYSIS OF VARIANCE

SOURCE OF VARIATION	SUM OF SQUARES	DF	MEAN SQUARE
Between People	13.45	9	1.49
Between Measures	.45	1	.45
Interaction	3.05	9	.34
Total	16.95	19	.89

People is symbolized as MS People and the mean square for Interaction as MS Interaction in formulas presented for calculating R. In Table 15.2, MS People = 1.49 and MS Interaction = .34. In other books, and using other computer programs, the sources of variation may be named differently than in Table 15.2. For example, the sources of variation "Between People" might be called "Rows" and "Interaction" might be called "Residual" or "Error."

In Table 15.1, two scorers were used in the pilot study so that objectivity could be determined. Most likely in the research study, the researcher would like to have one person score the test with assurance that the data obtained are basically the same data any well-trained scorer would award. The intraclass correlation coefficient can be calculated using several different formulas. In this case the intraclass correlation coefficient (R) is calculated as

$$R = \frac{\text{MS People} - \text{MS Interaction}}{\text{MS People} + \text{MS Interaction}} \tag{1}$$

where MS = mean square from a two-way analysis of variance (ANOVA) design; design is People × Scorers with two scorers; R = objectivity of a score for each participant which is from one scorer.

Applying formula (1) to the data in Table 15.2, $R = (1.49 - .34)/(1.49 + .34) = .63$ which is not high objectivity since R can be as high as 1.0.

If you don't understand the ANOVA technique, don't worry; the ANOVA values needed to calculate R are obtained using the computer. If the R formula seems a little overwhelming at this time, don't be too concerned. Formulas are presented so you can see that techniques differ as to the formula used. The important thing to know is that an intraclass R should be used, and the R formula is the one for this situation. Usually, objectivity is determined as presented in the example (data of two scorers in the pilot study; one scorer used in the research study). If this is the case, the researcher must indicate this when describing the procedures and findings for the research study. For example, since $R = .63$ using formula (1), the researcher might state that, using an intraclass R, the objectivity of the data of a single scorer was .63. The researcher stating that the objectivity was .63 is an inadequate description because neither the method of determining objectivity nor the score for which the objectivity is reported is indicated. If there are more than two scorers in the pilot study, and/or in the research study there are more than one scorer, the formula for R will change. There would be nothing wrong with having two scorers when determining objectivity in the pilot study and using two scorers during data collection in the research study. In this case the score for each participant in the research study would be the sum or mean of the participant's scores from the two scorers. In fact, as long as the number of scorers is the same in both the pilot study and the research study, the objectivity coefficient (R) would be calculated as

$$R = \frac{\text{MS People} - \text{MS Interaction}}{\text{MS People}} \tag{2}$$

See formula (1) for definitions of MS values; design is People $\times$ Scorers with two or more scorers; $R =$ objectivity of a score for each participant which is the sum or mean of the participant's scores from the scorers.

Using the data in Table 15.2 and formula (2), $R = (1.49 - 34)/(1.49) = .77$. Notice that formula (2) and formula (1) have the same numerator but different denominators. This is important since the formula for calculating R must be the correct one. The formula for R is dependent on the number of scorers used to determine objectivity in the pilot study and the number of scorers to be used when collecting the data in the research study. A common mistake is using a formula for R which is not consistent with the number of scorers used. Often researchers mistakenly use formula (2) with the pilot study data but have only one scorer in the research study. Again, when describing the procedures and findings for the research study, the researcher must indicate the method used to obtain R and the score for which R is reported. In fact, R can be calculated using information from a one-way ANOVA rather than the two-way ANOVA presented here, so the researcher should report that a two-way ANOVA was used. See Baumgartner, Jackson, Mahar, and Rowe (2007) for additional information on calculating R.

You may read a research report in which the researcher used a Pearson correlation coefficient (r) to determine objectivity. This is an outdated technique. Sometimes the author of a research report will determine objectivity by calculating **Cronbach's alpha,** sometimes called *coefficient alpha.* The coefficient alpha is the same as the R using formula (2). Note this R is not the objectivity coefficient for a

Cronbach's alpha
A correlation coefficient calculated as an estimate of objectivity and reliability; also called *coefficient alpha.*

single score (one scorer) during the research study data collection. Thus, coefficient alpha is not the correct value to calculate and report as the objectivity coefficient for a single scorer, but it is the correct value if in the research study the number of scorers will be the same number as in the pilot study. Earlier, you were cautioned to use and make sure authors of research reports use a formula for R which is consistent with the number of scorers used. Use of coefficient alpha as an objectivity coefficient is seldom appropriate because usually only one scorer is used in the research study.

Since the objectivity coefficient is influenced by the amount of agreement among scorers, characteristics of the group tested, like sex, age, experience, and such, usually have little influence on the objectivity coefficient. So a test documented as yielding data with objectivity for one group can be used with any group as long as the scorers are competent. The objectivity of data is dependent on the type of test. The more difficult the test to score accurately, the lower tends to be the objectivity coefficient. The minimal acceptable objectivity for a physical performance test is .70, but for knowledge tests and attitude scales the minimal value may be different. The minimal value is dependent on how much objectivity is needed, the objectivity obtained by other researchers, the objectivity obtained for similar tests, and so on.

The Reliability Analysis program in the SPSS package of statistical programs can be used to obtain an R as an estimate of objectivity. The program is quite versatile, calculating R for a score which is either a single scorer or the mean of several scorers and using either a one-way or two-way ANOVA model. The directions for this program are presented in section 13 of the Statistical Procedures part of Appendix A.

Reliability (Relative)

To determine reliability, each person must have at least two repeated measure scores. These scores might be (1) multiple trials (administrations) of a physical performance test within a day, (2) multiple administrations of a physical performance test with each administration on a different day, (3) multiple items on a knowledge test, (4) two different forms (A and B) of a knowledge test with both forms administered on different days or on the same day, or (5) other repeated measures. If the data are collected within a day, this allows a determination of **internal consistency reliability,** defined as consistency of the test scores within a day. If the data are collected on different days, this allows a determination of **stability reliability,** defined as consistency of the test scores across days. In all cases, some correlation coefficient is calculated to indicate the degree of relationship between the sets of scores. This correlation coefficient is called the **reliability coefficient.** Since it can vary from 0.00 to 1.00, 0.00 indicates no reliability and 1.00 indicates perfect reliability.

Internal consistency reliability
Consistency of test scores within a single day.

Stability reliability
Consistency of test scores across several days.

Reliability coefficient
A correlation coefficient indicating the relationship between the repeated measures or scores of a test.

Multiple Trials within a Day. This is typically multiple trials of a physical performance test administered within a day (internal consistency). The physical performance test must be one in which multiple trials can be administered without fatigue or learning changing performance from trial to trial. Multiple trials of a maximum exertion test, such as a treadmill test, would not be administered within a day. Administering a test before participants had sufficient time to learn how to take the test by practicing it would cause learning to change performance from trial to trial. An example of a multiple trial physical performance test would be when each person in turn is scored on a flexibility test and the group continues to rotate taking turns until all people in the group of 20 people have been scored five times (five trials). Another example would be when each person is administered five trials of the flexibility test, then another person is administered five trials, and so on, until all 20 people have five scores. So the data arrangement is as shown in Table 15.3. Usually, in this situation, the score of a participant is the sum or the mean of the participant's trial scores, and an intraclass correlation coefficient is calculated to estimate reliability using formula (2); R = reliability of a score for each participant which is the sum or mean of the participant's trial scores.

The data in Table 15.3 were analyzed using the Reliability Analysis program in the SPSS package of statistical programs, and the results of this analysis are presented in Table 15.4. Using this information and formula (2), $R = (20.70 - 1.62)/(20.70) = .92$. In this situation, the more trials, the higher tends to be the R. An R of .70 to .80 is usually the minimum accepted value. The R of .92 obtained

TABLE 15.3 Multiple Trial Data Arrangement

PERSON	TRIAL 1	TRIAL 2	TRIAL 3	TRIAL 4	TRIAL 5
1	8	7	9	7	9
2	10	9	9	12	12
3	7	7	7	8	9
4	7	10	12	9	9
5	10	7	11	11	8
6	10	6	8	10	11
7	6	6	6	6	6
8	9	11	12	8	8
9	9	9	8	10	8
10	6	6	6	7	5
11	8	10	10	9	11
12	7	9	6	7	6
13	5	8	6	7	6
14	5	5	5	5	5
15	6	5	6	7	6
16	5	6	5	5	5
17	10	10	12	12	12
18	10	10	10	12	8
19	12	14	11	12	11
20	7	7	11	9	11

TABLE 15.4 Means and ANOVA Summary Table for the Data in Table 15.3

	MEAN	STD. DEVIATION	CASE
Trial 1	7.85	2.06	20
Trial 2	8.10	2.31	20
Trial 3	8.50	2.50	20
Trial 4	8.65	2.32	20
Trial 5	9.30	2.43	20

ANALYSIS OF VARIANCE

SOURCE OF VARIATION	SUM OF SQUARES	DF	MEAN SQUARE
Between People	393.36	19	20.70
Between Measures	8.06	4	2.02
Interaction	122.74	76	1.62
Total	524.16	99	5.29

is quite good. Type of test, sex and age of the people tested, and so on, all influence the reliability of the data. Thus, a test which yields reliable data for one group may not yield reliable data for a group with different characteristics.

Multiple Days.   This is a typical situation with physical performance tests where the same test is administered to a group of people (30 or more) on two different days, usually one to seven days apart. Thus, this testing procedure allows stability reliability to be determined. The data arrangement is as presented in Table 15.5. Usually, in this situation, the reason the test was administered on two different days in the pilot study was to be able to determine reliability, but in the future the researcher would like to administer the test on one day with assurance that the data collected during the research study data collection have high stability reliability. An intraclass correlation coefficient is calculated to estimate stability reliability using formula (1); R = reliability of a score for each participant which is collected on one day.

The data for trials 1 and 2 in Table 15.3 were analyzed treating the trials as if they were day-one and day-two scores, so that an example calculation of R using formula (1) is possible. Based on the analysis of the trial 1 and trial 2 data which are presented in Table 15.6, $R = (7.97 - 1.63)/(7.97 + 1.63) = .66$. This is a low reliability coefficient.

There are differences between formulas (2) and (1) in terms of how the data are collected (within a day or between days), the denominator of the formula, and the score for which R is reported [sum (mean) of scores or one score]. If formula (2) was used on the values in Table 15.6, $R = (7.97 - 1.63)/(7.97) = .80$. This is an acceptable value for a reliability coefficient, but it requires that the score for each participant be based on scores for two trials or two days. Just reporting that the

TABLE 15.5 Multiple Day Data Arrangement		
PERSON	**DAY 1**	**DAY 2**
1	X	X
2	X	X
3	X	X
•	•	•
•	•	•
•	•	•
n	X	X

Note: n = number of people tested; X = a test score

TABLE 15.6 Means and ANOVA Summary Table for Trials One and Two in Table 15.3		
	MEAN	**STD. DEVIATION**	**CASES**
Trial 1	7.85	2.06	20
Trial 2	8.10	2.31	20

	ANALYSIS OF VARIANCE		
SOURCE OF VARIATION	**SUM OF SQUARES**	**DF**	**MEAN SQUARE**
Between People	151.48	19	7.97
Between Measures	.63	1	.63
Interaction	30.88	19	1.63
Total	182.99	39	4.69

reliability is a value (like .66) is a totally inadequate description of the test reliability. The ANOVA model (one way or two way) (see Baumgartner, Jackson, Mahar, and Rowe 2007 for more information), criterion score (one score or mean score), type of reliability (internal consistency or stability), and value of R must be reported to adequately describe the situation. Formula (1) is correct if in the pilot study the test was administered on two days to determine R and in the research study the test is administered on one day. There would be nothing wrong with administering the test on each of two days during both the pilot study and the research study data collection and the score for each participant being the sum or mean of the participant's day 1 and day 2 scores. In fact, as long as the number of days the test is administered is the same in both the pilot study and the research study, the stability coefficient (R) is determined by formula (2); R = reliability of a score for each participant which is the sum or mean of the participant's day scores.

General Case.   If the test was administered more than twice (three or more trials or days) to determine R, so each person has more than two scores, the formula changes, as presented by Baumgartner, Jackson, Mahar, and Rowe (2007). This formula is

$$R = \frac{\text{MS People} - \text{MS Interaction}}{\text{MS People} + (K/K' - 1)(\text{MS Interaction})} \tag{3}$$

where K = the number of times the test was administered and K' = the number of scores used to form the score of a person. See formula (1) for definitions of MS values.

This formula is important because it is a general formula which can be used in any reliability or objectivity situation. If the test was administered on three days in the pilot study to determine R and the score of a participant in the research study will be from one day, $K = 3$ and $K' = 1$ in formula (3). If, for internal consistency reliability, five trials of a test were administered in the pilot study to determine R and the score of a participant in the research study will be the sum or mean of the best three of the five trials, $K = 5$ and $K' = 3$ in formula (3). Also, if the test was administered on more than two days in the pilot study to determine R and the score of each participant in the research study will be the sum or mean of the scores from more than one day, the formula for R changes, as presented by Baumgartner, Jackson, Mahar, and Rowe (2007) and shown in formula (3).

The Reliability Analysis program in the SPSS package of programs can be used to obtain an R as an estimate of reliability. The program is quite versatile, calculating R for a score which is either a single score or the mean of several trials or days and using either a one-way or two-way ANOVA model. The directions for this program are presented in section 13 of the Statistical Procedures part of Appendix A.

Knowledge Test.   A knowledge test composed of many true-false and/or multiple-choice items is administered to a group in a pilot study in order to determine internal consistency reliability. Each item measures some part of a total construct. Notice that, for this type of test, each item is scored right (1 point) or wrong (0 point) and the total score of a person is the number of items correctly answered. The reliability of the total score is determined by calculating one of the **Kuder-Richardson** coefficients (20 or 21) or the Cronbach's alpha coefficient. These coefficients are correlation coefficients and they are easy to calculate, presented in most measurement books, and commonly found in packages of computer programs. Cronbach's alpha is the same as the R using formula (2) with items replacing trials in Table 15.3. The type of test, sex and age of the people tested, and so on, influences the magnitude of the reliability coefficient. To decide whether the reliability coefficient for the data of a test is large enough, compare it to reliability coefficients obtained by other researchers and/or for similar tests. Probably a reliability coefficient of .70 or higher is required for sufficient reliability.

Kuder-Richardson
A correlation coefficient calculated as an estimate of reliability.

Stability reliability is seldom if ever determined for knowledge tests. If a knowledge test is administered on each of two different days, most participants score better on the second day because they remembered answers to items from the first-day administration and/or obtained answers to items between the first-day and second-day administrations.

Questionnaire.   A questionnaire may have a number of different forms. If the questionnaire has many items with potential answers provided, it is much like a knowledge test. For example, the questionnaire may be for measuring attitudes, with each item a statement to which the research participant responds *strongly agree, agree, disagree,* or *strongly disagree.* The responses are numerically coded with *strongly agree* = 4, *agree* = 3, *disagree* = 2, and *strongly disagree* = 1. Notice that these are just codes and not real scores. The codes could be any numbers (for example, 9,8,3,1), as long as each response has a different code. Further, note that there are no right answers to the items and for many questionnaires the items are unrelated to each other, not measuring a total construct as for a knowledge test. Thus, although a total score—which is the sum of the codes for the item responses—is possible, a total score is usually inappropriate and meaningless. This being the case, determining reliability with techniques used with knowledge tests is incorrect. It is not uncommon when reading a research article to find that a Kuder-Richardson coefficient or coefficient alpha has been used inappropriately to determine the reliability of the data from a questionnaire.

Internal consistency reliability of questionnaire data could be determined by using several pairs of items in the questionnaire. For example, items 11 and 32, 25 and 41 are paired. If participants respond in a similar manner to the two items in a pair and this is true for each pair, this is acceptable evidence that each item in the questionnaire provides reliable data. Reliability for each pairing of items is probably determined by using the coefficient alpha, but an intraclass correlation coefficient (formula number 2) could be used. Again, characteristics of the questionnaire and the people tested influence the magnitude of the reliability coefficient. Reliability coefficients for questionnaire data are often not high; maybe .60 is an acceptable value. As with knowledge tests, stability reliability is seldom determined for questionnaires.

Dichotomously Scored Tests.   Some tests are scored pass or fail, proficient or nonproficient, and so on. For these tests there is some score (standard) which, if obtained or exceeded, results in a person being classified as passing; otherwise, the person fails. For example, to pass a 100-point knowledge test, a score of at least 90 is required. To determine reliability of the data, the test must be administered twice (two trials within a day or two days), and each time the test is administered, each person is assigned a score of one (1) if the person passes, or zero (0) if the person fails. Thus, there is a data arrangement as shown in Table 15.7.

Reliability for the data of this type may be estimated by several different methods. One simple method is **percent agreement,** which indicates the percentage

Percent agreement
An estimate of the reliability of dichotomous data.

TABLE 15.7 Dichotomously Scored Test Data Arrangement for Reliability

		SECOND ADMINISTRATION	
		1	0
FIRST ADMINISTRATION	1	n1	n2
	0	n3	n4

n1 = the number of people classified as a 1 for both administrations
n2 = the number of people classified as a 1 for the first administration but 0 on the second administration

of the group classified the same on both administrations. This value can vary from zero to one. The formula is

$$\text{Percent agreement} = \frac{n1 + n4}{n1 + n2 + n3 + n4} \tag{4}$$

Other methods commonly used are calculating the **kappa coefficient** and the **modified kappa** coefficient. These values are correlation coefficients, so positive values closer to 1.00 than 0.00 are indications of good reliability. The kappa and modified kappa coefficients are discussed in measurement books. Because the possible scores for dichotomously scored tests are one and zero rather than many different values, the reliability coefficient may not be high. The minimum score required to classify a person as passing influences the magnitude of the reliability coefficient. If the majority of the people receive the same classification, probably the reliability coefficient will be higher than the coefficient when about one-half the group receive each classification. Again, characteristics of the test and the group tested influence the magnitude of the reliability coefficient.

Kappa coefficient
Another estimate of the reliability of dichotomous data.

Modified kappa
A third estimate of the reliability of dichotomous data.

Reliability (Absolute)

The reliability techniques discussed so far have involved the use of a correlation coefficient or a percentage to indicate the degree of agreement between multiple-trial or multiple-day test scores of a group. If people who score high on one trial or on one day score high on all trials or days and people who score low on one trial or day consistently score low, the degree of agreement will be high. Sometimes it is desirable to express reliability in actual test score units, indicating how much the test score of a person might change from trial to trial or day to day due to measurement error.

If each person is administered multiple trials of a test within a day or tested on multiple days, a standard deviation for the multiple measures could be calculated for each person, and this standard deviation is the measurement error to expect for the person. However, if each person is administered only one trial or tested on only one day, the mean amount of measurement error in the data is estimated for the entire group by calculating the **standard error of measurement:**

$$SEM = s\sqrt{1 - R} \tag{5}$$

Standard error of measurement
An estimate of the amount of measurement error to expect in the score of any person in a group.

where SEM = standard error of measurement
s = standard deviation of the data
R = reliability coefficient for the data

For example, if $s = 10$ and $R = .84$, SEM $= 10(\sqrt{1 - .84}) = (10)(.4) = 4.0$. The standard error of measurement is an estimate of how much one should expect a test score to vary due to measurement error, lack of reliability.

If, from a practical standpoint, the SEM is small enough to be tolerated because it does not change the interpretation of the data, then the data are sufficiently reliable. Many books, like Nunnally and Berstein (1994), contain a lengthy discussion of measurement theory and the SEM. Note that the SEM is based on the data of a group, and all members of the group may not follow the scoring pattern of the group. Darracot (1995) found the standard error of measurement tends to be an overestimate of the standard deviation of the repeated measures for an individual.

Validity

If acceptable objectivity and reliability are determined for the data, then validity evidence is gathered. There are several basic types of validity evidence. Thus, each type is just an estimate or indication of the validity of the interpretations of the test scores. In the past people talked about types of validity. Presently, the use of validity types is no longer considered correct. The basic and commonly used types of validity evidence will be discussed so, as a researcher, you have a good understanding of what types of validity evidence are available to you and, as a consumer of research, you understand types of validity evidence used in a research article. All types of validity evidence can't be discussed, and the types of validity evidence presented can't be discussed in great detail. Thus, you may want to consult other sources, such as Baumgartner, Jackson, Mahar, and Rowe (2007), or other measurement books. A very comprehensive source is *Standards for Educational and Psychological Testing* (American Educational Research Association 1999).

Logical validity evidence
A statement based on knowledge that a test measures an attribute and yields scores that can be validly interpreted.

Logical Evidence. Physical educators and exercise scientists often use **logical validity evidence** when they state that a test provides test scores which allow valid interpretations of test scores, because based on all they know about the physical attribute to be measured and physical performance, the test measures that physical attribute. Note that this is usually a statement that the test yields test scores which can be validly interpreted with no reference to the degree of validity (high, medium, or low). Also, note that the person claiming logical validity evidence may be wrong and/or all people will not agree with her/him. Logical validity evidence is acceptable if there is no other evidence possible. Many measurement experts believe that several types of validity evidence should be provided for the data, and so using logical validity evidence and some other evidence would be acceptable. The term *content validity evidence* probably originated with knowledge tests. The researcher claims the knowledge test yields scores which allow valid interpretations of knowledge, because the test is a comprehensive coverage of the content of the course, unit, program, and such. Since the opinions of several people are usually better than the opinion of one person, it is quite common for a researcher to use a jury of experts when collecting logical validity evidence for a knowledge test, questionnaire, or any type of paper-and-pencil test. Basically the *jury of experts* examines the test and evaluates it as to whether it is a comprehensive coverage of the content to be tested, whether the test items are well constructed and understandable, whether the format of the test is conducive to obtaining test scores which lead to valid interpretations, and so on. The jury of experts may suggest improvements in the test or questionnaire and request to see the improved test before giving it approval. When a jury of experts is used, the number of people in the jury, and their qualifications, must be determined. A jury of experts composed of two available graduate students, faculty, or peers hardly seems sufficient. Depending on a number of factors, a jury of experts is composed of 3 to 12 persons knowledgeable about some if not all aspects of the test and the attribute to be tested. A jury with some test construction experts and some content experts is fine. The jury of experts doesn't have to be the authorities in the profession but members should have qualifications which the average person in the profession does not possess. A jury composed entirely of peers, colleagues, or members of the same academic department or unit seldom would be considered a strong jury of experts.

Criterion Evidence.

The use of **criterion validity evidence** is quite traditional. It involves determining the correlation between scores on a test and scores on a criterion measure or standard which is known or accepted as providing scores which can be validly interpreted. Thus, each person in a group has a score on both the test and the criterion. If the correlation coefficient (r) is high enough, the test yields scores which can be validly interpreted, since people who have good scores on the test have good scores on the criterion and people who have poor scores on the test have poor scores on the criterion. In other words, the test is providing the same information as the criterion. The correlation coefficient obtained is often called the *validity coefficient.* The criterion is supposed to be the *gold standard,* the standard that is recognized by all people as being the best. For example, some laboratory measures of aerobic capacity and body composition are recognized as the gold standard. Many times there is no gold standard, so one of the several good standards is used as the criterion. Thus, the magnitude of the validity coefficient obtained is influenced by the criterion selected. Sometimes there is disagreement among knowledgeable professionals as to which criterion to use. The criterion is a laboratory measure or some measure which is difficult, time-consuming, and/or

Criterion validity evidence
A correlation coefficient between scores on a test and scores on a criterion measure or standard.

expensive to obtain. The test for which validity evidence is being collected is a field-based test which is easier, quicker, and/or less expensive to administer than the criterion measure. For example, in physical education and exercise science, the field-based mile run test as a measure of aerobic capacity is compared to laboratory measures of oxygen consumption; the field-based skinfold test as a measure of body composition is compared to underwater weighing measures from the laboratory. Another example is a field-based test of anxiety which practitioners could use is compared to measures of anxiety which only a trained psychologist can obtain. There are situations where scores on a test are correlated with a criterion which is the sum of judges' ratings to obtain a validity coefficient. In this case several well-qualified judges independently rated each person in a group. Finding and assembling the judges is difficult and it is time-consuming for them to do the ratings. The test can be administered by a practitioner with limited expertise in a short period of time. If the test yields the same information as judges' ratings, it will be used in preference to judges' ratings.

There are numerous other criteria which could be used to collect validity evidence. The researcher must consider what possible criteria are available and how appropriate they are. In general, criteria are anything the researcher and others who read and evaluate the research think appropriate. Sometimes no acceptable criteria exist, so criterion validity evidence can't be collected.

The magnitude of the validity coefficient is influenced by the test, the sex, age, and experience of the people tested, and the criterion used. The minimum acceptable value of the validity coefficient is dependent on how much validity is necessary and what other researchers have obtained for the same or similar groups and/or tests. Seldom is a validity coefficient less than .70 considered acceptable in a research setting. In some nonresearch settings where great accuracy in the data and the classification of people based on the data are not required, validity coefficients less than .70 are acceptable.

Construct
Something which is known to exist although it may not be precisely defined and/or measured.

Construct validity evidence
Evidence that a test measures a construct and yields scores that can be validly interpreted.

Construct Evidence.

A **construct** is something which is known to exist although it may not be precisely defined and/or measured. A judge in a pornography trial said, "Pornography, I can't define it but I know it when I see it." Pornography is a construct. Feelings, attitudes, team work, total ability in a sport or job, and so on, are all potential constructs. The validity of the interpretations based on scores from a test designed to measure a construct may be determined in a variety of different ways. Any of the ways already discussed may be used. For this reason some measurement experts maintain that all validity evidence is **construct validity evidence.**

Forming groups which are known to differ in terms of the construct to be measured and comparing them in regard to test scores are accepted construct validity evidence. If the best group has the highest mean score on the test, and the second-best group has the second-highest mean score on the test, and so on, this is evidence that the test yields data which can be interpreted with at least some degree of validity. Groups which are known to differ might be formed based on sex, age, or any attribute which seems appropriate. However, comparing groups with extreme differences (for example, 6-year-old compared to 18-year-old individuals, professional athletes compared to nonathletes) may not make sense. Remember, the researcher is trying to determine if a test yields data which can be validly interpreted for a defined classification of people, so each person in the groups used to collect validity evidence basically must be a member of the defined classification of people (population). So, in the earlier example, if the researcher is trying to determine if a test yields data which allow valid interpretations for 18-year-old individuals, comparing the data of 6-year-old and 18-year-old individuals makes no sense. In this example, if, by using appropriate techniques, construct validity evidence is obtained, this indicates that the test has the ability to identify different levels of ability—that is, the better the test score, the more ability a person has.

Comparing an untrained group to a trained group or an uninstructed group to an instructed group in terms of mean test score is commonly done to obtain construct validity evidence. If the trained or instructed group has a better mean test score than the other group, this is construct validity evidence. Comparing the data of a group before and after training or instruction and finding that the group had a better mean test score after training or instruction is construct validity evidence.

Other Evidence.   Characteristics of dichotomously scored tests were discussed earlier in the reliability section of this chapter. Any of the techniques discussed up to this point could be used with dichotomously scored tests. However, two techniques to obtain criterion validity evidence commonly used by researchers and, thus, commonly found in research articles are discussed here. In this case the validity question is whether the data from a test will classify people the same way as a criterion. For example, if the test score of a person is good enough to classify the person as proficient, is the performance of the person on the criterion sufficient to classify the person as proficient? Thus, the data format is as presented in Table 15.8.

TABLE 15.8 Dichotomously Scored Test Data Arranged for Validity Estimation

		CRITERION	
		PROFICIENT	NONPROFICIENT
TEST	**PROFICIENT**	n1	n2
	NONPROFICIENT	n3	n4

where n1 = the number of people classified as proficient both on the test and on the criterion
      n2 = the number of people classified as proficient with the test but nonproficient based on the criterion

Phi
A correlation coefficient calculated as an estimate of validity for dichotomous data.

The percent agreement coefficient, discussed in the reliability section, could be used here. A correlation coefficient called **phi** is often used as the validity coefficient in this situation. The phi coefficient is presented in most introductory statistics books and measurement books, like Baumgartner, Jackson, Mahar, and Rowe (2007), and provided in many packages of statistical computer programs, like SPSS.

Reporting Validity. No matter how validity evidence was collected, the collection process needs to be well described in the research report. The type of participant, number of participants, and validity evidence must be presented no matter whether the researcher or another person conducted the validity estimation work.

OTHER MEASUREMENT CONSIDERATIONS

It should be noted that a desirable but not essential characteristic of a test is that it is economical. An economical test is inexpensive to purchase, and if it requires equipment, the equipment is not expensive to purchase. Also, the test is quick to administer. Further, administration of the test requires neither a large number of people nor people with great expertise. Finally, the time it takes to score the test and the cost of scoring the test is minimal.

There are some things which the researcher should do when preparing to test participants and actually collecting data on participants. These things will increase the chances of having acceptable objectivity and reliability for the data and validity of the interpretations of the data. Measurement books tend to have a chapter devoted to these topics. Experienced researchers tend to do these things and to describe them in the procedures section of the journal article.

Recognize that physical performance tests and paper-and-pencil tests may not be similar in terms of how participants are prepared to take the tests, how the tests are administered, and how participants perform the tests. Paper-and-pencil tests which include true-false items and/or multiple-choice items, and questionnaires with the possible responses provided (see closed-ended items in Chapter 9), are administered and taken in basically the same way, no matter what the content area of the test. Preparation for taking the test, test-taking strategy, and actual taking of the test are similar for all true-false or multiple-choice tests. However, each physical performance test has a unique set of directions and is administered in a unique manner. For example, a mile run test is different from a sit-up test. Having taken a mile run test does not prepare a person to take a sit-up test and certainly does not prepare a person to take a paper-and-pencil test.

There are some common elements with paper-and-pencil testing and physical performance testing. Participants need to be prepared to take the test. They need to know what the test is and to have had experience with the subject matter and, in physical performance, with the performance being tested. Participants need to know why they are being tested and what a test score indicates. There must be directions concerning test administration and scoring directions, which are presented to the participants in writing and/or verbally the day of the test. Sufficient time must be allowed for participants to take the test without feeling rushed. All participants must be encouraged to score at their highest level. Age often influences test performance, so one test or one set of procedures may not be appropriate for all people. Failure to address these things will likely decrease reliability of the data and validity of the data interpretations.

There are some unique elements with paper-and-pencil testing and physical performance testing. Generally, with paper-and-pencil testing, many participants can be tested at the same time, whereas with physical performance testing, often only one participant can be tested at a time. So testing time may be more of a concern and longer with physical performance tests than with paper-and-pencil tests. The reading level of participants is a concern with paper-and-pencil tests but not with physical performance tests. However, with physical performance tests, gender, height, and weight often influence the data but seldom influence paper-and-pencil data. As mentioned earlier, each physical performance test is unique and participants must have had prior experience with the test, where this is not a major problem with paper-and-pencil tests. Participants copying answers from the knowledge test paper of another person or not completing a questionnaire accurately or honestly are concerns with paper-and-pencil tests, but honesty is not a concern with a physical performance test if well-trained scorers are used (participants testing each other could be a problem). Again, failure to address these things will likely decrease reliability of the data and validity of the data interpretations.

If the researcher has found in a pilot study, or other researchers have found for the type of participant in the study, that the test yields reliable data and the interpretations of the data are valid, the researcher still must be careful to administer the test in a manner which will yield reliable data and valid interpretations of the data. With paper-and-pencil tests this may not be too difficult because both the tester and participants have had experience with the test. The tester knows how to administer and score the test. The participants know how to perform the test. This may not be true with physical performance tests.

Planning and experience are the key to having acceptable objectivity and reliability, for the data and valid interpretations of the data. Planning all aspects of the data collection is essential. When testing will occur, how long testing will take, what to do if measurement equipment malfunctions and/or participants don't take the test correctly, and preparing participants to be tested are just a few of the things which must be planned. No matter what the measurement and the characteristics of the participants, directions dealing with why the test is being administered, and how the test is administered, are essential. If people know why they are being tested and how to take the test, they are more likely to give their best effort, perform the test correctly, and receive a score approaching their best possible score. For example, physical performance tests each have different administrative procedures; people must have had experience with the test prior to being tested. Giving participants experience with the physical performance test in advance of the day they are tested is probably important for acceptable reliability of the data and valid interpretations of the data. For maximum exertion physical performance tests, participants have to be prepared physiologically and psychologically to give their maximum effort.

In order to obtain data which allows for valid interpretations of the data, the test administrator must have experience with the test used and the people tested. It is not enough to read the directions for a new test once. This is particularly true with physical performance tests, but generally true with all tests. Testing techniques appropriate for first-grade students, college students, and elderly individuals differ considerably. Lack of experience with the test and the people tested may jeopardize obtaining data which allows for valid interpretations of the data.

Summary of Objectives

1. **Discuss objectivity in terms of what it is, why it is important, and how it is estimated.** Objectivity means that two or more people could administer a test and achieve similar scores. Objectivity is important because it means that the data are consistent and not influenced by the person administering or scoring the test. Objectivity is estimated by duplication of test results by independent testers.

2. **Discuss reliability in terms of what it is, why it is important, and how it is estimated.** Reliability is the degree to which a measure is consistent and unchanged over a short period of time. Reliability helps the researcher ensure that the data collected are a true indication of the ability of the persons being tested and that the data would not be entirely different if collected at some other time.

3. **Discuss validity in terms of what it is, why it is important, and how it is estimated.** Validity is the degree to which interpretations based on the test scores lead to correct conclusions. Validity is the most important characteristic of data; it allows the researcher to make decisions based on the data.

4. **Identify things to consider both when preparing to test participants in a research study and when testing them.** Researchers must always recognize that physical performance tests differ from paper-and-pencil tests in terms of how prepared participants are to take the tests and how they perform on the tests. It is important that the test administrator be experienced and knowledgeable about the type of test being given in order to obtain data which can be interpreted with validity.

Part Four

Writing and Reporting

It is important to note that research is a shared enterprise among members of a professional group. Part Four of this book focuses on developing the research proposal and preparing a scientific paper describing the research results. These chapters do not contain direct information regarding how to conduct research, but focus on the writing associated with planning the research as well as reporting the results.

Chapter 16 focuses on preparing a research proposal. The proposal is used to present one's idea about a researchable problem to others, such as a faculty adviser, a thesis or dissertation committee, or a potential grant provider. Chapter 17 offers guidance on reporting one's findings through a variety of formats ranging from a thesis or dissertation to a journal article or conference presentation.

16

Developing the Research Proposal

OBJECTIVES

The preparation of a research proposal is a crucial step in the overall research process. In this chapter, we will review the essential elements of a research proposal and provide a general framework for writing a proposal.

After reading Chapter 16, you should be able to

1. Understand the purpose of the research proposal.
2. Recognize the basic parts of a research proposal.

As one contemplates conducting a research study, there comes a point at which the researcher will need to develop a written account of the proposed research, explaining the problem to be investigated, the rationale for the study, and the specific procedures that will be followed to investigate the problem. The preparation of the proposal is an important part of the overall research process. For the graduate student, the proposal typically serves as the primary basis for gaining approval from the student's thesis or dissertation committee to commence a study. For others, the proposal may serve as a formal document requesting funding support for a planned research project. In either case, the significance of the proposed study, the appropriateness of the research design, and the clarity in which the proposal has been communicated to the reader will go a long way toward its approval. Although the specific format may vary from institution to institution and from funding agency to funding agency, the generic parts of a research proposal discussed here are widely accepted.

Research proposal
Document presenting a researchable problem and a plan of attack and protocol for investigating the problem; often required by a potential funding agency or thesis/dissertation committee.

According to Locke, Spirduso, and Silverman (2007), a **research proposal** may function in at least three ways: as a means of communication, as a plan, and as a contract. It communicates to others, who may provide approval or support, the intent to pursue a particular research project; it provides a detailed description of the research plan and the procedures to guide the study; and, when approved, it serves as a "contract" between a student and his or her committee or between an investigator and a funding agency. The format for a research proposal may vary substantially from one department to another, from one institution to another, and among funding agencies. When specified, the precise guidelines and regulations governing student research as well as sponsored research should be followed. The following guidelines for developing a research proposal provide a general framework that has been widely used among many colleges and universities in the United States and are generally recognized by most faculty advisers. The final definition of the problem occurs when the graduate student develops a research proposal for the thesis or dissertation that is being planned. In most instances the proposal consists of three chapters: introduction, review of related literature, and procedures for collecting data, although the specific format and content may vary considerably. Those three chapters ultimately become the first three chapters of the thesis or dissertation. Before discussing the content of these chapters in detail, a few words about the title of the research project are appropriate.

PROPOSAL TITLE

All research proposals will be titled, but the name given to the project at this time is considered only temporary. It may be changed several times before being finalized. The title is important in that it is the first thing the reader sees. Based on the title, the reader will continue reading or lose interest. Moreover, the title will serve to identify the study for purposes of information retrieval. A brief title, one that is streamlined, is currently preferred. The following title is too long:

> An Analysis of the Specific Curriculum Content for the Preparation of Recreation Majors and the Relationship between the Details of the Curriculum and the Details of the Majors' On-the-Job Duties

Not only is this title overly long, but it also includes some redundancy and is confusing. The title should be long enough to cover the subject of the research, but short enough to be interesting. Usually, 12 to 15 words are sufficient. The beginning researcher should ask these questions when contemplating a project title:

1. Does the title precisely identify the area of the problem?
2. Is the title clear, concise, free from jargon, and adequately descriptive to permit indexing the study in its proper category?
3. Does the title identify the key variables and provide some information about the scope of the study?
4. Are unnecessary words, such as "a study of," "an investigation of," and "an analysis of" avoided? (*Note:* These words and other catchy, misleading, and vague phrases lengthen titles and do not add substance. They are superfluous.)
5. Do nouns, as opposed to adjectives, serve as the key words in the title?
6. Have words been selected that will aid computerized retrieval systems?
7. Are the most important words placed at the beginning of the title?

The following examples illustrate appropriate titles. Each title meets the criteria for a streamlined yet complete title. Moreover, each accurately reflects the research problem.

- "Leisure Participation of Urban Chinese Adolescents" (Wang 2000)
- "Psychological Factors Related to Eating Disorders among Female College Cheerleaders in Iowa" (Musser 2002)
- "Effects of Trampoline Training on Balance in Functionally Unstable Ankles" (Hess 2004)
- "Effects of Special Olympic Participation and Self-Esteem of Adults with Mental Retardation" (Major 1998)
- "Parental Influence on Children's Physical Activity" (Lambdin-Abraham 2009)

WRITING CHAPTER ONE: INTRODUCTION

Chapter one of the research proposal usually begins with a brief introduction. Customarily, the researcher includes a paragraph or two (perhaps more, depending on the nature of the problem) to help lead the reader into the problem. The researcher specifies the problem to be investigated, provides the underlying rationale, and establishes why it is important. How the researcher became interested in the problem is usually indicated. Some references to the literature should be made in the introduction, although it should not be so extensive to resemble a review of literature, which is more properly done in chapter two. The literature cited in the introduction, coupled with the researcher's own thoughts, should be used to stimulate interest and to establish the underlying rationale for the study. Again, it is not necessary that this section be long. Typically, the introduction section of a research proposal will be one to two pages in length. Following are two examples, both paraphrased from the completed research proposals, that illustrate the essence of introductory sections:

Example 1

Lateral ankle sprains are one of the most common injuries experienced in athletics. In the United States, 23,000 people a day are seen in doctors' offices for ankle injuries (Braun 1999). Eighty-five percent of these injuries are lateral ankle sprains typically involving the lateral ankle structures including the anterior talofibular ligament (ATF) and/or the calcaneofibular ligament (CF). These injuries range from very mild to complete rupture of the lateral ankle ligaments. Another result of an ankle sprain is functional ankle instability, which may be the result of damage to nervous tissue in and around the ankle (Ritchie 2001). In light of the prevalence of lateral ankle sprains and the associated disability, researchers and clinicians have sought to identify rehabilitation methods that are both effective and cost efficient. This study is designed to compare the effects of minitrampoline training (dynamic) versus solid floor training (static) on functional ankle instability. (Hess 2004)

Example 2

Obesity is prevalent in our society, and its treatment is constantly being explored. All proper weight loss programs for the moderately obese include aerobic exercise as well as dietary restriction. Obese individuals are often told to exercise two or three times a day for short periods in order to burn more calories. The goal of exercise is to mobilize fats from adipose tissue stores for energy production. It is, however, not known if this is the most effective method of achieving weight loss. The optimal exercise prescription for the moderately obese has not been determined. This study, then, examined the duration of exercise in an attempt to determine the most effective exercise prescription for moderately obese women. (Sun 1988)

Purpose of the Study

Immediately after the introductory comments, the **purpose statement** should appear. This will usually be a declarative statement that indicates the goals for the research project. The purpose of the study should be stated clearly, concisely, and definitively. All the key elements, including the variables to be studied, should be expressed in an orderly system of relationships. The statement results from the researcher's analysis of all the facts and explanations that might possibly be related to the problem.

Take care with your wording. "This study investigates" is not a good way to begin. Inanimate objects cannot take action; hence a study cannot investigate. Note that in the research proposal, the purpose statement is written in the present tense

purpose statement
A specific, definitive statement expressing the researcher's intent or goal for conducting the study.

since the study has not yet occurred. After completing the study, this will be changed to the past tense.

Following are a few examples of purpose statements in student thesis or dissertation proposals that meet the criteria for clarity and conciseness:

1. The purpose of this study is to investigate the psychological factors related to indicators of eating disorders among college female cheerleaders in Iowa. (Musser 2002)
2. The purpose of this study is to identify the general patterns of leisure participation of selected urban Chinese youth. (Wang 2000)
3. The purpose of the present study is to examine the effect of color (green, blue, red, and white) on the performance of a controlled target accuracy task. (Araki 2000)
4. The primary purpose of this study is to test the effectiveness of the Fire PALS program on fire and life safety knowledge and behavioral intent of elementary school students. (Vander Werff 2003)

Significance of the Study

This section of chapter one in the research proposal follows the statement of purpose, and its function is to elaborate why the study is needed. Moreover, this section serves to further establish the underlying rationale for the study and to justify its need. Use the literature to help show why the study is needed, to explain why it is significant, or to justify its content. This is the place to present examples of how the problem has manifested itself in society. The development of this section will attempt to show that one or more of the following are true:

1. Knowledge gaps exist between the theoretical and practical aspects of the problem.
2. More and better knowledge is needed in the problem areas.
3. Present knowledge in the problem area needs validation.
4. Current practices concerning the problem need to be found.
5. There is conflicting knowledge about the problem area that needs to be resolved.

The following example of a "significance of the study" section appeared in a research proposal in which the purpose of the study was to determine the impact of a preventive education program on the knowledge and behavioral intent of young children:

> Schools provide important opportunities for injury prevention. Every year, millions of children benefit from the education they receive in school. Many students, however, are not provided with the injury prevention education they need. Unintentional injuries have been a major cause of premature death for children and teenagers for many years (IDPH 2000). Recognizing the need for injury prevention, educating children at an early age will help prevent problems later in life (Eichel and Goldman 2001). In order to decrease the number of deaths and injuries due to unintentional injury, it is important to provide quality preventive education to the populations most effected. Waterloo Fire Rescue's Fire PALS school-based injury prevention program is one example of providing preventive education. Prior to this study, the Fire PALS program had not formally been evaluated. The results of this study will determine the program's effectiveness in changing the fire and life safety knowledge and behavioral intentions of elementary school students in Waterloo, IA. The findings of this study will inform those responsible for preventive education for elementary school students regarding the efficacy of the Fire PALS injury prevention program, and thus provide meaningful information for curriculum modification and implementation. (Vander Werff 2003)

Delimitations

In research circles, **delimitations** refer to the scope of the study. It is in this section of chapter one of the research proposal that the researcher draws a line around the study and, in effect, fences it in. This section identifies what is included in the research. Delimitations spell out the population studied and include those things the researcher can control. It establishes the parameters in such characteristics of the study as (1) number and kinds of research participants, (2) number and kinds of variables, (3) tests, measures, or instruments utilized in the study, (4) special equipment, (5) type of training program, (6) the time and duration of the study (e.g., date, number of weeks, time of year), and (7) analytical procedures. These are the ingredients that the researcher uses to attack the problem. If an item does not appear in the list of delimitations, then it is of no concern in the research. A particular population is targeted on which selected variables will be studied. The variables will be measured by specific test instruments. A certain training program may be involved, and the study will be conducted over a specified period of time.

Delimitations
Characteristics specified by the investigator that define the scope of the research study, effectively "fencing it in."

The section on delimitations in the research proposal does not have to be excessively long, but it should specify those parameters of the research proposal that the researcher can control. Typically, a proposal would list 5 to 10 delimitations. An example of delimitations taken from a research proposal to ascertain the relationship between self-esteem, eating behaviors, and eating attitudes among female collegiate swimmers is presented below:

1. Twenty-four female collegiate swimmers, age 18 to 21.
2. A purposive sample consisting of members of the University of Northern Iowa's women's swimming team during spring 1998.
3. The use of the Rosenburg Self-Esteem Scale to measure self-esteem.
4. The use of the Eating Attitudes Tests (EAT-26) of the National Eating Disorders Screening Program to measure the construct and concerns characteristic of an eating disorder.
5. Administration of the data collection instruments during a single testing session held during a team meeting of the swimming team immediately following completion of the collegiate swimming season. (Fey 1998)

The format for presenting the delimitations (as well as the limitations and assumptions) in a research proposal often includes an introductory phrase, such as, "This study is delimited to the following:" followed by a listing or numeration of the applicable delimitations as illustrated above.

Limitations

Limitations
Aspects of a research study for which the investigator cannot control that represent weaknesses to the study and may negatively affect the results.

In research terminology **limitations** refer to weaknesses of the study. All studies have them because compromises frequently have to be made in order to conform to the realities of a situation. Limitations are those things the researcher could not control, but may have an influence on the results of the study. The reader of a research report should always know at the outset those conditions of the study that could reflect negatively on the work in some way. Only those things that might affect the acceptability of the research data should be presented. The researcher will, of course, try to eliminate extremely serious weaknesses before the study is commenced. Among the items that typically involve statements of limitation are the following:

1. The research approach, design, method(s), and techniques
2. Sampling problems
3. Uncontrolled variables
4. Faulty administration of tests or training programs

5. Generalizability of the data
6. Representativeness of the data
7. Compromises to internal and external validity
8. Reliability and validity of the research instruments

It is important that all statements of limitation sound like, or imply, weakness. The statement, "The sample size was small," is not sufficient, because a small sample does not necessarily assume a weakness of the study. However, the statement, "The sample size of the study ($N = 30$) is small, necessitating caution in extrapolation of the data to a larger obese population," implies a possible weakness of the study. Whereas the number of limitations listed will vary depending upon the nature of the study, the research design, and the methodology utilized, it is generally recommended that the number of limitations be less than the number of delimitations presented. While it is important that the researcher recognize from the outset potential weaknesses of the study, an exceedingly long list of limitations raises serious questions about why so many facets of the research were not controlled, thus questioning the overall veracity of the research. The following limitations were adapted from those included in a proposal for studying an obesity problem:

1. The sample size of this study is small ($N = 30$) necessitating caution in extrapolation of the data to a larger obese population.
2. Daily activities of the subjects other than the exercise program are not controlled.
3. Although subjects are requested to stay on a diet that is well balanced and restricted by 500 calories a day, occasional variance from this may occur. In addition, due to the nature of the diet analyses performed, changes in caloric intake may not be detected.
4. The investigator is unable to personally conduct all of the maximal graded exercise tests in pretraining and posttraining as well as the exercise sessions. To ensure standardization in testing and training, the investigator will meet with all research assistants in order to discuss the testing and training procedures.
5. Resting metabolic rate will not be measured following the exercise sessions and lipolytic changes during this time will not be determined.
6. Since plasma FFA, glycerol, and lipolytic hormones can be affected by conditions other than exercise, it is possible that such conditions may exist.
7. Plasma FFA do not reflect FFA flux in adipose or skeletal muscle tissue, and, therefore, conclusions concerning fat metabolism must be interpreted with caution. (Sun 1988)

Assumptions

Assumptions
Facts or conditions that are presumed to be true, yet not actually verified, that become underlying basics in the planning and implementation of the research study.

Assumptions are derived primarily from the literature. Assumptions then become the basis for the hypotheses, or predictions of eventual outcomes, of the study. In other words, what does the literature tell the researcher about what can be assumed to be true for purposes of planning the study? The information gleaned from the literature frequently serves as the basis for much of the development of the research project. The literature provides information about a particular behavior being investigated and the various conditions influencing that behavior, and sometimes contains factual evidence explaining the behavior. The researcher undertakes a study with certain assumptions about this information. Assumptions are also made about the way the instrumentation, procedures, methods, and techniques will contribute to the study.

The researcher may also assume that certain things that could not be controlled or documented may occur in the study. The following are examples of this type of assumption:

1. All research participants will answer the questionnaire honestly and correctly.
2. The research participants will comply with the researcher's request to perform maximally on all trials of the test.
3. The test instrument is a reliable and valid measure of the desired construct.

The following provides an example of assumptions made by the author of a study designed to investigate the effects of participation in Special Olympics on the self-esteem of adults with mental retardation:

1. The test instrument, as modified, is appropriate for the target population and is a valid and reliable measure of self-esteem.
2. The subjects will be able to understand the directions as they are intended.
3. The subjects will complete the self-esteem inventory to the best of their ability.
4. The subjects are a representative sample of adults with mental retardation who reside in the state of Iowa.
5. The interviewers will be sufficiently trained and capable of utilizing the recommended survey administration procedures. (Major 1998)

Hypotheses

This section of chapter one permits the researcher to predict the outcome of the study in advance and to present tentative explanations for the solution of the problem.

The assumptions made by the researcher provide the launching pad for hypotheses. A simple research hypothesis can be written as a single sentence in which the researcher describes the expected outcome. Consider the following examples of simple research hypotheses:

- There is a positive relationship between the level of intrinsic motivation and performance on a test of cardio-respiratory function.
- There is a difference in the self-reported alcohol usage of male collegiate athletes compared to female collegiate athletes.

Normally, a statement of hypothesis will be declared for each research question posed, although some descriptive questions may not warrant hypotheses. It is important to note that because of space limitations in some professional journals, authors often do not explicitly present their research hypotheses in the published research reports, although such hypotheses may be implied in the paper and undoubtedly have been made by the researcher. On the other hand, graduate students, preparing their research proposal or writing their dissertation or thesis, are normally expected to explicitly state their research hypotheses in clear, unambiguous terms. Stating hypotheses helps make a researcher's thought process about the research situation more concrete. If a prediction of a specific outcome is made, this forces more thorough consideration of which research techniques, methods, test instruments, and data-collecting procedures should be employed. It is extremely important that the hypotheses be testable. Hypotheses also help set up the way the data will be analyzed and how the final report will be organized and written. Following is an example of hypotheses presented in a research proposal to determine the effect of sea kayak touring on the self-concept of patients with low-level spinal cord injuries (SCI):

1. Patients with a low level of SCI of at least one-year duration exhibit an increased self-concept after participation in a two-week sea kayak tour.
2. Increased self-concept changes are significantly greater for those patients participating in the sea kayak tour than patients participating in a two-week camping experience or a regular rehabilitation program.
3. Self-concept does not change for those patients participating in a two-week camping experience or in a regular rehabilitation program.
4. For those patients participating in the sea kayak tour, self-concept remains elevated for six months after completion of the tour. (Pate 1987)

Definition of Terms

Definition of terms is a necessity since many terms and concepts have multiple meanings. The researcher should define terms as they will be interpreted and used throughout the study. Always define operational and behavioral terms and concepts, and check special terms in technical dictionaries or have them reviewed by experts in the field. An operational definition gives meaning to a concept or term by indicating what operation has to be accomplished so as to be able to measure the concept. In experimental studies a researcher will cause a particular result to occur by using a certain procedure or operation. An operational definition of personality might refer to the "scores on the Cattell 16 Personality Factor Inventory" or some other personality test selected by the researcher. Directly quoted or accurately paraphrased time-honored definitions, if they fit the research situation, are considered superior to definitions made up or "coined" by the researcher. Once defined, a term should be applied consistently throughout the study so as not to confuse the reader. It is customary to alphabetize the terms in a list of operational definitions. Following is an example of a partial list of terms defined in a research proposal related to assessment practices in school physical education:

Authentic assessment. Assessment that uses multiple scoring systems to measure students' habits and repertoires on significant task related to life outside the classroom.

Constructivism. A theory that posits that learners construct their own knowledge through conversation, hands-on activity or experience.

Extent of authentic assessment use. Proportion of teachers who use authentic assessment techniques.

Motivation. The driving force or the inner-thrust behind behavior.

Skill achievement. The resulting outcome of a student's actions or technique accomplished through great effort, perseverance or courage. (Mintah 2001)

WRITING CHAPTER TWO: REVIEW OF RELATED LITERATURE

After the literature has been thoroughly reviewed, the researcher will then organize the notes and transpose them into a chapter two, which is usually called the "Review of Related Literature," "Related Literature," or "Literature." This section should be a well-organized chapter that consists of an insightful analy-sis and evaluation of each research source as it relates to the objectives of the current study. The literature review helps to justify the study. A careful analysis of related studies is important in verifying the worth of the study and in helping to establish the overall justification. Only those studies that have a significant relationship to the current problem should be included. It is also important to note that all references located will not be included in this chapter. Some will not be used at all or will be used in other chapters of the proposal.

The review of literature should not merely present previous studies in chrono-logical order, leaving it to the reader to assimilate the facts and to draw relationships between the cited research and the problem. Above all, the literature review should not be presented as a series of abstracts of various studies. Facts and theories should be presented and their relationships shown. Gaps in the existing knowledge in the problem area should surface.

Researchers vary in the way they organize the literature, but two methods are more common than others. In one, the sources are divided into literature related to the present study in content and literature related in method. Discussion of the content literature will present relevant facts, theories, hypotheses, and background information. Method-related literature covers such items as design, techniques, instrumentation, and analysis. A second method is to sort and classify the literature according to topics. It is generally recommended that the literature be organized around topical areas. The ability to read related literature and synthesize this infor-mation into a meaningful treatise is a good indication that the researcher under-stands the problem area. For example, in a study related to the "Female Athlete Triad" (Billings 2002), the literature reviewed was organized under the following topic headings:

1. Disordered Eating
2. Eating Disorders
   a. Anorexia Nervosa
   b. Bulimia Nervosa
   c. Compulsive Overeating
   d. Eating Disorders in Athletes
   e. Factors Influencing Eating Disorders
3. Normal Menstrual Cycle
4. Amenorrhea
   a. Prevalence of Amenorrhea
   b. Incidence of Amenorrhea in Athletes
   c. Consequences of Amenorrhea

    5. Osteoporosis

        a. Bone Loss

        b. Types of Osteoporosis

        c. Osteoporosis in the Triad

    6. Summary

The introduction to chapter two should always contain an opening paragraph that relates the literature to the problem being studied and explains how the chapter is organized. Often, the introductory paragraph will include a restatement of the problem that was presented in chapter one of the research proposal. Consider the following example:

> The literature related to perception of bodily attractiveness in American culture is reported in this chapter. For organizational purposes, the literature is presented under the following topics: (1) Body Image and Self-Esteem, (2) Attractiveness in American Culture, (3) Influence of the Mass Media, (4) The Thin Standard of Bodily Attractiveness for Women, (5) Impact of the Thin Standard, (6) Body Dissatisfaction in Nonclinical Populations, (7) Measurement of Body Image, and (8) Summary. (Collins 1989)

Chapter two is the only chapter in the research proposal that may need a summary. It appears as the last section of the chapter and should be relatively brief. An attempt should be made to summarize the key findings and indicate what the literature has told us about the problem area. What is it that we know? Don't know? What gaps need to be filled? The summary should not be used to report or present any additional specific references to the literature; this should already have been done in detail. Instead, the summary should be a series of statements that tie all the previous reporting together. The following example illustrates the function of a summary.

> There has been a substantial amount of research conducted relating to disordered eating and eating disorders. In general, there has also been a substantial amount of research conducted on athletes and eating disorders as a whole, especially involving the sports of gymnastics and figure skating. Although many athletes may not be clinically diagnosed with eating disorders, many take part in unhealthy weight loss practices such as disordered eating. The highest prevalence of disordered eating and eating disorders is seen among female athletes, especially female athletes

participating in lean body appearance sports or in sports in which leanness and/or specific weight are considered important factors. However, there is a lack of research pertaining to disordered eating and eating disorders in the sport of college cheerleading, a sport in which body appearance and leanness is highly desired.

It is known that many athletes use extreme measures when dealing with the insecurities about their body weight and turn to disordered eating and/or eating disorders to meet their goals of low body weight and body fat percentage. Although there are many factors contributing to the onset of disordered eating and eating disorders, perceived body image of the athlete can play a major role in the onset of these illnesses.

It appears that cheerleading can be considered an "at-risk sport" for the development of eating disorders. Therefore, it is the purpose of this study to investigate the specific factors which may influence eating disorders among this special population of females. (Musser 2002)

The author concisely summarizes the literature related to eating disorders and disordered eating among female athletes and points out a large gap in the literature concerning college female cheerleaders, a group at high risk for developing eating orders. The author concluded that more research must be done to investigate the factors that might influence eating behaviors of college female cheerleaders.

WRITING CHAPTER THREE: PROCEDURES

The third chapter of a research proposal deals with the procedures for collecting data. Alternative titles for chapter three are "Procedures," "Methodology," "Experimental Procedures," and "Survey Procedures." All proposals must include a detailed and appropriate **data collection plan** for attacking the problem. Earlier in the proposal (primarily in chapter one), the rationale for selecting certain methods, techniques, and procedures was presented as background information for the problem. However, a more detailed rationale is needed in chapter three. The entire research proposal is like a contract between the student researcher and a faculty committee. If the research study is conducted as proposed, the committee cannot seriously complain about the procedures at the final defense meeting. Hence the procedures section becomes extremely critical. The soundness of the study will depend on the appropriateness of the planned attack on the research problem. The reader will analyze this section closely and relate the

Data collection plan Detailed procedure for acquiring the information needed to attack the research problem.

methods, techniques, and procedures to the relative quality of the research data to be obtained.

The procedures chapter is considered to be the "cookbook" or "recipe" portion of the proposal or research report. Its presentation requires much attention to detail as the researcher illuminates the reader about where the data came from (sources), how the data were gathered (collection methods), and how the data were analyzed (treatment). This step-by-step set of instructions for conducting the investigation should be so detailed that if another researcher wanted to replicate the study, there would be no trouble in doing so. The reader should not have to make any assumptions about what or how something was done in the research situation.

Normally, chapter three of the research proposal will consist of an introductory paragraph, which restates the purpose of the study and foretells the organization of the chapter, and then specific sections related to the research participants, research design, instrumentation, procedures, and data analysis. The following items provide a framework for determining the content of chapter three:

1. A discussion of the research participants and the sampling techniques used for obtaining them.
2. A discussion of the tests, instruments, or measures that were used to collect the data.
3. A discussion of the design of the study within which the data were collected.
4. A discussion of the administrative procedures used to collect the data.
5. A discussion on how the data were treated or analyzed.

Depending upon the nature of the study, the advice of the faculty adviser, and the whims of the researcher, these five items are translated into a variety of section topics. Following are some topic headings typically found in this section:

- Arrangements for Conducting the Study
- Selection of Participants
- Selection of the Test Instrument(s)
- Development of the Test Instrument(s)
- Instrumentation
- Design of the Study
- Training Program
- Administration of Test

- Procedures for Testing and Gathering Data
- Data Collection Procedures
- Preliminary Investigation
- Pilot Study
- Treatment of Data
- Data Analysis Procedures

The format of the various topical headings selected will depend upon the style manual used at the various institutions. While some sections, "Treatment of Data," for example, do not have to be unduly long, they should clearly describe the procedures and methods that the researcher plans to follow in the conduct of the study. As stated earlier, chapter three constitutes a "recipe for conducting research" and should be written with enough detail and specificity that another researcher having similar expertise would be able to follow the procedures and conduct the study in the same manner by which it was originally done. The following questions can be used as a guide to evaluate the appropriateness of content found in chapter three:

1. Was the population clearly specified?
2. Is the design appropriate to the problem?
3. Were the sampling procedures clearly specified and the total sample adequate?
4. If a control group was involved, was it selected from the same population?
5. Were the various treatments (including control) assigned at random?
6. Were appropriate statistical treatment procedures selected, and was the level of significance selected in advance?
7. Were the reliability and validity of the data-gathering instruments and procedures established and reported?
8. Were the treatments and/or methods of the collection of data described so clearly and completely that an independent investigator could replicate the study?
9. Are the characteristics of the research participants clearly representative of the population?
10. Were extraneous sources of error either held constant or randomized among groups?

See Examples 16.1 through 16.5 for illustrations of the various content areas of chapter three of a research proposal. These examples are taken from research proposals for either a thesis or dissertation developed by former students of the authors of this textbook.

EXAMPLE 16.1
An Opening Paragraph for
Chapter Three

The purpose of this study is to describe selected characteristics of certified substance abuse counselors in the state of Kansas. Specifically, the following characteristics will be considered: education, experience, age, gender, length of time in profession, salary range, and if the counselor considers himself/ herself recovering or not. Also, substance abuse treatment approaches, knowledge, and experiences of the substance abuse counselors were compiled. A description of the research design, subject selection, research instrument, survey procedure, and methods of analysis are discussed in this chapter. (Vogt 2001)

EXAMPLE 16.2
Selection of Research
Participants

Three hundred and ninety-six physical education teachers will be randomly sampled from the population of school physical education teachers currently employed at public or parochial schools in the state of Iowa. The target population of teachers will be classified as either elementary or middle/ junior high or high school physical education teachers. A stratified random sampling technique will be used to select 132 female and male teachers from each grade level. The stratified random sampling technique will ensure equal representation of subjects by gender and by grade level (Huck and Cormier 1996; Krathwohl 1993). In addition, the equal representation of subjects is designed to minimize potential standard error of the difference (Rossi, Wright, and Anderson 1989) and for accurate comparisons by gender and grade level. (Mintah 2001)

EXAMPLE 16.3
Research Design

This study will utilize a pretest-posttest control group, quasi-experimental design. Four intact groups will include college-age females enrolled in (a) an aerobics only course, (b) a course consisting of aerobic training and weight training, (c) a skill only course, and (d) a weight training only course. The control groups will consist of college-age females enrolled in physical activity classes that are not involved in weight training (aerobics only and skills courses). The independent variable is the type of activity (weight training, aerobic conditioning, personal conditioning, and skill courses), and the dependent variable is physical self-concept as measured by the Physical Self-Concept Subscale (PSCS) of the Tennessee Self-Concept Scale (Fitts 1965). (Glew 2001)

EXAMPLE 16.4
Instrumentation

A self-report questionnaire will be used as a means of data collection. The questionnaires to be used in this study consist of the Rosenburg Self-Esteem Scale (1965), the Eating Attitude Test (EAT-26) (Garner et al. 1982), and four open-ended questions designed by the researcher.

Rosenburg's (1965) 10-item self-report questionnaire is designed to measure feelings about the self directly. All items on the questionnaire employ a four-point Likert scale response format with potential responses including (a) strongly agree = 1 point, (b) agree = 2 points, (c) disagree = 3 points, and (d) strongly disagree = 4 points. Questions 3, 5, 8, 9, and 10 are reverse scored items. The total score ranges from 10 to 40, with the lower number representing high self-esteem. The reliability and validity of the Rosenburg Self-Esteem Scale has been examined by a variety of researchers who report acceptable measures for the inventory. Silber and Tippett (1965) reported a test-retest correlation of .85 for 28 subjects after a 2-week interval. Fleming and Courtney (1984) reported a test-retest correlation of .82 for 259 male and female subjects with a 1-week interval. Internal consistency was measured by Dobson, Goudy, Keith, and Powers (1979) who obtained a Cronbach alpha level of .77 for their sample. Measure from the Rosenburg Self-Esteem Scale correlated .72 with the Lerner Self-Esteem Scale, and .27 with peer rating for an adolescent sample (Savin-Williams and Jaquish 1981).

The Eating Attitude Test (EAT-26) (Garner et al. 1982) will be used to examine symptoms commonly associated with anorexia nervosa. The EAT-26 consists of 9 demographic questions, 26 Likert-type questions, and 5 "yes" or "no" questions. The Likert-type scale consists of six potential responses, including 3 points for "always," 2 points for "usually," 1 point for "often," and 0 points for either "sometimes," "rarely," or "never." Question 26 is reverse scored and weighted in the opposite manner. The total EAT-26 score is the sum of all items. This shortened version of the original Eating Attitudes Test-40 has been shown to be a reliable substitute (r = .98) (Wilkins et al. 1989). Furthermore, internal consistency was shown to be Cronbach's alpha = .90 (Wilkins et al. 1989).

Four open-ended questions developed by the researcher will be used to obtain information on subjects' desires or triggers to lose weight. The questions were written in accordance with the guidelines by Gulbrium and Hostein (1997), *The New Language of Qualitative Methods.* (Fey 1998)

EXAMPLE 16.5
Data Treatment and
Analysis

The data collected from the self-report questionnaire will consist of two separate scores from the Rosenburg Self-Esteem Scale and the EAT-26 test, and qualitative responses from the four open-ended questions. A total score above 20 on the EAT-26 is considered to be in the "at risk" range for developing eating disorders according to Garner et al. (1982). Total scores on the Rosenburg Self-Esteem Scale can range from 10–40, with the lower score representing higher self-esteem. Body mass index (BMI) will also be computed for each subject based on the self-reported height and weight.

A Pearson product-moment correlation will be used to examine the relationship among the scores on the Rosenburg Self-Esteem Scale, the EAT-26, current weight, and BMI. A .05 probability level will be used to determine significance. Furthermore, descriptive statistics will be calculated for all dependent variables. All analyses will be performed using SPSS 9.0 software (PC version). (Fey 1988)

Summary of Objectives

1. **Understand the purpose of the research proposal.**
The research proposal provides a written account of the proposed research, explaining the problem under investigation, the rationale for the study, and the procedures that will be followed in the investigation. The proposal typically serves as the primary basis of approval of a research project, be it from a dissertation committee, the editor of a publication, or a funding agency.

2. **Recognize the basic parts of a research proposal.** While formats vary from institution to institution, there are four generally accepted parts in a research proposal. The title alerts readers to what lies ahead, and is an important part of the proposal. Chapter one is usually an introduction that leads the reader into the problem. Chapter two offers a review of existing literature, and chapter three details the procedures and methodology that will be used in the research.

Writing the Research Report

17

OBJECTIVES

This chapter offers a basic overview of the research report. The function of a research report is to communicate a set of ideas and facts to those who are interested in the problem area in which the research was undertaken. Whereas there is no universally accepted format for the research proposal and resultant research report, most tend to follow a similar style.

After reading Chapter 17, you should be able to

1. Determine the characteristics of a good research report.
2. Understand the format for a report and the kinds of information required in each division of the report.
3. Differentiate between the style of writing in a research report for a thesis or dissertation and a research report for publication in a journal.

The culmination of the research process is the disclosure of the findings to other professionals or interested persons. The researcher may present her or his findings through a journal article, a report to a sponsoring agency, a thesis or dissertation, an online publication, or a presentation at a professional conference. Traditionally, a written **research report** has been the option of choice. The purpose of the written research report, whether a master's thesis, doctoral dissertation, or journal article, is to convey ideas and facts generated by the research to those who will read the report. To be effective, the information must be communicated in a manner that is clear and easily understood. Clarity is fundamental. The process of writing a research report is essentially the same as writing the proposal, except in this case the report is written in past tense and new information is added that describes the findings and what they mean.

> **Research report**
> A scientific paper completed at the culmination of a research project in which the results of the investigation are presented to others.

The reader should not be required to guess how the research was performed or have to make any assumptions about what was found. The reader should hold no doubts or questions about the meaning of any statement included in the report. Besides clarity, other important characteristics of the report include (1) organization, or the logic underlying the order in which the various parts of the report appear and the degree to which the transition between parts is clear and smooth; (2) good and correct presentation, which includes adherence to proper spelling, grammar, diction, punctuation, and the mechanics of a systematic format for presentation of the research material; (3) completeness, meaning that the total body of facts should be presented to enhance clarity; and (4) conciseness, an elimination of any material adding unnecessary length to the report rather than adding to its completeness and clarity.

FORMAT OF THE REPORT

Thesis format
Traditional, generic format of a research report prepared by graduate students in which the body of the report is organized within specific chapters, such as, introduction, review of literature, procedures or methods, results and discussion, and conclusions.

Graduate students completing a thesis or dissertation are often required by their respective colleges or universities to follow a particular **thesis format** for organizing and presenting the report. If the institution has no established requirement, then the college, school, division, or department of kinesiology probably will. Various published and standardized formats are used, although special modifications are frequently made by the institution or department. Before commencing the written report, students are expected to become familiar with the prescribed style and format required at their institution.

Published research reports must conform to the style and format specified by the selected journal. The researcher is expected to check the format required and carefully follow the prescribed guidelines. The most frequently used style manuals include the *Publication Manual of the American Psychological Association,* 6th ed. (2010), *MLA Handbook for Writers of Research Papers,* 7th ed. (Gibaldi 2009), the *Chicago Manual of Style,* 16th ed. (2010), *Form and Style: Research Papers, Reports, Theses,* 11th ed. (Salde and Perrin 2009), and *A Manual for Writers of Term Papers, Theses, and Dissertations,* 7th ed. (Turabian 2007).

DIVISIONS OF A THESIS OR DISSERTATION

Preliminary items
Front matter of a thesis or dissertation that includes items such as a title page, approval page, acknowledgments page, table of contents, list of tables and figures, and an abstract; introductory material in a published research report; may include title, author, institution, acknowledgments, and abstract.

Usually, a research report, such as a thesis or dissertation, is arranged in three major parts: preliminary items, the text or body of the report, and supplementary items.

Preliminary Items

The **preliminary items** usually included are the title page, approval page, acknowledgments page, table of contents, list of tables, list of figures, and abstract. Examples 17.1 to 17.4 provide samples of these items completed by former students of the authors of this textbook.

EXAMPLE 17.1
Title Page
From Fey (1998).

RELATIONSHIP BETWEEN SELF-ESTEEM, EATING BEHAVIORS, AND EATING ATTITUDES AMONG FEMALE COLLEGIATE SWIMMERS

A Thesis Submitted
in Partial Fulfillment
of the Requirements for the Degree
Master of Arts

Melissa Ann Fey
University of Northern Iowa
July 1998

EXAMPLE 17.2
Approval Page
From Fey (1998).

This Study by: Melissa A. Fey

Entitled: Relationship between Self-Esteem, Eating Behaviors, and Eating Attitudes among Female Collegiate Swimmers

Has been approved as meeting the thesis requirement for the

Degree of Master of Arts in Physical Education

_____

Date   Chair, Thesis Committee

_____

Date   Thesis Committee Member

_____

Date   Thesis Committee Member

_____

Date   Dean, Graduate College

EXAMPLE 17.3
Acknowledgments Page

Acknowledgments

I would like to express my sincere gratitude to Dr. _____,
Dr. _____, and Dr. _____
for their assistance and guidance in this investigation. The author is
especially indebted to Dr. _____ whose help and
encouragement were invaluable to the completion of this study.

Special thanks are offered to the author's new young friends and their
teachers who provided their time and energy so generously during the
data-collection process.

EXAMPLE 17.4
Abstract

Abstract

The general purpose of this study was to investigate the role of parental influence on children's physical activity (PA) behaviors. The specific purposes were to (1) determine the relationship between parental attitudes and their children's PA, (2) determine if parental exercise habits are related to their children's PA participation, (3) determine if parental knowledge of physical activity recommendations is related to their children's PA participation, (4) examine the nature of parenting practices on their children's PA participation, and (5) investigate the mediating effect of socio-economic status on the influence parents have on their children's PA participation.

Questionnaires were obtained from 5th and 6th grade parents and children at two schools in Iowa. To assess the physical activity behaviors of the participants, children completed the Physical Activity Questionnaire for Children, PAQ(C). Parents completed a questionnaire consisting of five sections: demographics, parental exercise behavior, parenting practices scale, physical activity knowledge scale, and exercise benefits and barriers scale.

Data were collected on 57 fifth and sixth grade parents and students during fall semester 2010. The study sample included 28 girls and 29 boys. Students ranged in age from 9 to 12 years, with a mean age of 10.6 years. The parents ranged from 29–52 years, with a mean age of 34.9 years.

The results of the study showed that parental influences do not have a large impact on children's physical activity. No significance was found between parental physical activity behaviors or attitude/beliefs and children's physical activity behavior. The majority of the parenting practice items did illustrate a weak, positive correlation while parental knowledge results showed a weak negative correlation with children's physical activity behavior. Socioeconomic status did not impact the correlations between the parental variables and children's physical activity behavior. There are many factors that influence the physical activity behaviors of children outside of parents and future research should investigate other potential factors.

(Eshelman 2010)

Abstract

Example 17.4 is a sample of an abstract for a master's thesis. Most institutions require an abstract varying in length from 250 to 350 words. The abstract is one of the preliminary items of the thesis or dissertation. Most research journals also require an abstract when researchers submit an article for publication. Though the length requirement varies among the journals, 150 to 200 words is typical. The researcher should use all of whatever abstract length is allowed, because the more that can be reported to the reader, the greater the chance for good understanding of the research. Often abstracts are written as a single paragraph but sometimes may include separate paragraphs for each section.

An abstract must be concise but should include enough detail to enable the reader to determine whether or not the entire research report, article, thesis, or dissertation needs to be read. The abstract should be brief and contain the overall essence of the information included in the larger work. The reader should be able to glean from the abstract all the main ideas of the original research investigation.

An appropriate abstract will usually include comments concerning each of the following elements:

1. The *problem* that was investigated, including the rationale from which the problem was developed.
2. The *methods* by which the data for the problem were collected. Included here will be an identification of the variables studied, the procedure used in carrying out the research and collecting the data, and a discussion of how the data were analyzed.
3. A brief report of the *findings* resulting from the study. These results are usually not given in tables, figures, and graphs due to the limitations placed on the length of an abstract.
4. The *conclusions* made by the researcher based upon the findings. If room in the abstract exists, it could also include the researcher's interpretation of the possible implementation of the results or recommendations for further research in the problem area.

The Body or Text of the Report

In the traditional thesis or dissertation format, the text or body of the report for most descriptive and experimental studies usually consists of five chapters. The first three chapters (introduction, review of related literature, and procedures or methods) were discussed in detail earlier in Chapter 16. Under ideal conditions, the first three chapters of the research proposal will serve as the opening chapters of the final thesis or dissertation (Locke, Spirduso, and Silverman 2007). Converting the first three chapters of the proposal into the opening chapters of the final report may require only a changing of the tense of verbs, updating the review of literature, and, if necessary, altering the procedures section to reflect exactly what took place in the study. Chapter four, covering the results and discussion, and chapter five, which includes the summary, conclusions, and recommendations, make up the remainder of the body of the thesis or dissertation. Note that some institutions and faculty advisors prefer that chapter four merely present the results, with no discussion, and that chapter five include a discussion of the findings along with the conclusions and recommendations. A brief overview of the first three chapters is presented below, followed by a more detailed description of chapters four and five, including several examples illustrating their content.

Chapter One: Introduction.   The introduction chapter of the thesis or dissertation is designed to present the research question to the reader, including the underlying rationale for the study. A specific purpose statement will clearly and concisely identify the goals for the research study. The chapter will also contain information about the scope of the study (delimitations), assumptions that are made by the researcher, limitations or weaknesses of the study, as well as research hypotheses, if appropriate. In addition, key terms as they are interpreted and used throughout the study are defined.

Chapter Two: Review of Related Literature.   This is a report of previous investigations related to the problem being studied. Theoretical formulations from other studies, the major issues of methodology, instrumentation, interpretation, and background information are presented. It is a well-organized chapter that shows how the present study may differ from previous ones and, at the same time, add to their contributions. Knowledge gaps in the problem area are noted. Through a review of the literature, a theoretical basis and justification for the present study are formed.

Chapter Three: Procedures or Methods.   This is a systematic and careful plan for attacking the problem. The procedures, methods, and techniques are detailed in a step-by-step set of instructions for conducting the study. The topics frequently included are selection of research participants, instrumentation, design of the study, administrative procedures for collecting the data, and treatment of the data.

Chapter Four: Results and Discussion.   This is the reporting chapter of the thesis or dissertation in which the researcher (1) presents the data and (2) discusses and interprets those data. This chapter should begin with an opening paragraph that restates the purpose of the study and may also include information regarding the content and organization of the chapter (Example 17.5). Following that paragraph will be several sections in which the data analysis and/or findings will be reported. Typical items that need to be included in these sections are the following: (1) demographic information pertaining to the research participants, (2) descriptive information for the various measures, and

(3) the results of the data analysis. Tables are often used to present statistical information that supplement the written narrative. See Examples 17.6 to 17.8.

EXAMPLE 17.5
Opening Paragraph
Adapted from Visker (1986).

The problem of the study was to determine if the psychological factors of self-consciousness and physical self-efficacy discriminate between female adults who adhere to exercise programs and female adults who do not adhere to exercise programs. Included in the study was an attempt to identify the reasons exercise adherers give for continuing an exercise program and the reasons exercise nonadherers give for discontinuing exercise programs. The analysis of the data is presented in this chapter according to the following topics: (1) data-gathering instrument distribution, (2) demographic data, (3) chi-square analysis, (4) discriminant analysis data, (5) multiple regression data, (6) reasons for continuing or discontinuing an exercise program, and (7) discussion of findings.

Note that the emphasis in the first section of chapter four is usually on reporting only, with no editorializing, discussion, or interpretation included. The standard procedure is to introduce a table containing data, present the table, and point out the significant findings in the table. The report of the data and findings should be followed by a detailed discussion and interpretation of the findings. This final

EXAMPLE 17.6
Reporting Participant
Characteristics
Adapted from Kwon (2006).

Characteristics of Participants

The physical characteristics of the research participants are shown in Table 1. Mean (with SD in parentheses) age was 13.1 (0.6) years, mean BMI was 21.8 (5.2) kg/m^2. There were no significant differences in age and BMI by sex ($p > .05$).

TABLE 1 Characteristics of Participants

VARIABLES	BOYS ($N = 66$)		GIRLS ($N = 74$)		TOTAL ($N = 140$)		
	M	SD	M	SD	M	SD	P
Age (years)	13.00	0.60	13.20	0.70	13.10	0.60	.09
Height (m)	1.59	1.00	1.59	0.65	1.59	0.83	.83
Weight (kg)	56.30	16.40	54.30	12.90	55.20	14.70	.44
BMI (kg/m^2)	22.20	5.70	21.40	4.70	21.80	5.20	.37

EXAMPLE 17.7
Data Reporting
Adapted from Crimi (2007).

Reporting Descriptive Information

Psychosocial values for each gender group are shown in Table 4. The results of the ANOVA indicate no interaction between grade and gender for any of the psychosocial factors. Perceived competence [$F(1,161) = 24.09$, $p < .05$, $ES = 0.14$], liking of games [$F(1,161) = 9.34$, $p < .05$, $ES = 0.06$], fun of exertion [$F(1,161) = 7.23$, $p < .05$, $ES = 0.05$], and self-esteem [$F(1,161) = 6.88$, $p < .05$, $ES = .01$] were significantly different between genders. For all of these factors, the mean scores for boys were significantly higher than girls, although effect size values would be considered small for each.

TABLE 4 Descriptive Statistics for Psychosocial Subscales by Gender

PSYCHOSOCIAL VARIABLE	BOYS $M \pm SD$	GIRLS $M \pm SD$	TOTAL $M \pm SD$
Likes games/sports	3.63 ± .57	3.26 ± .75	3.43 ± .70
Fun of physical exertion	3.44 ± .66	3.15 ± .56	3.28 ± .62
Likes exercise	3.51 ± .57	3.41 ± .62	3.46 ± .60
Importance of exercise	3.59 ± .53	3.61 ± .49	3.60 ± .51
Peer acceptance	3.25 ± .71	2.96 ± .80	3.09 ± .77
Perceived competence	3.38 ± .50	2.88 ± .68	3.11 ± .65
Self-esteem	3.43 ± .64	3.07 ± .75	3.23 ± .72
Parental role-modeling	2.82 ± .64	2.96 ± .68	2.90 ± .66
Parental support	3.12 ± .51	3.05 ± .53	3.08 ± .52
Parental encouragement	3.44 ± .45	3.40 ± .46	3.42 ± .45

section of the chapter may be labeled "Discussion of Findings." Here are some questions and thoughts concerning this section:

1. Are there any explanations for any of the findings? If so, these thoughts should be shared with the reader.

2. Do some findings defy explanation? Are some really surprising? If so, what are they? Speculate why these particular results may have come about in this way.

3. In answering the questions posed in 1 and 2 above, the element of hindsight in the procedure sometimes enters the discussion. The hindsight may be clear to the researcher, but not to the reader; so share that hindsight with the reader.

4. Are the findings consistent with findings in similar studies? Do the findings differ?

EXAMPLE 17.8
Analysis Reporting
Adapted from Crimi (2007).

Correlations

Correlational analyses indicated that all ten psychosocial variables were significantly related to children's physical activity (see Table 5). The subscale with the single highest correlation for boys was "likes exercise" with an $r = 0.61$, whereas "likes sports/games" had the highest correlation for girls with $r = 0.44$. In addition, the inter-relationships among the ten psychosocial variables were low to moderate, ranging from 0.28 to 0.66.

TABLE 5 Correlations Between Psychosocial Variables and Physical Activity Scores

PSYCHOSOCIAL VARIABLE	BOYS	GIRLS
Likes games/sports	.38**	.44**
Fun of physical exertion	.37**	.25*
Likes exercise	.61**	.41**
Importance of exercise	.42**	.41**
Peer acceptance	.41**	.28**
Perceived competence	.50*	.41**
Self-esteem	.31**	.28**
Parental role-modeling	.27*	.23*
Parental support	.39**	.32**
Parental encouragement	.45**	.31**

* $p < .05$; ** $p < .01$

This part of the research report is often difficult to accomplish, but a feeling of satisfaction accompanies its completion. For an excellent example illustrating how some researchers have incorporated the information included in the comments made above, see Example 17.9.

Chapter Five: Summary, Conclusions, and Recommendations. This is the final and, typically, the shortest chapter in a thesis or dissertation. A summary of the study as well as the general conclusions and recommendations resulting from the research should be placed in this chapter. Only material mentioned earlier in the report may be included in the summary.

In the summary, the purpose of the study should be restated, a general overview of the sources of data and the methods used should be provided, and the more

EXAMPLE 17.9
Discussion of Findings
Adapted from Visker (1986).

The consistency in determining the significant contribution of perceived physical ability in the study was similar to the findings of other studies using perceived physical ability as a variable. Snyder and Spreitzer (1984), Spreitzer and Snyder (1983), and Spreitzer (1981) found significant correlations between perceived athletic ability and involvement in vigorous physical activities. The finding of the present study reiterates the position that the higher an individual perceives her physical abilities to be, the more likely she will be to continue with an exercise program.

The findings of the study also supported Sonstroem's Physical Activity Model (1978, 1976, 1974). Sonstroem theorized that as one's estimation of physical ability increases, so will one's attraction to physical activity, which will result in an increase in physical activity. In the present study, the subjects who scored higher in perceived physical ability also were engaged in more minutes per week of vigorous physical activity than subjects who scored lower in perceived physical ability.

Since the data in the study were analyzed using multivariate correlational techniques, it would be inappropriate to suggest that a woman's perception of her physical abilities caused her to adhere to or discontinue an exercise program. All that can be inferred from this finding is that a significant positive relationship does exist between a woman's perceived physical ability and the likelihood that she will continue with an exercise program.

The lack of scientific inquiry into reasons for adhering to a program of exercise makes it difficult to draw parallels to other investigations. However, several of the reasons given for adhering to an exercise program have been investigated in other studies. Many of the reasons address the situational factors in which the exercise program is carried out. This alone provides credence to Dishman's (1984) conceptual model for exercise adherence which posits that whether a person stays with an exercise program or not is determined by an interaction between the exerciser and his or her environment. Specially the social reason of exercising with others has been found to be significant in other studies. Heinzelman and Bagley (1970) found that 90 percent of the subjects in their investigation preferred to exercise with others. Massie and Shepard (1971) found that exercise adherence was higher for subjects who exercised as a group than for subjects who exercised alone.

EXAMPLE 17.9
Concluded

Exercise and mental health have been the subject of many research investigations (Sach 1984; Folkins and Sime 1981; Morgan 1981). It has consistently been shown that regular vigorous physical activity will enhance one's mental health. The frequency of the response of enhancing mental health found in this investigation is consistent with that found in other studies.

The exercise environment was also cited as a reason for adhering to an exercise program. One factor in the exercise environment which was specifically mentioned was the use of music. The use of music in an exercise setting is a dissociative technique which focuses the exerciser's attention away from the discomfort of exercise, resulting in more enjoyable exercise bouts. Martin et al. (1984) found dissociative intervention strategy to be effective in increasing exercise adherence.

Several studies have investigated the reasons individuals give for discontinuing exercise programs (Lee and Owen 1985; Andrew et al. 1981; Boothy, Tungatt, and Townsend 1981). Two of the reasons exercise nonadherers cited in the present study are consistent with earlier findings. Perhaps the most frequent reason given for discontinuing an exercise program is lack of time. The frequency of this reason in the present study is parallel to studies by Boothby, Tungatt, and Townsend (1981); Gettman, Pollock, and Ward, (1983); and Lee and Owen (1985).

The distance traveled to the exercise setting was also cited as a reason for dropping out of an exercise program. While the frequency of this response is not as high as the response of lack of time, this response is consistent with other studies (Lee and Owen 1985; Andrew and Parker 1979; and Morgan 1977).

Because the present investigation was composed entirely of women, some of the reasons given for adhering to or discontinuing an exercise program were unique to this investigation. Many of these reasons deal with traditional female roles. For example some of the reasons given for adhering to an exercise program are the availability of babysitting services and reversing the effects of childbirth.

However, the fact that the response of demands of employment was one of the most frequent responses given for discontinuing an exercise program is, perhaps, an indication of the changing nature of women's roles in society.

important findings should be listed. For this reporting of the findings, brief statements will suffice rather than repeating the details already discussed.

General conclusions drawn from the findings should be presented in the same order as the hypotheses stated at the beginning of the research. The conclusions should be definitive and bring the study to an end. Conclusions should not be repetitions or summaries of findings but should answer this question: The data (findings) say this, so what does this tell me as to the conclusion that is warranted? Conclusions beyond the data obtained (i.e., the findings) should not be made. In stating the conclusions, avoid the use of "hedging" phrases, such as "It seems as though" or "It appears that." The data tell the researcher what is or is not, and the conclusion statements should reflect such definitiveness. The distinction between a finding and the conclusion should be made abundantly clear.

The recommendation section should appear last in the chapter, and the recommendations may be of more than one type. The researcher may recommend that certain specified actions be taken in light of the findings. How can the findings be used in a practical situation, or in what ways would the findings make a contribution to professional practice? This reflects how the researcher envisions the findings being applied. In addition, the researcher may recommend that further study be made of the problem by using either the same data or a different sample or that a study be made of a related problem or of the same problem in greater detail or after a certain length of time has elapsed. A typical chapter five of a thesis or dissertation is illustrated in Example 17.10.

References

The body of the text is always followed by a list of references organized according to the prescribed style manual required by the students' college or university or academic unit. With a relatively short list of sources to be referenced, different types of literary pieces may be incorporated. However, if the list of sources is quite long, they may be grouped according to type, such as books, documents, manuscripts, newspapers, pamphlets, and periodicals. The usual convention is to include only those sources that were referenced in the text. Occasionally, it may be necessary to include a source that was not cited, but the usual caution is not to pad the list of references.

Supplementary Items

Supplementary items
Back matter of a thesis or dissertation that includes items such as questionnaires, consent documents, instructions to research participants, diagrams of research settings, and tables of raw data.

The appendixes serve as the repository for **supplementary items** that are unnecessary for inclusion in the body of the text, but can be used by the reader to clarify various aspects of the thesis or research report. They provide additional

Summary

The problem of the study was to determine if the psychological factors of self-efficacy discriminate between female adults who adhere to exercise programs and female adults who do not adhere to exercise programs. Included in the study was an attempt to identify the reasons exercise adherers give for continuing an exercise program and the reasons exercise nonadherers give for discontinuing an exercise program.

The subjects of the study were 168 females who had enrolled in physical fitness classes at the Monroe County YMCA, Bloomington, Indiana, during the spring of 1985. All subjects completed a survey instrument consisting of the self-consciousness scale, the physical self-efficacy scale, and questions designed to determine demographic data and exercise habits. The data for the study were collected during the months of May and June 1986.

The data were analyzed using four statistical techniques. Chi-square test of association was used to test the differences in fitness class attended, education level, and marital status between exercise adherers and nonadherers. Discriminant analysis was used to determine if the independent variables of private self-consciousness, perceived physical self-efficacy, age, and income could significantly predict the dependent variables of group membership (exercise adherer or nonadherer). Multiple regression analysis was used to determine if the independent variables of the study could significantly predict the number of minutes per week spent in vigorous physical activity. Finally, a frequency distribution of the reasons exercise adherers gave for continuing an exercise program and the reasons exercise nonadherers gave for discontinuing an exercise program was done. The Statistical Package for the Social Sciences (SPSS) was used for all statistical analysis except the frequency distributions.

The analysis of the data revealed the following significant findings:

1. The independent variables of private self-consciousness, public self-consciousness, social anxiety, self-consciousness, perceived physical ability, physical self-presentation confidence, physical self-efficacy, age, and income significantly predicted group membership as an exercise adherer or nonadherer.

2. The independent variable of perceived physical ability and physical self-efficacy accounted for most of the function which discriminated between exercise adherers and nonadherers.

EXAMPLE 17.10
Sample of a Chapter Five
Adapted from Visker (1986).

EXAMPLE 17.10
Continued

3. The optimal linear combination of the independent variables of private self-consciousness, social anxiety, perceived physical ability, physical self-presentation confidence, physical self-efficacy, age, education level, marital status, and income, taken altogether, significantly predicted the number of minutes per week spent in vigorous physical activity.

4. By itself, only perceived physical ability significantly predicted the number of minutes per week spent in vigorous physical activity.

5. The most frequent reasons given by exercise adherers for continuing an exercise program were to maintain health, social status, enhance mental health, relieve stress, and appearance.

6. The most frequent reasons given by exercise nonadherers for discontinuing an exercise program were lack of time, demands of employment, schedule conflicts, demands of children, and illness or injury.

Conclusions

Within the limitations of the study the following conclusions are warranted:

1. Significant psychological differences exist between female exercise adherers and nonadherers.

2. Females who adhere to a program of exercise perceive their physical abilities at a higher level than do females who discontinue a program of physical exercise.

3. Self-consciousness is not an important factor in the psychological differences between female exercise adherers and nonadherers.

4. Females who have a higher perception of their physical abilities exercise more than do females who have a lower perception of their physical abilities.

Recommendations

The following recommendations are made for further research in the area of exercise adherence:

1. The present study should be replicated using both male and female participants.

EXAMPLE 17.10
Concluded

2. The relationship of self-consciousness and physical self-efficacy to exercise adherence should be examined in an experimental type of study. This would permit more control in the variable of exercise adherence since it would not rely on the subjects' truthfulness regarding their exercise habits.

3. A study should be conducted to determine the cause-and-effect relationship between perceived physical ability and exercise adherence.

4. Additional studies identifying other psychological variables which could be related to exercise adherence are needed.

5. The present investigation should be replicated in other communities to gain a large cross-section of the adult population from which data can be obtained.

6. The psychological variables of self-consciousness and physical self-efficacy related to exercise adherence should be investigated in a nonstructured exercise program setting.

7. Additional studies identifying reasons exercise adherers give for continuing an exercise program are needed to corroborate the findings of the present study.

The findings of the study may be implemented into either a professional practice situation or a research setting in the following ways:

1. The significance of perceived physical ability to discriminate between female exercise adherers and nonadherers should be considered in developing psychological profiles of exercise.

2. Adherence to an exercise program could be enhanced by the use of intervention strategies designed to increase the participants' perception of their physical ability. Programs involving the use of progression in skills and intensity of training could increase one's self-perception of physical ability and thereby increase the likelihood of an individual continuing in those exercise programs.

3. If exercise adherence is one of the major goals in physical activity programs, the enhancement of one's self-perceived physical abilities should be a major concern in elementary and secondary physical education programs. Exposure to a variety of skills will increase the likelihood of finding an activity in which the skills can be mastered, thus increasing the chance for regular lifelong participation in that activity.

specific information if the reader desires it. Typically appendixes include the following types of items:

1. Copies of the instruments (e.g., questionnaires, interview guides)
2. Instructions to participants on how to engage in physical performance tests (e.g., fitness, skill tests)
3. Letters and similar documents
4. Human participant consent forms
5. Raw data from both a pilot study and the actual study
6. Diagrams of testing settings
7. Tables from related research
8. Supplementary reference lists
9. Credentials of the members of a jury of experts or committee of authorities
10. Interview and other data collection schedules
11. Legal codes

All such materials should be clearly labeled and lettered for quick and easy reference. Each appendix should bear a descriptive title of what is included.

THESIS FORMAT VERSUS PUBLISHED ARTICLE FORMAT

On the foregoing pages, the format for a thesis or dissertation was described in some detail. The major difference between a thesis or dissertation and a published research report is the length of the document. Researchers who publish articles are limited by the established publishing criteria of particular journals in the amount of detail they can submit. A six- to eight-page article, as prescribed by a specific publication, cannot possibly include all the information contained in a 150-page thesis or dissertation. Although the precise **article format** may vary depending upon the nature of the research, a published research report typically includes the following elements:

Article format
Alternative form of a research report prepared by graduate students whose format is based upon the style specified by the journal in which the student hopes to publish the manuscript.

1. Preliminary information
   a. Title
   b. Author and organizational affiliation
   c. Acknowledgments (if any)
   d. Abstract

2. Introduction
   a. Background information and literature review
   b. Rationale for study
   c. Purpose statement
   d. Hypotheses or research questions
3. Methods
   a. Participants
   b. Instrumentation
   c. Procedures
   d. Statistical analysis
4. Results
   a. Presentation of data
5. Discussion
   a. Conclusions
   b. Recommendations
6. References
7. Appendix (if appropriate)

The style in which the published article is written will also be determined by whatever style manual is followed by the journal. Quite frequently, the style will be different from that found in a thesis or dissertation. Capitalization may differ, as will punctuation, the spelling of numbers, and abbreviations.

Theses or dissertations written by graduate students are considered "final" manuscripts. They usually have a long life span and will be read and referred to over a long time. A journal manuscript tends to be a "copy" manuscript that, in turn, becomes a typeset article. Copy manuscripts have a relatively short life. They are read by reviewers, editors, and typeset experts. The original content can sometimes be changed dramatically as a result of the publication process.

Students who complete a thesis or dissertation are encouraged to publish one or more articles derived from their study. Preparation of an article entails transposing selected thesis content to journal material according to the publishing restrictions of the journal in which the article will appear. This is not a particularly difficult task, although some people find it to be a laborious chore. Some confuse transposition with creating a whole new document. Students who write a thesis under one format are sometimes confused in following the guidelines imposed by the journal format requirements.

In recent years, some institutions, including those of the authors of this textbook, have adopted regulations that enable students to write their theses and dissertations in the form required by those journals in which the students hope to publish articles based upon their research. This would result in documents of 20 to 30 pages in length and containing only the essential information from the literature, procedures, and results sections. The more detailed information from the other thesis sections would become part of appendices. The underlying idea is to make it quicker and easier for the student to create a journal article for publication from a document written to fulfill a degree requirement. Relatively few theses or dissertations written using the traditional format end up being published. This alternative format for a thesis or dissertation may enhance the likelihood that research conducted to satisfy a degree requirement will contribute new knowledge to the field. Readers are encouraged to read the excellent article by Thomas, Nelson, and Magill (1986), who advocate for use of the journal format for theses and dissertations. Whether or not the movement away from the traditional thesis format will become large scale is yet to be seen.

PREPARING A MANUSCRIPT FOR PUBLICATION

The decision to prepare a manuscript for publication represents a commitment to building the body of knowledge within a given subject area. A published manuscript serves as a primary communication document for a profession and, as such, has the potential to advance theory and inform professional practice. Publishing a manuscript based upon one's own research can be one of the most exciting and professionally rewarding experiences for both young scholars and seasoned veterans. The process is often challenging and requires perseverance. We have outlined below several suggestions that should be considered as you begin the task of preparing a manuscript for publication.

Before Writing

Prior to starting to prepare a manuscript for publication, the researcher should do several things. One, the researcher needs to select the journal to which the manuscript will be submitted. Two, the researcher needs to examine articles published in that journal to get a general idea of the format used and needs to read the guidelines for submitting manuscripts to the journal. Guidelines are published in the journal. Select the journal primarily on its orientation and type of reader. Some journals are geared primarily toward researchers; others are more for practitioners. Some journals are highly specialized, while others are for a general audience. There is no use in submitting a manuscript to a journal that does not publish the type of research described in the manuscript. Also, the researcher should try to determine the manuscript acceptance rate of the journal.

Acceptance rates vary from 10 percent for very prestigious and specialized research journals to as high as 70 percent or more for practical, general-audience state association journals.

By looking at articles in the selected journal, the researcher may discover a useful model to follow. Certainly the researcher will be able to determine whether an abstract is required as part of the manuscript, what organization and major headings are required in the manuscript, and the typical length of a manuscript based on the length of articles in the journal.

During Writing

Any manuscript starts with the title of the research study. The title needs to be short yet represent the research well and stimulate a person to read the entire article. If an abstract is required, that element appears next in the manuscript; it should be one to three paragraphs long. The abstract will contain the statement of purpose for the study, description of the research participants, major procedures, major results, and conclusions.

The manuscript for most published articles begins with an introduction and brief review of the most important related literature. Somewhere, wherever appropriate, there should be a statement of the purpose of the study. This part of the manuscript is typically three to six paragraphs. Next in a manuscript is a procedures or methods section. Typically included in this section are descriptions of research participants, how the research was conducted, data collection techniques, and data analysis procedures. The content and length of this section is dependent on the type of research conducted and the complexity of describing how the research was conducted. Tables and figures in this section are commonly used to clearly and economically present information. Not every small point concerning the conduct of the research can be presented, or the manuscript could not be kept to a reasonable length.

A results section follows the procedures section. This section usually makes up a relatively large portion of the manuscript because it includes all the major data analysis and findings of the research study. Much of this information is presented in text form; however, the use of tables and figures is also common. The recommended organization when using tables and figures is to introduce a table or figure, present it, and then discuss it. This is not always possible, but the recommendation is a good rule of thumb. The discussion following the table or figure may be just a short sentence or two with the extensive discussion in a later section, or it may be quite extensive. The decision to present major discussion in this section or in a later section is left to the researcher. The majority of researchers probably place the extensive discussion in the next section.

The discussion and conclusions section are where the results previously reported are discussed at length and conclusions based on the results are stated. This part of the manuscript is usually of considerable length. The discussion may include comments on each finding followed by a discussion of all the findings as a whole. However, if each finding was discussed at length when introduced in the results section, then the discussion is reserved for the findings as a whole. Often included in the discussion of findings is a comparison of how the findings agree with those in the literature cited at the beginning of the manuscript. Usually, in the discussion are statements concerning the importance and application of the findings. No matter how the discussion is structured, the conclusions follow it. Anytime the research involves a population from which one or more samples were drawn, conclusions consist of statements concerning what the researcher thinks is true at the population level based on the findings from the samples used in the study.

The last section in a manuscript is a list of references. Included in the list are all sources cited in the manuscript. The length of this section is dependent on the number of sources cited. Normally, it is not a lengthy section and will contain from 10 to 20 listings.

After Writing

After writing the first draft of the manuscript, one must spend considerable time proofing it. Correctness of manuscript form, correctness of content, economy and clarity of presentation, and correctness of spelling and grammar are important. The more prestigious the journal where the manuscript will be submitted, the more important the proofreading.

The spell check and grammar check options on most word processing computer programs are often quite helpful in revising the manuscript. However, they do not catch all problems, and the final responsibility for correctness rests with the writer. Spell check will not catch words left out, the wrong word, confusing sentences, or homonyms. When the manuscript is ready to be submitted to a journal, send the required number of copies and the necessary cover sheet containing author name(s) and contact information. If there are multiple authors, names are listed in order from major contribution to minor contribution to the research and manuscript. Major contributions would include such items as developing the problem, formulating hypotheses, developing the research design, selecting the data analysis procedures, interpreting the findings, and writing the majority of the report.

All manuscripts submitted to a journal are typically evaluated by two to four reviewers or associate editors for the journal. This evaluation takes one to three months. After the manuscript has been evaluated, the journal editor sends copies of the reviews to the author indicating whether the manuscript is accepted, needs revision, or is rejected. Authors should expect that the manuscript will not be acceptable in the form submitted. Thus, when the reviews are returned, revise the manuscript and return it to the original journal, or send it to another journal.

GUIDES TO PREPARATION OF THE RESEARCH REPORT

There exist a plethora of guidebooks and references that are designed to assist in the preparation of both the research proposal and the research report. Many sources are available from the Internet as well. The following list highlights some of our favorites.

Frequently Asked Questions about APA style, www.apastyle.org/.

A Guide for Writing Research Papers, webster.commnet.edu/apa/apa_intro.htm.

Cone, J. D., and Foster, S. L. (2006). *Dissertations and Theses from Start to Finish* (2nd ed.). Washington, DC: American Psychological Association.

Day, R. A., and Gastel, B. (2011). *How to Write and Publish a Scientific Paper* (7th ed.). Westport, CT: Greenwood Press.

Dees, R. (2003). *Writing the Modern Research Paper* (4th ed.). Toronto: Pearson Education Canada.

Locke, L., Spirduso, W., and Silverman, S. (2007). *Proposals That Work: A Guide for Planning Dissertations and Grant Proposals* (5th ed.). Newbury Park, CA: Sage Publications.

Summary of Objectives

1. **Determine the characteristics of a good research report.**
   A well-written report will provide readers with all the information they need to fully understand the nature of the research and findings. The report must be clear, well organized, with proper grammar, spelling, and punctuation. It must also be fairly concise.

2. **Understand the format for a report and the kinds of information required in each division of the report.**
   A research report begins with a few preliminary items, including the title page, approval page, acknowledgments, table of contents, lists of tables and figures, and abstract. The body (or text) of the report offers several chapters, including an introduction to the subject, a review of related literature, procedures or methods, and a discussion of the results. Also included here are the summary, conclusions,

and recommendations, as well as references, and any supplementary items.

3. **Differentiate between the style of writing in a research report for a thesis or dissertation and a research report for publication in a journal.** Students completing research are usually required to follow a style of reporting selected by the university or the students' department. The style for published research will follow a format required by the journal to which the report is submitted for publication. The documents also differ in terms of length: while a thesis or dissertation typically runs over 100 pages, journal articles are generally more restrictive in terms of length.

Appendix A

SPSS for Windows Basics

1. Getting into SPSS (several methods possible)

   A. You should save your data on a data storage device or the computer, so insert a data storage device if needed.
   B. Click on **Start** in the lower left hand corner of the screen and then click on **Program** in the drop down menu.
   C. Click on **SPSS for Windows** in the next menu.
   D. In the SPSS Windows dialog box:
      (1) Click on **Tutorial** and then **OK** if you want information on using SPSS.
      (2) Click on **Type in Data** and then **OK** if you want to enter data.
      (3) Click on **Open an Existing File** and then **OK** if the data is already saved.
   E. Alternative to D.:
      (1) **SPSS Data Editor** window is displayed.
      (2) Click on **File.**
      (3) Select the data entry option desired.

2. Entering the data

   A. Click on the **SPSS Data Editor** window title bar to make it the active window if it is not already highlighted. At the bottom of the window are two tabs: (1) Data View—to enter the data, edit the data, and see the data; and (2) Variable View—to name variables, and define variables. When you click on a tab it is displayed in dark letters. Define all variable names before entering the data.
   B. To define all variable names, click on the **Variable View** tab. Or to define one variable name, double click on the dimmed title *var* at the top of the column you want to name. This displays the headings (Name, Type, etc.) under which information can be entered.
   C. Enter a name for each variable under **Name.** [*Note:* The following rules apply to valid variable names: (1) one word, (2) maximum 8 characters, (3) no special characters (!,*,?,-, etc).] You may backspace to correct typos. Make sure for

each variable under Type the term is Numeric. Click on the right side of the cell if you need to change it. Also, for each variable it is suggested that under Width the number is 8 and under Decimals the number is 2. Then click on the **Data View** tab and the entered names appear at the top of the columns. [*Note:* The first column you have not named is labeled **var00001.**]

D. After defining all variable names, put the cursor on the first empty cell (square) in the first column and click once. Type a score which is displayed in the space below the **SPSS Data Editor** menu. Each time you press **Enter,** the value appears in the cell with the default or selected number of decimal places, and the cursor will move down. If you press **Tab** rather than **Enter** the cursor will move to the right.

E. If a person has no score for a variable (score is missing), enter it as a blank (enter no score and press **Enter** or **Tab**). The missing score is represented by a period (.).

F. After entering all the data for a column or row, select the first cell in the next column (the next defined variable) or row (next person) by using the mouse to click on the cell or using the arrow keys on the keyboard or using the arrow keys on the right and bottom margin of the **SPSS Data Editor** to move to the cell.

G. Do step D and E until all data are entered.

H. Additional information: in the SPSS Data Editor window, note the buttons at the top of the window for doing special things like inserting cases and variables.

I. Additional information: when naming a variable, in addition to a title for the variable, labels for each level of the variable, changing the position of the decimal point, etc. are possible.

J. Example: variable is sex with 1 = female and 2 = male.

   (1) In the Data Editor window click on the **Variable View** tab or click twice on **var** to name a column.

   (2) The headings (Name, Type, etc.) are displayed.

   (3) Click on **Name** and type in the name of the variable: Sex.

   (4) Click on **Label** and type in the title of the variable: Sex of Person.

   (5) Click on **Values,** then the button for Values, and then type in the following:

      Value: 1

      Value Label: Female

      click on **Add**

      Value: 2

      Value Label: Male

      click on **Add**

      click on **OK**

   (6) This information will be shown in the output of any analysis (Frequencies used).

   Sex of Person

	Frequency
Female	35
Male	45

K.   Additional information: to remove a variable (column) or case (row) in a data file, first highlight the column or row, then click on **Edit** on the menu bar, then click on **Cut.**

3. Saving the data

A.   To save the entered data in a file, Save does not have to be after the last score is entered. Click on **File** in the **SPSS Data Editor** menu and then click on **Save.** This opens the **Save Data As** dialog box. Enter a name for the data file in the **File name:** text box. Select the drive where the data are to be saved in the **Save in:** dialog box.

B.   At the **Save as type:** make sure the file is **SPSS(*.sav).** Click on **Save.**

C.   [*Note:* The untitled window will be changed to the drive and file name which you entered in 3-A.] The **SPSS Data Editor** window is still displayed. If this does not happen, save the data again.

D.   After a file is named, more data can be saved in it by clicking on **Save File** in the **SPSS Data Editor** menu.

4. Editing the data

A.   You can change data values which are incorrect, so the data entered should be still displayed on the screen.

B.   Where there are mistakes, click on the cell with the incorrect score or use the arrow keys to move to the incorrect score. Type in the correct value and press the **Enter** key. After editing, save the data again by clicking on **File** in the **SPSS Data Editor** menu and then clicking on **Save.** Make sure the **SPSS Data Editor,** and not an **Output** or **Syntax** window, is active because **Save** will save the active window. The **SPSS Data Editor** window is still displayed.

C.   If you type in a score twice you may want to delete it rather than change it. If you leave out a score you may want to insert it. This may require deleting or inserting a row of data. To delete a row, click on the row to be deleted. The entire row will be highlighted. From the **SPSS Data Editor** menu click on **Edit** and then **Clear.** To insert a row (case) click on the row where you want to insert a row. Click on **Data** in the **SPSS Data Editor** menu. Click on **Insert Case,** the row you clicked on and all rows below it will be moved down, then enter the data. [*Note:* See SPSS guides in the Reference or the SPSS Help menu for more details.]

5. Analyzing the data

A.   After doing steps 2–4 to enter the data, or the existing data file has been identified, click the analysis you want and then click on what options you want in the drop down menus. For data analysis, click **Analyze.** For graphs of the data, click **Graph.** For transformation of the data, click **Transform.**

B.   Since usually data analysis (Analyze) is desired, the options for Analyze are Report, Descriptive Statistics, Compare Means, etc. [*Note:* Put the cursor (no need to click) on any of these options and the screen will display a drop down menu of available options.]

C.   For specific information on using the options, see the SPSS for Windows Statistical Procedures later in this document.

D. The results of the analysis are displayed on the screen. After this you can print the output if desired or do another analysis on the same data. You can also enter another set of scores and analyze it or retrieve another set of saved scores and analyze it.

6. Printing output of the analysis

A. To print the contents of the output of the analysis, make sure the **SPSS Output Statistics Viewer** is the active window at the top left of the screen. If it is not the active window, click on **Window** in the menu bar and then **SPSS Output Viewer.** The content of the active window is displayed on the right hand side of the screen (content pane) and the output objects on the left hand side of the screen (outline pane). Use the arrow keys to move around the screen.

B. Before printing, indicate whether the entire contents (the default) or just part of the contents are to be printed. SPSS tends to produce many partially full pages of printout. To decrease the number of printed pages, select just the output desired.

   (1) In the left pane of Output Viewer highlight what contents of Output Viewer are to be printed.

   (2) From the Output Viewer click on **File** and then click on **Print.**

C. The name of the file is shown in the dialog box. The printer name is also displayed. Click on the print option desired (All Visible Output or Selection). By default, one copy is printed. If you want multiple copies, enter the number of copies you want to print. If there are too many columns (>7–8) to get on one vertical page (Portrait), or a line for the output can't be seen in full on the screen, select **Landscape** to print a horizontal page. To select Landscape print, click on **Properties,** click on **Landscape,** and then click on **Continue.** To print the contents, click on **OK.**

D. Example:

   (1) Suppose the Descriptives and Frequencies programs have been run on scores for each person called jump, pullups, and run. The output from both programs is in Output Viewer.

   (2) The left pane of Output Viewer will look like this:

   SPSS Output
       Descriptives
           Title
           Notes
           Descriptive Statistics
       Frequencies
           Title
           Notes
           Statistics
           Jump
           Pullups
           Run

   (3) If SPSS Output in B. is clicked on, everything in B. will be highlighted and the entire output will be printed.

       (4) If Descriptives in B. is clicked on, the Descriptives title and the three things under it will be highlighted and only that content will be printed.

       (5) If Run which is under Frequencies in B. is clicked on, it will be highlighted and that content will be printed.

  E. Situations for the example in D.

       (1) If Descriptives is run, the Descriptives output is printed, and then Frequencies is run, all that needs to be printed is the Frequencies output by highlighting Frequencies in the left pane of Output Viewer.

       (2) If Descriptives is run, and Frequencies is run, all of the output needs to be printed by highlighting **SPSS Output** in the left pane of Output Viewer.

  F. Useful information and hints on printing.

       (1) What is highlighted in the left pane is enclosed with a dark line box in the right pane of Output Viewer. If only part of the contents of Output Viewer is selected to be printed in the print menu, make sure Selection is highlighted as the print range.

       (2) If both the Data Editor and Output Viewer are on the screen, be sure to click **File** or **Print** under Output Viewer to print the output.

       (3) At the bottom of the screen both of the windows, Data Editor and Output, are shown. Click on one of them to make it the active window displayed on the screen.

       (4) The content of the Output Viewer window can be eliminated by clicking on **File** for the Output Viewer window, then **Close,** and finally **No** (don't save content). This is useful when there is a lot of content no longer needed. The same thing can be accomplished by clicking on the **X** box in the upper right hand corner of the Output Viewer window.

  G. If you want to print the contents of the **SPSS Data Editor** window, do steps B and C after activating the **SPSS Data Editor** window (see A and F-3).

7. Getting out of SPSS

  A. To end an SPSS session, click on **File** under the **SPSS Data Editor** or **Output Viewer** and then click on **Exit SPSS** in the drop down menu.

  B. [*Note:* SPSS will ask whether you want to save the contents of the **Output Viewer** and **SPSS Data Editor** windows. If you want to save them, click on **Yes.** If not, click on **No.** Only if you want to keep the output and/or you have not previously saved the data do you need to click on **Yes.**]

8. Retrieving saved data (data entered using **SPSS for Windows**)

  A. If just getting into SPSS, see l-D-(3).

  B. If opening a saved data file, from the **SPSS Data Editor** menu click on **File** and then on **Open.**

  C. Click on the drive to use from the **Look in:** dialog box and then click on **SPSS(*.sav)** in the **Files of type** list. You can click on a file from the list to use it or you can type in a filename. Then click on **Open.**

  D. The retrieved data file is displayed on the screen.

9. Importing and exporting data

  A. Importing data is using data not entered in SPSS (e.g., in Excel).

  B. Exporting data is using data entered in SPSS in some other program (e.g., Excel).

C. A file format may have to be selected when importing or exporting data. The file format can be either fixed field or free field. With fixed field the scores must be kept in specified columns and decimal points do not have to be entered whereas with free field the scores only have to be separated by one blank space and decimal points must be entered.

D. [*Note:* For more detailed procedures on importing and exporting data, see guides in Reference.]

Reference

Green, S. B., and Salkind, N. J. (2005). *Using SPSS for Windows and Macintosh: Analyzing and understanding data* (4th ed). Upper Saddle River, NJ: Prentice-Hall. (It has 458 pages, with good coverage of topics.)

Pavkov, T. W., and Pierce, K. A. (2003). *Ready, set, go! A student guide to SPSS 11.0 for Windows.* New York: McGraw-Hill. (Short and inexpensive.)

Prentice-Hall distributes SPSS Student Version for Windows and other SPSS publications. At the website the local Prentice-Hall representative can be identified. At the website, search on SPSS to identify many SPSS publications: www.prenhall.com.

The SPSS website has a wealth of information about the program, manuals, etc.: www.spss.com.

SPSS for Windows Statistical Procedures

Table of Contents for the SPSS programs described in this document.

1. Frequencies

2. Descriptives

3. One-Sample T Test

4. Independent-Samples T Test (two independent groups)

5. Paired-Samples T Test (dependent groups and repeated measures)

6. One-Way ANOVA

7. Repeated Measures ANOVA

8. Two-Way Factorial ANOVA

9. One-Way Chi-Square

10. Two-Way Chi-Square

11. Correlation

12. Linear Regression

13. Reliability Analysis

14. Percentiles

15. Percentile Ranks

16. Standard Scores (z-scores)

17. Transformation

18. Histograms

19. Line Chart (similar to frequency polygon)

20. Scatterplot

Note: Click on **Analyze** or **Graphs** or **Transform** under the **SPSS Data Editor** menu and all of the sub-headings for it will be displayed. Click on one of the sub-headings and all of the procedures under the sub-heading will be displayed.

SPSS has a **Help** feature which can be clicked on from the **SPSS for Windows** menu or any procedure menu. **Help** is excellent for learning about a statistical procedure or what to do in a procedure. To quit **Help,** click on **Cancel.**

1. Frequencies

   A. Click on **Analyze** under the **SPSS Data Editor** menu. Click on **Descriptive Statistics.** Click on **Frequencies** which opens the **Frequencies** dialog box.
   B. Click on one or more variables from the left variable box. The variable(s) is highlighted. Click on the arrow button and the variable(s) will show in the Variables box. By default, frequency tables are displayed with the data listed in ascending order (small to large). If small score is a good score, the data should be displayed in descending order. Click on **Format,** then on **Descending** (value), and finally click on **Continue** when through.
   C. To get optional descriptive and summary statistics, click on **Statistics** in the **Frequencies** dialog box. Click on the statistics desired. The **median** statistic is not provided by the Descriptives program, but is provided here. Many people use the Frequencies program to get descriptive statistics. When using Frequencies to get descriptive statistics, if you don't want frequencies for each variable, turn off the **Display Frequencies Tables** option before analyzing the data. Click on **Continue** when through.
   D. To get optional bar charts or histograms, click on **Charts** in the dialog box. Click on the charts or histograms desired in the dialog box. Click on **Continue** when through.
   E. Click on **OK** when ready to analyze the data.

2. Descriptives

   A. To get descriptive statistics, click on **Analyze** under the **SPSS Data Editor** menu. Click on **Descriptive Statistics.** Click on **Descriptives.** This opens the **Descriptives** dialog box.
   B. Click on one or more variables from the left variable box. The variable(s) is highlighted. Click on the arrow button and the variable(s) will show in the Variables box. By default, mean, standard deviation, minimum score, and maximum score will be displayed.

C. If you want to get additional statistics, click on **Options** under the Descriptive dialog box. This opens the **Descriptives:Options** dialog box.

D. Click on one or more options from the box. [*Note:* The **median** statistic is not an option, but it can be obtained under optional statistics in the Frequencies program (see directions for Frequencies).] Click on **Continue** when through.

E. Click on **OK** when ready to analyze the data.

3. One-Sample T Test

A. Click on **Analyze** under the **SPSS Data Editor** menu. Click on **Compare Means.** Then click on **One-Sample T Test.**

B. Click on one or more variables from the left variable box to use in the analysis. The variable(s) is highlighted. Click on the arrow button to put the variables in the **Test Variable(s)** box. Click on the value in **Test Value** and enter a number which is the value of the mean against which the variable is tested (the hypothesized population mean).

C. By default, the confidence interval is 95%. If you want to change this value, click on **Options** in the dialog box then type the numeric value for the confidence interval. Click on **Continue** when through.

D. Click on **OK** when ready to analyze the data.

E. The mean is provided automatically in the analysis output.

4. Independent-Samples T Test (two independent groups)

A. Click on **Analyze** under the **SPSS Data Editor** menu. Click on **Compare Means.** Click on **Independent-Samples T Test.**

B. Click on one or more variables from the left variable box to use in the analysis. The variable(s) is highlighted. Click on the arrow button to put the variable(s) in the **Test Variable(s)** box.

C. Click on a variable to form the two groups and then click on the arrow button for **Grouping Variable.**

D. You must define a value of the grouping variable for each groups. To define groups, click on **Define Groups.** Enter a value of the **Grouping Variable** which identified (is the code for) **Group 1.** Click on **Group 2** and enter a value for the grouping variable. Click on **Continue** when through.

E. By default, the confidence interval is 95% (alpha = .05). Click on **Options** to change it (see 3-C).

F. Click on **OK** when ready to analyze the data. Landscape print is suggested.

G. The means for the groups are provided automatically in the analysis output.

5. Paired-Samples T Test (dependent groups and repeated measures)

A. Click on **Analyze** under the **SPSS Data Editor** menu. Click on **Compare Means.** Click on **Paired-Samples T Test.**

B. Click on (highlight) one of the variables from the left variable box and click on the arrow button. It appears as **Variable 1** under **Paired Variables.** Click on another variable from the left variable box and click on the arrow button. It appears as **Variable 2.** Other pairs can be entered.

C. To change the confidence interval, click on **Options** (see 3-C).

   D.   Click on **OK** when ready to analyze the data. Landscape print is suggested.

   E.   The means for the repeated measures are provided automatically in the analysis output.

6. One-Way ANOVA

   A.   Click on **Analyze** under the **SPSS Data Editor** menu. Click on **Compare Means.** Click on **One-Way ANOVA.**

   B.   Click on (highlight) one or more variables from the left variable box to test (analyze). Click on the arrow button to put the variable(s) in the **Dependent List:** box.

   C.   Click on a variable for forming groups and click on the arrow button to put it in the **Factor** box.

   D.   Click on **Options, Descriptive,** and any other options desired. You *must* select descriptive statistics like the mean and standard deviation for each group. When through click on **Continue.**

   E.   If you want post hoc tests, click on **Post Hoc** and click on one of the 18 tests. When through, click on **Continue.**

   F.   Click on **OK** when ready to analyze the data.

7. Repeated Measures ANOVA

   A.   Click on **Analyze** under the **SPSS Data Editor** menu. Click on **General Linear Model.** Click on **Repeated Measures.**

   B.   A screen, Repeated Measures Define Factors, is displayed.
      (1) Within-Subject Factor Name: "factor1" is provided by SPSS so use it.
      (2) Number of Levels; enter the number of repeated measures.
      (3) Click the **Add** button.
      (4) Click the **Define** button.

   C.   A screen, Repeated Measures, is displayed.
      (1) On the left side, the variables available in the data set are listed in a box.
      (2) Put the repeated measure variables to be used into the Within-Subject Variable box by clicking a variable and then clicking the arrow to put the variable in the box.
      (3) Click on **Options** and select Descriptive Statistics.
      (4) Click on **Continue** to return to the Repeated Measures menu.
      (5) Click on **OK** to analyze the data.

8. Two-Way Factorial ANOVA

   A.   Click on **Analyze** under the **SPSS Data Editor** menu. Click on **General Linear Model.** Click on **Univariate.** (Only Univariate is in the student version.)

   B.   On the left side, the variables available in the data set are listed in a box.

   C.   On the right side are: Dependent Variable, Fixed Factors, Random Factors, and Covariance boxes.

   D.   Put the variable to be the data analyzed in the Dependent Variable box.

   E.   Put the variables for the rows and columns in the Fixed Factors box.

   F.   Example: If the variables in the data set are named Row, Column, and Score, put Score in the Dependent Variable box, and Row and Column in the Fixed Factors box.

G. Click on **Options** to get the means for rows, columns, and cells.

    (1) On the left side, in the Factors box, are listed Overall, the name of the row variable, the name of the column variable, and the name of the row $\times$ column interaction.

    (2) On the right side is the Display Means box.

    (3) Put everything from the Factors box into the Display Means box.

    (4) Click on **Continue** to return to the GLM-General Factorial menu.

H. Also, post hoc tests, effect size, observed power, etc. are available in Options. If post hoc tests are selected, it must be identified whether the post hoc tests are for rows, columns, or both.

I. Click on **OK** to analyze the data.

9. One-Way Chi-Square

A. Click on **Analyze** under the **SPSS Data Editor** menu. Click on **Nonparametric Tests.** Click on Legacy Dialogs. Click on **Chi-Square.** This opens the **Chi-Square Test** dialog box.

B. Click on (highlight) a variable from the left variable box and then click on the arrow button to put it in the **Test Variable List.** Do this for each variable to be analyzed.

C. Under **Expected Range** the **Get from Data** should already be selected (marked; the default). If it is not selected, click on it.

D. Under **Expected Values, All Categories Equal** will be marked (the default). If you do not want all categories equal, click on **Values** and enter an expected value for each category by typing in a value and then clicking on **Add.** The expected values are used with all the variables in the **Test Variable List.**

E. Click on **Options** and then click on **Descriptives** in the dialog box. When through selecting values you want, click on **Continue.**

F. Click on **OK** when ready to analyze the data. If the output is more than five columns, landscape print is suggested.

10. Two-Way Chi-Square

A. Click on **Analyze** under the **SPSS Data Editor** menu. Click on **Descriptive Statistics.** Click on **Crosstabs.** This opens the Crosstabs dialog box.

B. Click on (highlight) the variables in the left variable box you want to use as the row and column variables. Click on a variable to highlight it and then click on the arrow button for **Row(s)** or for **Column(s).**

C. Click on **Statistics** in the **Crosstabs** dialog box. Click on Chi-square, Contingency coefficient, Correlation, and anything else you want. When through, click on **Continue.**

D. Click on **Cell** in the **Crosstabs** dialog box. Click on **Observed, Expected,** and all three options under **Percentages.** When through, click on **Continue.**

E. Click on **OK** when ready to analyze the data.

11. Correlation

A. Click on **Analyze** under the **SPSS Data Editor** menu. Click on **Correlate.** Click on **Bivariate.**

B. Click on (highlight) two or more variables from the left variable box in the **Bivariate Correlations** dialog box. Click on the arrow button and the variable(s) will show in the **Variables** box.

C. Click on one or more of the correlation coefficients in the box (usually Pearson).

D. If you want a significance test, click on the type of significant test: **One-tailed** or **Two-tailed** (usually two-tailed).

E. Click on options. Click on mean and standard deviation. Click on continue.

F. Click on **OK** when ready to analyze the data.

12. Linear Regression

A. Click on **Analyze** under the **SPSS Data Editor** menu. Click on **Regression.** Click on **Linear.**

B. Click on (highlight) a variable from the left variable box for the dependent score (the Y-score). Click on the arrow button to put the variable in the **Dependent** box. Click on (highlight) a variable(s) from the left variable box for the independent variable (the X-score(s)). Click on the arrow button to put the variable(s) in the **Independent** box.

C. Click on one of the regression methods (usually **Enter**).

D. Click on Statistics. Under Regression Coefficients click on Estimates, Model Fit, and Descriptives. Click on continue when through.

E. Click on **OK** when ready to analyze the data.

13. Reliability Analysis

A. This analysis is in the SPSS standard version and now in the SPSS student version.

B. Click on **Analyze** under the **SPSS Data Editor** menu. Click on **Scale.** Click on **Reliability Analysis.**

C. Click on (highlight) a variable from the left variable box and then click on the arrow button to put it in the **Items:** box. Do this for at least two variables. These are the repeated measure like trials or days.

D. The **Model:** box should have **Alpha** in it. If it does not, click on the down arrow in **Model:** and click on **Alpha.**

E. Click on **Statistics** in the **Reliability Analysis** dialog box. Click on **Item** under **Descriptives** to get item means and **F Test** under **ANOVA Table** to get the ANOVA summary table.

F. Also, in **Statistics,** click on **Intraclass Correlation Coefficient.** Set Model to One-Way or Two-Way Mixed depending on which ANOVA model is desired. **Confidence Interval** and **Test Value** can be changed but usually the default values are used. Click on **Continue** when through.

G. Click on **OK** when ready to analyze the data.

14. Percentiles

A. Analyze the data using the Frequencies procedure (see number 1 in this document). Click on **Analyze.** Click on **Descriptive Statistics.** Click on **Frequencies.**

B. Percentiles are calculated assuming a large score is good whether this is true or not. If frequency tables are not desired, click on **Display Frequency Tables** to eliminate that option.

C. Click on **Statistics** and then on mean, standard deviation, and then on **Percentile(s).**

D. The percentiles desired must be indicated by typing a number between 0 and 100 into the percentile box and then clicking on **Add.** Do this for each percentile desired. After indicating the percentiles desired, click on **Continue** to get out of **Statistics.**

Example: if the percentiles 5th, 10th, 15th, . . ., 100th are desired

Percentile Box	Add
5	click
10	click
•	•
•	•

E. The default for **Cut Points,** which is an alternative to typing in percentiles, is 10 equal groups yielding the 10th, 20th, etc. percentiles.
F. Click on **OK** when ready to analyze the data.

15. Percentile Ranks

A. Analyze the data using the **Frequencies** procedure (see number 1 in this document). Click on **Analyze.** Click on **Descriptive Statistics.** Click on **Frequencies.**
B. After getting into **Frequencies,** make sure that the scores are listed from worst to best (ascending order if large score is good).
C. The output from the analysis will look like this example.

Value	Frequency	Percent	Valid Percent	Cum. Percent
15	4	20	20	20
16	6	30	30	50
17	8	40	40	90
19	2	10	10	100
	20	100	100	

D. Calculate percentile ranks for a score (Value) by the formula:

$$PR = (\text{Cum. Percent above the score}) + (.5)(\text{Percent for the score})$$

$$PR \text{ for score} = 15: PR = 0 + (.5)(20) = 10$$

$$PR \text{ for score} = 16: PR = 20 + (.5)(30) = 35$$

16. Standard Scores (z-scores)

A. A z-score for each variable analyzed is calculated assuming a large score is good whether or not the data is listed in ascending or descending order. If a small score is good, the sign of the z-score is reversed (e.g., −2.0 should be 2.0).
B. Analyze the data using the **Descriptives** procedure (see number 2 in this document) by clicking on **Analyze,** then **Descriptive Statistics,** and finally **Descriptives.**
C. Click on **Save standardized values as variables** in the **Descriptives** dialog box. Highlight the variables you want z-scores for in the left hand box. Click the arrow to move the variables into the right hand box. Click on **OK** when ready to analyze the data. The z-scores are calculated, and added to the file

containing the original data. A message does appear in the output that this occurred. The names of the z-scores will be the names of the original data with a z in front of them (e.g., for the original variable CAT the z-score is ZCAT). Z-score can be seen by displaying the data file on the screen and printing it if desired. The data file must be saved again for the z-scores to be saved with the data. In most cases, saving the z-scores is not necessary. If saving the z-scores, it might be good to save them as a new file so the original data file is retained as one file, and the original data with z-scores are another file. When saving the z-scores as a new file, use **Save As.**

D. Sum of the z-scores can be obtained by using the Transformation procedure (presented in this document) and writing the formula for obtaining the sum of the z-scores allowing for the fact that some z-scores have the wrong sign (z-scores for scores when small score is good will have the wrong sign.) For example, if the original data were X1, X2, and X3 the z-scores are ZX1, ZX2, and ZX3, and if ZSUM is the name used for the sum of the z-scores:

$$ZSUM = ZX1 + ZX2 - ZX3 \text{ (for X3, small score is good)}$$

17. Transformation

A. See the guides in the Reference section for more information.

B. Many things can be done with transformations such as changing the values of variables, grouping variables, creating new variables, etc. First, creating a new variable is presented. Then other examples are presented.

C. Click on **Transform** and then **Compute.** In the **Compute Variable** dialog box the name of the variable to be computed is typed in the **Target Variable:** box and the numeric expression or equation for calculating the target variable is typed in the **Numeric Expression:** box. Click on **OK** when ready to do the analysis. The computed variable is displayed on the screen and saved with the original data.

D. Example 1, creating a new variable: There are 3 scores named X1, X2, and X3 on each person and for all three scores a large score is good.

(1) The sum (to be named SUMX) of the 3 scores is desired.
     Target Variable: SUMX
     Numerical Expression: X1 + X2 + X3

(2) The data have already been analyzed calculating z-scores for each score (see Standard Score in this document). These z-scores are named ZX1, ZX2, and ZX3. The sum of the z-scores (to be named ZSUM) is desired.
     Target Variable: ZSUM
     Numerical Expression: ZX1 + ZX2 + ZX3
     [*Note:* The target variable is added to the file containing the original data (and z-scores in the case of ZSUM). The data file must be saved again for the target variable to be saved with the rest of the file (see 16-D for save procedures).]

E. Example 2, creating new variables by computing and by recoding: Each person has an X, Y, and ZZ score. X score values are from 1 to 10; Y score values are from 0 to 3; and ZZ score values are from 10 to 29.

(1) Analysis 1: Calculate a new score for each person (Ratio) where Ratio = X/Y.
     (a) Click on **Transform** and then on **Compute.**

(b) Fill the Boxes:
   1. Target Variable Box: type in Ratio (name of new score).
   2. Numeric Expression Box: click on the box and type in X/Y or highlight X, click on the right arrow to put it in the box, click on /, highlight Y, and click on the right arrow to put it in the box.
   3. Click on **OK.**

(c) The new score (Ratio) is added to the data file as the last score for each person so now each person has an X, Y, ZZ, and Ratio score.

(d) [*Note:* (1) When Y is zero, Ratio = X/Y will be set to missing value (period)(.) since division by zero is undefined; (2) The Ratio score is not saved on the data disk at this time. If Ratio should be saved, save the file (File, Save) or save the file with a new name (File, Save As) to preserve the original data file. If multiple transformations are to be done, saving could be done after doing all the transformations.]

(2) Analysis 2: Calculate a new score for each person (Newz) using the ZZ scores and the Recode option as follows: (1) if ZZ = 10–14, Newz = 1; (2) if ZZ = 15–19, Newz = 2; (3) if ZZ = 20–24, Newz = 3, and if ZZ = 25–29, Newz = 4.

(a) Click on **Transform** and then on **Recode.**

(b) Click on **Into Different Variable.**

(c) Fill the Boxes:
   1. Numeric Variable Box: click on ZZ (the variable recoded), and click on the right arrow to put it in the box.
   2. Output Variable Box: click on it, and type in Newz (the name of the new variable).

(d) Click on **Old** and **New Values.**
   1. Under Old Value, click on **Range,** enter 10, tab or click to the **Through Box,** and enter 14
   2. Under New Value, click on **Value** and enter 1
   3. Click on **Add**
   4. Do this for each variable change

ZZ	Newz
15–19	2
20–24	3
25–29	4

   5. Click on **Continue**
   6. Click on **Change**
   7. Click on **OK**

(e) The new score (Newz) is added to the data file as the last score for each person.

(f) [*Note:* The Newz score is not saved on the data disk at this time. Save it if necessary.]

18. Histogram

   A. See the Help feature or the guides in Reference section for more information.
   B. Click on **Graphs,** Legacy Dialogs, and then on **Histograms.**

C. In the **Histogram** dialog box, click on (highlight) a variable from the left variable box and then click on the arrow button so the variable is listed under the **Variable:** box. Note a variable can be removed from the **Variable:** box by clicking on it and then on the arrow button.

D. If the default format for histogram is acceptable, click on **OK** to obtain the graph. The histogram is displayed in the **SPSS Viewer.** If you want to display the normal curve with the histogram, click on **Display normal curve** before clicking on **OK.** A normal curve will be superimposed over the histogram.

E. [*Note:* Double click on a graph in the **SPSS Viewer** to bring it in the **SPSS Chart Editor.** Double clicking on a graph created from interactive graphics activates the chart manager. The **SPSS Chart Editor** on the chart manager can be used to edit the chart.]

F. By default the histogram has bars showing the data divided into about 10 evenly spaced intervals. Usually 10–20 intervals are used with continuous data putting 2–5 different scores in an interval (e.g., 15–17 is interval size = 3). The base intervals of the histogram in the **SPSS Chart Editor** can be changed.

19. Line Chart (similar to frequency polygon)

A. See the Help feature or the guides in Reference section for more information.

B. Click on **Graphs,** Legacy Dialogs, and then on **Line.**

C. In the Line Charts dialog box click on **Simple** line chart and **Summaries for Groups of Cases.** Then click on **Define,** click on (highlight) the variable from the left variable box to use, click on the arrow button to put the highlighted variable in the **Category Axis:** box, and click on **N of cases.** Click on **OK** when ready to obtain the graph. The line chart is displayed in the **SPSS Viewer** (see Histogram for details on the editing chart).

D. By default the line chart has the data divided into about 15 intervals for the X-axis. Usually 10–20 labels (intervals) are used with continuous data putting 2–5 different score values in an interval (e.g., 15–17 is interval size = 3). The labels (intervals) for the X-axis can be altered.

20. Scatterplot

A. See the Help feature for more information.

B. Click on **Graphs,** Legacy Dialogs, then **Scatter/Dot,** and then **Simple** Scatter in the **Scatterplot** dialog box.

C. Now click on **Define.** Click on (highlight) a variable from the left variable box and then click on the arrow button to put it in the **X Axis:** box. Do the same thing for a second variable to put it in the **Y Axis:** box.

D. Click on **OK** when ready to obtain the graph.

E. The scatterplot is displayed in the **SPSS Viewer** (see Histogram for details on the editing charts).

Acknowledgment

Instructions for using SPSS were developed for earlier versions of SPSS by Suhak Oh and Ted Baumgartner. This document is an edited version of these instructions for SPSS.

Appendix B

	LEVEL OF SIGNIFICANCE FOR ONE-TAILED TEST					
	.10	.05	.025	.01	.005	.0005
	LEVEL OF SIGNIFICANCE FOR TWO-TAILED TEST					
df	.20	.10	.05	.02	.01	.001
1	3.078	6.314	12.706	31.821	63.657	636.619
2	1.886	2.920	4.303	6.965	9.925	31.598
3	1.638	2.353	3.182	4.541	5.841	12.941
4	1.533	2.132	2.776	3.747	4.604	8.610
5	1.476	2.015	2.571	3.365	4.032	6.859
6	1.440	1.943	2.447	3.143	3.707	5.959
7	1.415	1.895	2.365	2.998	3.499	5.405
8	1.397	1.860	2.306	2.896	3.355	5.041
9	1.383	1.833	2.262	2.821	3.250	4.781
10	1.372	1.812	2.228	2.764	3.169	4.587
11	1.363	1.796	2.201	2.718	3.106	4.437
12	1.356	1.782	2.179	2.681	3.055	4.318
13	1.350	1.771	2.160	2.650	3.012	4.221
14	1.345	1.761	2.145	2.624	2.977	4.140
15	1.341	1.753	2.131	2.602	2.947	4.073
16	1.337	1.746	2.120	2.583	2.921	4.015
17	1.333	1.740	2.110	2.567	2.898	3.965
18	1.330	1.734	2.101	2.552	2.878	3.922
19	1.328	1.729	2.093	2.539	2.861	3.883

Critical Values of t

Critical Values of *t*—*Concluded*

	LEVEL OF SIGNIFICANCE FOR ONE-TAILED TEST					
	.10	.05	.025	.01	.005	.0005
	LEVEL OF SIGNIFICANCE FOR TWO-TAILED TEST					
df	.20	.10	.05	.02	.01	.001
20	1.325	1.725	2.086	2.528	2.845	3.850
21	1.323	1.721	2.080	2.518	2.831	3.819
22	1.321	1.717	2.074	2.508	2.819	3.792
23	1.319	1.714	2.069	2.500	2.807	3.767
24	1.318	1.711	2.064	2.492	2.797	3.745
25	1.316	1.708	2.060	2.485	2.787	3.725
26	1.315	1.706	2.056	2.479	2.779	3.707
27	1.314	1.703	2.052	2.473	2.771	3.690
28	1.313	1.701	2.048	2.467	2.763	3.674
29	1.311	1.699	2.045	2.462	2.756	3.659
30	1.310	1.697	2.042	2.457	2.750	3.646
40	1.303	1.684	2.021	2.423	2.704	3.551
60	1.296	1.671	2.000	2.390	2.660	3.460
120	1.289	1.658	1.980	2.358	2.617	3.373
∞	1.282	1.645	1.960	2.326	2.576	3.291

Appendix B is taken from Table III of Fisher & Yates, *Statistical Tables for Biological, Agricultural and Medical Research.* Published by Longman Group UK Ltd., 1974. Reprinted by permission of Addison Wesley Longman Ltd.

Appendix C

Critical Values of F
.05 level (light type) and .01 level (bold type) points for the distribution of F

DEGREES OF FREEDOM FOR DENOMINATOR	DEGREES OF FREEDOM FOR NUMERATOR											
	1	2	3	4	5	6	7	8	9	10	11	12
1	161	200	216	225	230	234	237	239	241	242	243	244
	4052	**4999**	**5403**	**5625**	**5764**	**5859**	**5928**	**5981**	**6022**	**6056**	**6082**	**6106**
2	18.51	19.00	19.16	19.25	19.30	19.33	19.36	19.37	19.38	19.39	19.40	19.41
	98.49	**99.01**	**99.17**	**99.25**	**99.30**	**99.33**	**99.34**	**99.36**	**99.38**	**99.40**	**99.41**	**99.42**
3	10.13	9.55	9.28	9.12	9.01	8.94	8.88	8.84	8.81	8.78	8.76	8.74
	34.12	**30.81**	**29.46**	**28.71**	**28.24**	**27.91**	**27.67**	**27.49**	**27.34**	**27.23**	**27.13**	**27.05**
4	7.71	6.94	6.59	6.39	6.26	6.16	6.09	6.04	6.00	5.96	5.93	5.91
	21.20	**18.00**	**16.69**	**15.98**	**15.52**	**15.21**	**14.98**	**14.80**	**14.66**	**14.54**	**14.45**	**14.37**
5	6.61	5.79	5.41	5.19	5.05	4.95	4.88	4.82	4.78	4.74	4.70	4.68
	16.26	**13.27**	**12.06**	**11.39**	**10.97**	**10.67**	**10.45**	**10.27**	**10.15**	**10.05**	**9.96**	**9.89**
6	5.99	5.14	4.76	4.53	4.39	4.28	4.21	4.15	4.10	4.06	4.03	4.00
	13.74	**10.92**	**9.78**	**9.15**	**8.75**	**8.47**	**8.26**	**8.10**	**7.98**	**7.87**	**7.79**	**7.72**
7	5.59	4.74	4.35	4.12	3.97	3.87	3.79	3.73	3.68	3.63	3.60	3.57
	12.25	**9.55**	**8.45**	**7.85**	**7.46**	**7.19**	**7.00**	**6.84**	**6.71**	**6.62**	**6.54**	**6.47**
8	5.32	4.46	4.07	3.84	3.69	3.58	3.50	3.44	3.39	3.34	3.31	3.28
	11.26	**8.65**	**7.59**	**7.01**	**6.63**	**6.37**	**6.19**	**6.03**	**5.91**	**5.82**	**5.74**	**5.67**
9	5.12	4.26	3.86	3.63	3.48	3.37	3.29	3.23	3.18	3.13	3.10	3.07
	10.56	**8.02**	**6.99**	**6.42**	**6.06**	**5.80**	**5.62**	**5.47**	**5.35**	**5.26**	**5.18**	**5.11**
10	4.96	4.10	3.71	3.48	3.33	3.22	3.14	3.07	3.02	2.97	2.94	2.91
	10.04	**7.56**	**6.55**	**5.99**	**5.64**	**5.39**	**5.21**	**5.06**	**4.95**	**4.85**	**4.78**	**4.71**

From G. W. Snedecor and W. G. Cochran, *Statistical Methods,* 7th edition, Table of Critical Values of F, 1980. Copyright © 1980 Iowa State University Press, Ames, Iowa. Reprinted by permission.

14	16	20	24	30	40	50	75	100	200	500	∞
245	246	248	249	250	251	252	253	253	254	254	254
6142	**6169**	**6208**	**6234**	**6258**	**6286**	**6302**	**6323**	**6334**	**6352**	**6361**	**6366**
19.42	19.43	19.44	19.45	19.46	19.47	19.47	19.48	19.49	19.49	19.50	19.50
99.43	**99.44**	**99.45**	**99.46**	**99.47**	**99.48**	**99.48**	**99.49**	**99.49**	**99.49**	**99.50**	**99.50**
8.71	8.69	8.66	8.64	8.62	8.60	8.58	8.57	8.56	8.54	8.54	8.53
26.92	**26.83**	**26.69**	**26.60**	**26.50**	**26.41**	**26.35**	**26.27**	**26.23**	**26.18**	**26.14**	**26.12**
5.87	5.84	5.80	5.77	5.74	5.71	5.70	5.68	5.66	5.65	5.64	5.63
14.24	**14.15**	**14.02**	**13.93**	**13.83**	**13.74**	**13.69**	**13.61**	**13.57**	**13.52**	**13.48**	**13.46**
4.64	4.60	4.56	4.53	4.50	4.46	4.44	4.42	4.40	4.38	4.37	4.36
9.77	**9.68**	**9.55**	**9.47**	**9.38**	**9.29**	**9.24**	**9.17**	**9.13**	**9.07**	**9.04**	**9.02**
3.96	3.92	3.87	3.84	3.81	3.77	3.75	3.72	3.71	3.69	3.68	3.67
7.60	**7.52**	**7.39**	**7.31**	**7.23**	**7.14**	**7.09**	**7.02**	**6.99**	**6.94**	**6.90**	**6.88**
3.52	3.49	3.44	3.41	3.38	3.34	3.32	3.29	3.28	3.25	3.24	3.23
6.35	**6.27**	**6.15**	**6.07**	**5.98**	**5.90**	**5.85**	**5.78**	**5.75**	**5.70**	**5.67**	**5.65**
3.23	3.20	3.15	3.12	3.08	3.05	3.03	3.00	2.98	2.96	2.94	2.93
5.56	**5.48**	**5.36**	**5.28**	**5.20**	**5.11**	**5.06**	**5.00**	**4.96**	**4.91**	**4.88**	**4.88**
3.02	2.98	2.93	2.90	2.86	2.82	2.80	2.77	2.76	2.73	2.72	2.71
5.00	**4.92**	**4.80**	**4.73**	**4.64**	**4.56**	**4.51**	**4.45**	**4.41**	**4.36**	**4.33**	**4.31**
2.86	2.82	2.77	2.74	2.70	2.67	2.64	2.61	2.59	2.56	2.55	2.54
4.60	**4.52**	**4.41**	**4.33**	**4.25**	**4.17**	**4.12**	**4.05**	**4.01**	**3.96**	**3.93**	**3.91**

Critical Values of F—Continued

DEGREES OF FREEDOM FOR DENOMINATOR	DEGREES OF FREEDOM FOR NUMERATOR											
	1	2	3	4	5	6	7	8	9	10	11	12
11	4.84	3.98	3.59	3.36	3.20	3.09	3.01	2.95	2.90	2.86	2.82	2.79
	9.65	**7.20**	**6.22**	**5.67**	**5.32**	**5.07**	**4.88**	**4.74**	**4.63**	**4.54**	**4.46**	**4.40**
12	4.75	3.88	3.49	3.26	3.11	3.00	2.92	2.85	2.80	2.76	2.72	2.69
	9.33	**6.93**	**5.95**	**5.41**	**5.06**	**4.82**	**4.65**	**4.50**	**4.39**	**4.30**	**4.22**	**4.16**
13	4.67	3.80	3.41	3.18	3.02	2.92	2.84	2.77	2.72	2.67	2.63	2.60
	9.07	**6.70**	**5.74**	**5.20**	**4.86**	**4.62**	**4.44**	**4.30**	**4.19**	**4.10**	**4.02**	**3.96**
14	4.60	3.74	3.34	3.11	2.96	2.85	2.77	2.70	2.65	2.60	2.56	2.53
	8.86	**6.51**	**5.56**	**5.03**	**4.69**	**4.46**	**4.28**	**4.14**	**4.03**	**3.94**	**3.86**	**3.80**
15	4.54	3.68	3.29	3.06	2.90	2.79	2.70	2.64	2.59	2.55	2.51	2.48
	8.68	**6.36**	**5.42**	**4.89**	**4.56**	**4.32**	**4.14**	**4.00**	**3.89**	**3.80**	**3.73**	**3.67**
16	4.49	3.63	3.24	3.01	2.85	2.74	2.66	2.59	2.54	2.49	2.45	2.42
	8.53	**6.23**	**5.29**	**4.77**	**4.44**	**4.20**	**4.03**	**3.89**	**3.78**	**3.69**	**3.61**	**3.55**
17	4.45	3.59	3.20	2.96	2.81	2.70	2.62	2.55	2.50	2.45	2.41	2.38
	8.40	**6.11**	**5.18**	**4.67**	**4.34**	**4.10**	**3.93**	**3.79**	**3.68**	**3.59**	**3.52**	**3.45**
18	4.41	3.55	3.16	2.93	2.77	2.66	2.58	2.51	2.46	2.41	2.37	2.34
	8.28	**6.01**	**5.09**	**4.58**	**4.25**	**4.01**	**3.88**	**3.71**	**3.60**	**3.51**	**3.44**	**3.37**
19	4.38	3.52	3.13	2.90	2.74	2.63	2.55	2.48	2.43	2.38	2.34	2.31
	8.18	**5.93**	**5.01**	**4.50**	**4.17**	**3.94**	**3.77**	**3.63**	**3.52**	**3.43**	**3.36**	**3.30**
20	4.35	3.49	3.10	2.87	2.71	2.60	2.52	2.45	2.40	2.35	2.31	2.28
	8.10	**5.85**	**4.94**	**4.43**	**4.10**	**3.87**	**3.71**	**3.56**	**3.45**	**3.37**	**3.30**	**3.23**
21	4.32	3.47	3.07	2.84	2.68	2.57	2.49	2.42	2.37	2.32	2.28	2.25
	8.02	**5.78**	**4.87**	**4.37**	**4.04**	**3.81**	**3.65**	**3.51**	**3.40**	**3.31**	**3.24**	**3.17**
22	4.30	3.44	3.05	2.82	2.66	2.55	2.47	2.40	2.35	2.30	2.26	2.23
	7.94	**5.72**	**4.82**	**4.31**	**3.99**	**3.76**	**3.59**	**3.45**	**3.35**	**3.26**	**3.18**	**3.12**
23	4.28	3.42	3.03	2.80	2.64	2.53	2.45	2.38	2.32	2.28	2.24	2.20
	7.88	**5.66**	**4.76**	**4.26**	**3.94**	**3.71**	**3.54**	**3.41**	**3.30**	**3.21**	**3.14**	**3.07**
24	4.26	3.40	3.01	2.78	2.62	2.51	2.43	2.36	2.30	2.26	2.22	2.18
	7.82	**5.61**	**4.72**	**4.22**	**3.90**	**3.67**	**3.50**	**3.36**	**3.25**	**3.17**	**3.09**	**3.03**
25	4.24	3.38	2.99	2.76	2.60	2.49	2.41	2.34	2.28	2.24	2.20	2.16
	7.77	**5.57**	**4.68**	**4.18**	**3.86**	**3.63**	**3.46**	**3.32**	**3.21**	**3.13**	**3.05**	**2.99**
26	4.22	3.37	2.98	2.74	2.59	2.47	2.39	2.32	2.27	2.22	2.18	2.15
	7.72	**5.53**	**4.64**	**4.14**	**3.82**	**3.59**	**3.42**	**3.29**	**3.17**	**3.09**	**3.02**	**2.96**
27	4.21	3.35	2.96	2.73	2.57	2.46	2.37	2.30	2.25	2.20	2.16	2.13
	7.68	**5.49**	**4.60**	**4.11**	**3.79**	**3.56**	**3.39**	**3.26**	**3.14**	**3.06**	**2.98**	**2.93**
28	4.20	3.34	2.95	2.71	2.56	2.44	2.36	2.29	2.24	2.19	2.15	2.12
	7.64	**5.45**	**4.57**	**4.07**	**3.76**	**3.53**	**3.36**	**3.23**	**3.11**	**3.03**	**2.95**	**2.90**
29	4.18	3.33	2.93	2.70	2.54	2.43	2.35	2.28	2.22	2.18	2.14	2.10
	7.60	**5.42**	**4.54**	**4.04**	**3.73**	**3.50**	**3.33**	**3.20**	**3.08**	**3.00**	**2.92**	**2.87**

14	16	20	24	30	40	50	75	100	200	500	∞
2.74	2.70	2.65	2.61	2.57	2.53	2.50	2.47	2.45	2.42	2.41	2.40
4.29	**4.21**	**4.10**	**4.02**	**3.94**	**3.86**	**3.80**	**3.74**	**3.70**	**3.66**	**3.62**	**3.60**
2.64	2.60	2.54	2.50	2.46	2.42	2.40	2.36	2.35	2.32	2.31	2.30
4.05	**3.98**	**3.86**	**3.78**	**3.70**	**3.61**	**3.56**	**3.49**	**3.46**	**3.41**	**3.38**	**3.36**
2.55	2.51	2.46	2.42	2.38	2.34	2.32	2.28	2.26	2.24	2.22	2.21
3.85	**3.78**	**3.67**	**3.59**	**3.51**	**3.42**	**3.37**	**3.30**	**3.27**	**3.21**	**3.18**	**3.16**
2.48	2.44	2.39	2.35	2.31	2.27	2.24	2.21	2.19	2.16	2.14	2.13
3.70	**3.62**	**3.51**	**3.43**	**3.34**	**3.26**	**3.21**	**3.14**	**3.11**	**3.06**	**3.02**	**3.00**
2.43	2.39	2.33	2.29	2.25	2.21	2.18	2.15	2.12	2.10	2.08	2.07
3.56	**3.48**	**3.36**	**3.29**	**3.20**	**3.12**	**3.07**	**3.00**	**2.97**	**2.92**	**2.89**	**2.87**
2.37	2.33	2.28	2.24	2.20	2.16	2.13	2.09	2.07	2.04	2.02	2.01
3.45	**3.37**	**3.25**	**3.18**	**3.10**	**3.01**	**2.96**	**2.89**	**2.86**	**2.80**	**2.77**	**2.75**
2.33	2.29	2.23	2.19	2.15	2.11	2.08	2.04	2.02	1.99	1.97	1.96
3.35	**3.27**	**3.16**	**3.08**	**3.00**	**2.92**	**2.86**	**2.79**	**2.76**	**2.70**	**2.67**	**2.65**
2.29	2.25	2.19	2.15	2.11	2.07	2.04	2.00	1.98	1.95	1.93	1.92
3.27	**3.19**	**3.07**	**3.00**	**2.91**	**2.83**	**2.78**	**2.71**	**2.68**	**2.62**	**2.59**	**2.57**
2.26	2.21	2.15	2.11	2.07	2.02	2.00	1.96	1.94	1.91	1.90	1.88
3.19	**3.12**	**3.00**	**2.92**	**2.84**	**2.76**	**2.70**	**2.63**	**2.60**	**2.54**	**2.51**	**2.49**
2.23	2.18	2.12	2.08	2.04	1.99	1.96	1.92	1.90	1.87	1.85	1.84
3.13	**3.05**	**2.94**	**2.86**	**2.77**	**2.69**	**2.63**	**2.56**	**2.53**	**2.47**	**2.44**	**2.42**
2.20	2.15	2.09	2.05	2.00	1.96	1.93	1.89	1.87	1.84	1.82	1.81
3.07	**2.99**	**2.88**	**2.80**	**2.72**	**2.63**	**2.58**	**2.51**	**2.47**	**2.42**	**2.38**	**2.36**
2.18	2.13	2.07	2.03	1.98	1.93	1.91	1.87	1.84	1.81	1.80	1.78
3.02	**2.94**	**2.83**	**2.75**	**2.67**	**2.58**	**2.53**	**2.46**	**2.42**	**2.37**	**2.33**	**2.31**
2.14	2.10	2.04	2.00	1.96	1.91	1.88	1.84	1.82	1.79	1.77	1.76
2.97	**2.89**	**2.78**	**2.70**	**2.62**	**2.53**	**2.48**	**2.41**	**2.37**	**2.32**	**2.28**	**2.26**
2.13	2.09	2.02	1.98	1.94	1.89	1.86	1.82	1.80	1.76	1.74	1.73
2.93	**2.85**	**2.74**	**2.66**	**2.58**	**2.49**	**2.44**	**2.36**	**2.33**	**2.27**	**2.23**	**2.21**
2.11	2.06	2.00	1.96	1.92	1.87	1.84	1.80	1.77	1.74	1.72	1.71
2.89	**2.81**	**2.70**	**2.62**	**2.54**	**2.45**	**2.40**	**2.32**	**2.29**	**2.23**	**2.19**	**2.17**
2.10	2.05	1.99	1.95	1.90	1.85	1.82	1.78	1.76	1.72	1.70	1.69
2.86	**2.77**	**2.66**	**2.58**	**2.50**	**2.41**	**2.36**	**2.28**	**2.25**	**2.19**	**2.15**	**2.13**
2.08	2.03	1.97	1.93	1.88	1.84	1.80	1.76	1.74	1.71	1.68	1.67
2.83	**2.74**	**2.63**	**2.55**	**2.47**	**2.38**	**2.33**	**2.25**	**2.21**	**2.16**	**2.12**	**2.10**
2.06	2.02	1.96	1.91	1.87	1.81	1.78	1.75	1.72	1.69	1.67	1.65
2.80	**2.71**	**2.60**	**2.52**	**2.44**	**2.35**	**2.30**	**2.22**	**2.18**	**2.13**	**2.09**	**2.06**
2.05	2.00	1.94	1.90	1.85	1.80	1.77	1.73	1.71	1.68	1.65	1.64
2.77	**2.68**	**2.57**	**2.49**	**2.41**	**2.32**	**2.27**	**2.19**	**2.15**	**2.10**	**2.06**	**2.03**

Critical Values of F—Continued

DEGREES OF FREEDOM FOR DENOMINATOR

DEGREES OF FREEDOM FOR NUMERATOR

	1	2	3	4	5	6	7	8	9	10	11	12
30	4.17	3.32	2.92	2.69	2.53	2.42	2.34	2.27	2.21	2.16	2.12	2.09
	7.56	**5.39**	**4.51**	**4.02**	**3.70**	**3.47**	**3.30**	**3.17**	**3.06**	**2.98**	**2.90**	**2.84**
32	4.15	3.30	2.90	2.67	2.51	2.40	2.32	2.25	2.19	2.14	2.10	2.07
	7.50	**5.34**	**4.46**	**3.97**	**3.66**	**3.42**	**3.25**	**3.12**	**3.01**	**2.94**	**2.86**	**2.80**
34	4.13	3.28	2.88	2.65	2.49	2.38	2.30	2.23	2.17	2.12	2.08	2.05
	7.44	**5.29**	**4.42**	**3.93**	**3.61**	**3.38**	**3.21**	**3.08**	**2.97**	**2.89**	**2.82**	**2.76**
36	4.11	3.26	2.86	2.63	2.48	2.36	2.28	2.21	2.15	2.10	2.06	2.03
	7.39	**5.25**	**4.38**	**3.89**	**3.58**	**3.35**	**3.18**	**3.04**	**2.94**	**2.86**	**2.78**	**2.72**
38	4.10	3.25	2.85	2.62	2.46	2.35	2.26	2.19	2.14	2.09	2.05	2.02
	7.35	**5.21**	**4.34**	**3.86**	**3.54**	**3.32**	**3.15**	**3.02**	**2.91**	**2.82**	**2.75**	**2.69**
40	4.08	3.23	2.84	2.61	2.45	2.34	2.25	2.18	2.12	2.07	2.04	2.00
	7.31	**5.18**	**4.31**	**3.83**	**3.51**	**3.29**	**3.12**	**2.99**	**2.88**	**2.80**	**2.73**	**2.66**
42	4.07	3.22	2.83	2.59	2.44	2.32	2.24	2.17	2.11	2.06	2.02	1.99
	7.27	**5.15**	**4.29**	**3.80**	**3.49**	**3.26**	**3.10**	**2.96**	**2.86**	**2.77**	**2.70**	**2.64**
44	4.06	3.21	2.82	2.58	2.43	2.31	2.23	2.16	2.10	2.05	2.01	1.98
	7.24	**5.12**	**4.26**	**3.78**	**3.46**	**3.24**	**3.07**	**2.94**	**2.84**	**2.75**	**2.68**	**2.62**
46	4.05	3.20	2.81	2.57	2.42	2.30	2.22	2.14	2.09	2.04	2.00	1.97
	7.21	**5.10**	**4.24**	**3.76**	**3.44**	**3.22**	**3.05**	**2.92**	**2.82**	**2.73**	**2.66**	**2.60**
48	4.04	3.19	2.80	2.56	2.41	2.30	2.21	2.14	2.08	2.03	1.99	1.96
	7.19	**5.08**	**4.22**	**3.74**	**3.42**	**3.20**	**3.04**	**2.90**	**2.80**	**2.71**	**2.64**	**2.58**
50	4.03	3.18	2.79	2.56	2.40	2.29	2.20	2.13	2.07	2.02	1.98	1.95
	7.17	**5.06**	**4.20**	**3.72**	**3.41**	**3.18**	**3.02**	**2.88**	**2.78**	**2.70**	**2.62**	**2.56**
55	4.02	3.17	2.78	2.54	2.38	2.27	2.18	2.11	2.05	2.00	1.97	1.93
	7.12	**5.01**	**4.16**	**3.68**	**3.37**	**3.15**	**2.98**	**2.85**	**2.75**	**2.66**	**2.59**	**2.53**
60	4.00	3.15	2.76	2.52	2.37	2.25	2.17	2.10	2.04	1.99	1.95	1.92
	7.08	**4.98**	**4.13**	**3.65**	**3.34**	**3.12**	**2.95**	**2.82**	**2.72**	**2.63**	**2.56**	**2.50**
65	3.99	3.14	2.75	2.51	2.36	2.24	2.15	2.08	2.02	1.98	1.94	1.90
	7.04	**4.95**	**4.10**	**3.62**	**3.31**	**3.09**	**2.93**	**2.79**	**2.70**	**2.61**	**2.54**	**2.47**
70	3.98	3.13	2.74	2.50	2.35	2.23	2.14	2.07	2.01	1.97	1.93	1.89
	7.01	**4.92**	**4.08**	**3.60**	**3.29**	**3.07**	**2.91**	**2.77**	**2.67**	**2.59**	**2.51**	**2.45**
80	3.96	3.11	2.72	2.48	2.33	2.21	2.12	2.05	1.99	1.95	1.91	1.88
	6.96	**4.88**	**4.04**	**3.56**	**3.25**	**3.04**	**2.87**	**2.74**	**2.64**	**2.55**	**2.46**	**2.41**
100	3.94	3.09	2.70	2.46	2.30	2.19	2.10	2.03	1.97	1.92	1.88	1.85
	6.90	**4.82**	**3.98**	**3.51**	**3.20**	**2.99**	**2.82**	**2.69**	**2.59**	**2.51**	**2.43**	**2.36**
125	3.92	3.07	2.68	2.44	2.29	2.17	2.08	2.01	1.95	1.90	1.86	1.83
	6.84	**4.78**	**3.94**	**3.47**	**3.17**	**2.95**	**2.79**	**2.65**	**2.56**	**2.47**	**2.40**	**2.33**
150	3.91	3.06	2.67	2.43	2.27	2.16	2.07	2.00	1.94	1.89	1.85	1.82
	6.81	**4.75**	**3.91**	**3.44**	**3.14**	**2.92**	**2.76**	**2.62**	**2.53**	**2.44**	**2.37**	**2.30**

14	16	20	24	30	40	50	75	100	200	500	∞
2.04	1.99	1.93	1.89	1.84	1.79	1.76	1.72	1.69	1.66	1.64	1.62
2.74	**2.66**	**2.55**	**2.47**	**2.38**	**2.29**	**2.24**	**2.16**	**2.13**	**2.07**	**2.03**	**2.01**
2.02	1.97	1.91	1.86	1.82	1.76	1.74	1.69	1.67	1.64	1.61	1.59
2.70	**2.62**	**2.51**	**2.42**	**2.34**	**2.25**	**2.20**	**2.12**	**2.08**	**2.02**	**1.98**	**1.96**
2.00	1.95	1.89	1.84	1.80	1.74	1.71	1.67	1.64	1.61	1.59	1.57
2.66	**2.58**	**2.47**	**2.38**	**2.30**	**2.21**	**2.15**	**2.03**	**2.04**	**1.98**	**1.94**	**1.91**
1.98	1.93	1.87	1.82	1.78	1.72	1.69	1.65	1.62	1.59	1.56	1.55
2.62	**2.54**	**2.43**	**2.35**	**2.26**	**2.17**	**2.12**	**2.04**	**2.00**	**1.94**	**1.90**	**1.87**
1.96	1.92	1.85	1.80	1.76	1.71	1.67	1.63	1.60	1.57	1.54	1.53
2.59	**2.51**	**2.40**	**2.32**	**2.22**	**2.14**	**2.08**	**2.00**	**1.97**	**1.90**	**1.86**	**1.84**
1.95	1.90	1.84	1.79	1.74	1.69	1.66	1.61	1.59	1.55	1.53	1.51
2.56	**2.49**	**2.37**	**2.29**	**2.20**	**2.11**	**2.05**	**1.97**	**1.94**	**1.88**	**1.84**	**1.81**
1.94	1.89	1.82	1.78	1.73	1.68	1.64	1.60	1.57	1.54	1.51	1.49
2.54	**2.46**	**2.35**	**2.26**	**2.17**	**2.08**	**2.02**	**1.94**	**1.91**	**1.85**	**1.80**	**1.78**
1.92	1.88	1.81	1.76	1.72	1.66	1.63	1.58	1.56	1.52	1.50	1.48
2.52	**2.44**	**2.32**	**2.24**	**2.15**	**2.06**	**2.00**	**1.92**	**1.88**	**1.82**	**1.78**	**1.75**
1.91	1.87	1.80	1.75	1.71	1.65	1.62	1.57	1.54	1.51	1.48	1.46
2.50	**2.42**	**2.30**	**2.22**	**2.13**	**2.04**	**1.98**	**1.90**	**1.86**	**1.80**	**1.76**	**1.72**
1.90	1.86	1.79	1.74	1.70	1.64	1.61	1.56	1.53	1.50	1.47	1.45
2.48	**2.40**	**2.28**	**2.20**	**2.11**	**2.02**	**1.96**	**1.88**	**1.84**	**1.78**	**1.73**	**1.70**
1.90	1.85	1.78	1.74	1.69	1.63	1.60	1.55	1.52	1.48	1.46	1.44
2.46	**2.39**	**2.26**	**2.18**	**2.10**	**2.00**	**1.94**	**1.86**	**1.82**	**1.76**	**1.71**	**1.68**
1.88	1.83	1.76	1.72	1.67	1.61	1.58	1.52	1.50	1.46	1.43	1.41
2.43	**2.35**	**2.23**	**2.15**	**2.06**	**1.96**	**1.90**	**1.82**	**1.78**	**1.71**	**1.66**	**1.64**
1.86	1.81	1.75	1.70	1.65	1.59	1.56	1.50	1.48	1.44	1.41	1.39
2.40	**2.32**	**2.20**	**2.12**	**2.03**	**1.93**	**1.87**	**1.79**	**1.74**	**1.68**	**1.63**	**1.60**
1.85	1.80	1.73	1.68	1.63	1.57	1.54	1.49	1.46	1.42	1.39	1.37
2.37	**2.30**	**2.18**	**2.09**	**2.00**	**1.90**	**1.84**	**1.76**	**1.71**	**1.64**	**1.60**	**1.56**
1.84	1.79	1.72	1.67	1.62	1.56	1.53	1.47	1.45	1.40	1.37	1.35
2.35	**2.28**	**2.15**	**2.07**	**1.98**	**1.88**	**1.82**	**1.74**	**1.69**	**1.62**	**1.56**	**1.53**
1.82	1.77	1.70	1.65	1.60	1.54	1.51	1.45	1.42	1.38	1.35	1.32
2.32	**2.24**	**2.11**	**2.03**	**1.94**	**1.84**	**1.78**	**1.70**	**1.65**	**1.57**	**1.52**	**1.49**
1.79	1.75	1.68	1.63	1.57	1.51	1.48	1.42	1.39	1.34	1.30	1.28
2.26	**2.19**	**2.06**	**1.98**	**1.89**	**1.79**	**1.73**	**1.64**	**1.59**	**1.51**	**1.46**	**1.43**
1.77	1.72	1.65	1.60	1.55	1.49	1.45	1.39	1.36	1.31	1.27	1.25
2.23	**2.15**	**2.03**	**1.94**	**1.85**	**1.75**	**1.68**	**1.59**	**1.54**	**1.46**	**1.40**	**1.37**
1.76	1.71	1.64	1.59	1.54	1.47	1.44	1.37	1.34	1.29	1.25	1.22
2.20	**2.12**	**2.00**	**1.91**	**1.83**	**1.72**	**1.66**	**1.56**	**1.51**	**1.43**	**1.37**	**1.33**

Critical Values of *F—Concluded*

**DEGREES OF
FREEDOM FOR
DENOMINATOR**

DEGREES OF FREEDOM FOR NUMERATOR

	1	2	3	4	5	6	7	8	9	10	11	12
200	3.89	3.04	2.65	2.41	2.26	2.14	2.05	1.98	1.92	1.87	1.83	1.80
	6.76	**4.71**	**3.88**	**3.41**	**3.11**	**2.90**	**2.73**	**2.60**	**2.50**	**2.41**	**2.34**	**2.28**
400	3.86	3.02	2.62	2.39	2.23	2.12	2.03	1.96	1.90	1.85	1.81	1.78
	6.70	**4.66**	**3.83**	**3.36**	**3.06**	**2.85**	**2.69**	**2.55**	**2.46**	**2.37**	**2.29**	**2.23**
1000	3.85	3.00	2.61	2.38	2.22	2.10	2.02	1.95	1.89	1.84	1.80	1.76
	6.66	**4.62**	**3.80**	**3.34**	**3.04**	**2.82**	**2.66**	**2.53**	**2.43**	**2.34**	**2.26**	**2.20**
∞	3.84	2.99	2.60	2.37	2.21	2.09	2.01	1.94	1.88	1.83	1.79	1.75
	6.64	**4.60**	**3.78**	**3.32**	**3.02**	**2.80**	**2.64**	**2.51**	**2.41**	**2.32**	**2.24**	**2.18**

14	16	20	24	30	40	50	75	100	200	500	∞
1.74	1.69	1.62	1.57	1.52	1.45	1.42	1.35	1.32	1.26	1.22	1.19
2.17	**2.09**	**1.97**	**1.88**	**1.79**	**1.69**	**1.62**	**1.53**	**1.48**	**1.39**	**1.33**	**1.28**
1.72	1.67	1.60	1.54	1.49	1.42	1.38	1.32	1.28	1.22	1.16	1.13
2.12	**2.04**	**1.92**	**1.84**	**1.74**	**1.64**	**1.57**	**1.47**	**1.42**	**1.32**	**1.24**	**1.19**
1.70	1.65	1.58	1.53	1.47	1.41	1.36	1.30	1.26	1.19	1.13	1.08
2.09	**2.01**	**1.89**	**1.81**	**1.71**	**1.61**	**1.54**	**1.44**	**1.38**	**1.28**	**1.19**	**1.11**
1.69	1.64	1.57	1.52	1.46	1.40	1.35	1.28	1.24	1.17	1.11	1.00
2.07	**1.99**	**1.87**	**1.79**	**1.69**	**1.59**	**1.52**	**1.41**	**1.36**	**1.25**	**1.15**	**1.00**

Appendix D

Critical Values of Chi-Square

PROBABILITY UNDER H_0 THAT $X^2 \geq$ CHI-SQUARE

df	.99	.98	.95	.90	.80	.70	.50	.30	.20	.10	.05	.02	.01	.001
1	.00016	.00063	.0039	.016	.064	.15	.46	1.07	1.64	2.71	3.84	5.41	6.64	10.83
2	.02	.04	.10	.21	.45	.71	1.39	2.41	3.22	4.60	5.99	7.82	9.21	13.82
3	.12	.18	.35	.58	1.00	1.42	2.37	3.66	4.64	6.25	7.82	9.84	11.34	16.27
4	.30	.43	.71	1.06	1.65	2.20	3.36	4.88	5.99	7.78	9.49	11.67	13.28	18.46
5	.55	.75	1.14	1.61	2.34	3.00	4.35	6.06	7.29	9.24	11.07	13.39	15.09	20.52
6	.87	1.18	1.64	2.20	3.07	3.83	5.35	7.23	8.56	10.64	12.59	15.03	16.81	22.46
7	1.24	1.56	2.17	2.83	3.82	4.67	6.35	8.38	9.80	12.02	14.07	16.62	18.48	24.32
8	1.65	2.03	2.73	3.49	4.59	5.53	7.34	9.52	11.03	13.36	15.51	18.17	20.09	26.12
9	2.09	2.53	3.32	4.17	5.38	6.39	8.34	10.66	12.24	14.68	16.92	19.68	21.67	27.88
10	2.56	3.06	3.94	4.86	6.18	7.27	9.34	11.78	13.44	15.99	18.31	21.16	23.21	29.59
11	3.05	3.61	4.58	5.58	6.99	8.15	10.34	12.90	14.63	17.28	19.68	22.62	24.72	31.26
12	3.57	4.18	5.23	6.30	7.81	9.03	11.34	14.01	15.81	18.55	21.03	24.05	26.22	32.91
13	4.11	4.76	5.89	7.04	8.63	9.93	12.34	15.12	16.98	19.81	22.36	25.47	27.69	34.53
14	4.66	5.37	6.57	7.79	9.47	10.82	13.34	16.22	18.15	21.06	23.68	26.87	29.14	36.12
15	5.23	5.98	7.26	8.55	10.31	11.72	14.34	17.32	19.31	22.81	25.00	28.26	30.58	37.70
16	5.81	6.61	7.96	9.31	11.15	12.62	15.34	18.42	20.46	23.54	26.30	29.83	32.00	39.29
17	6.41	7.26	8.67	10.08	12.00	13.53	16.34	19.51	21.62	24.77	27.59	31.00	33.41	40.75
18	7.02	7.91	9.39	10.86	12.86	14.44	17.34	20.60	22.76	25.99	28.87	32.35	34.80	42.31
19	7.63	8.57	10.12	11.65	13.72	15.35	18.34	21.69	23.90	27.20	30.14	33.69	36.19	43.82
20	8.26	9.24	10.85	12.44	14.58	16.27	19.34	22.78	25.04	28.41	31.41	35.02	37.57	45.82
21	8.90	9.92	11.59	13.24	15.44	17.18	20.34	23.86	26.17	29.62	32.67	36.34	38.93	46.80
22	9.54	10.60	12.34	14.04	16.31	18.10	21.34	24.94	27.30	30.81	33.92	37.66	40.29	48.27
23	10.20	11.29	13.09	14.85	17.19	19.02	22.34	26.02	28.43	32.01	35.17	38.97	41.64	49.73
24	10.86	11.99	13.85	15.66	18.06	19.94	23.34	27.10	29.55	33.20	36.42	40.27	42.98	51.18
25	11.52	12.70	14.61	16.47	18.94	20.87	24.34	28.17	30.68	34.38	37.65	41.57	44.31	52.62
26	12.20	13.41	15.38	17.29	19.82	21.79	25.34	29.25	31.80	35.58	38.88	42.86	45.64	54.05
27	12.88	14.12	16.15	18.11	20.70	22.72	26.34	30.32	32.91	36.74	40.11	44.14	46.96	55.48
28	13.56	14.85	16.93	18.94	21.59	23.65	27.34	31.39	34.03	37.92	41.34	45.42	48.28	56.89
29	14.26	15.57	17.71	19.77	22.48	24.58	28.34	32.46	35.14	39.09	42.56	46.69	49.59	58.30
30	14.95	16.31	18.49	20.60	23.36	25.51	29.34	33.53	36.25	40.26	43.77	47.96	50.89	59.70

From Table IV of Fisher & Yates, *Statistical Tables for Biological, Agricultural and Medical Research.* Published by Longman Group UK Ltd., 1974. Reprinted by permission of Addison Wesley Longman Ltd.

Glossary

abstract Preliminary item in a research report that provides a brief summary of the research study.

acknowledgments Preliminary item in a research report in which the author lists the contributions of others who have assisted with the research.

action planning A unique stage within the action research process whereby the researcher identifies local actions that take place based on the findings of the study.

action research A distinct type of applied, practical research often seen in education in which the focus is on local needs, problems, or issues.

alpha level Probability level selected that warrants rejection of the null hypothesis.

analysis of covariance (ANCOVA) A statistical technique to gain control by adjusting for initial differences among groups.

analysis of variance (ANOVA) A statistical test with two or more groups.

applied research Research whose primary aim is toward the solution of practical problems, yet seeks to make inferences beyond the study setting.

article format Alternative form of a research report prepared by graduate students whose format is based upon the style specified by the journal in which the student hopes to publish the manuscript.

assent Statement of consent or agreement made by a child regarding his or her involvement in a research project.

assumptions Facts or conditions presumed to be true, yet not actually verified, that become underlying basics in the planning and implementation of the research study.

attributable risk Percentage of cases in the total group that occur in the group with a risk factor.

authorship The primary method through which researchers receive recognition for their research efforts.

background information Important literature on the topic being investigated that is cited in the introductory section of a research report, thus establishing the foundation for the study.

basic research Research whose primary aim is the discovery of new knowledge through theory development or evaluation.

bell-shaped curve *See* **normal curve.**

Belmont Report The fundamental document that provides current federal regulations for the protection of human participants in research in the United States.

Beneficence Ethical principle obligating researchers to protect persons from harm and to maximize possible benefits and minimize possible harms.

beta (β) Probability of making a type II error.

block design An extension of matched pairs design with three or more groups.

boolean search strategy A strategy for searching electronic literature databases by using AND, OR, and NOT between search words.

case study Study that provides an intensive, holistic, and in-depth understanding of a single unit or bounded system. Also involves studying an event, activity, program, process, or one or more individuals.

causal-comparative research Research that seeks to investigate cause-and-effect relationships that explain differences that already exist in groups or individuals; also called *ex post facto research.*

cell A row-column intersection in a two-dimensional data layout.

central tendency A descriptive value that indicates the point at which scores tend to be concentrated.

central tendency error A tendency to rate most participants in the middle of the rating scale.

closed-ended item Same definition as for multiple-choice item.

cluster sampling A type of probability sampling in which the sampling unit is a naturally occurring group or cluster (such as classrooms) of members of the population.

coefficient alpha *See* **Cronbach's alpha.**

coefficient of determination A value that indicates the amount of variability in one measure that is explained by the other measure.

common rule The general name for federal law 45 C.F.R. 46 that establishes regulations governing research involving human participants in the United States.

completion item Question for which answer is left blank and participant fills in the blank.

conceptual literature The conjectural, often abstract, literature that provides the theoretical underpinnings for a research study.

conclusions A closing portion of a research report in which the author provides an answer to the research problem.

confidentiality The ability to link information or data collected during a research study to a person's identity.

confirmability A form of objectivity associated with qualitative research.

constant comparison A qualitative analysis technique for recording, coding, and analyzing data.

construct Something which is known to exist although it may not be precisely defined and/or measured.

construct validity evidence Evidence that a test measures a construct and yields scores that can be validly interpreted.

content analysis A process in which a researcher examines a class of social artifacts, typically written documents, to describe specific characteristics of a message.

continuous scores Scores that have a potentially infinite number of values.

control group In a research study, the group which receives no treatment that should change its ability.

correlation A mathematical technique for determining the relationship between two sets of scores.

correlation coefficient A value indicating the degree of relationship between two sets of scores.

correlational research Type of research that seeks to investigate the extent of the relationship between two or more vaiables.

counterbalanced design Method of gaining control by all participants receiving all treatments but in different orders.

covariate Score used to adjust for initial differences among groups in ANCOVA.

credibility A form of internal validity associated with qualitative research.

criteria for critiquing an article Basic standards or guidelines for evaluating a research report or proposal.

criterion validity evidence A correlation coefficient between scores on a test and scores on a criterion measure or standard.

criterion-referenced standards Minimum proficiency or pass-fail standards.

critical reading The process of reading a large amount of literature while thinking about, reflecting upon, and critically analyzing what is being said.

critical region The region at which all values of the statistical test are at or beyond the critical value.

critical value The tabled value of the statistical test needed to reject the null hypothesis.

Cronbach's alpha A correlation coefficient calculated as an estimate of objectivity and reliability; also called *coefficient alpha*.

cross-sectional approach Method for testing many groups and assuming each group is representative of all other groups when they are at the point in time.

cross-validation Method for checking the accuracy of a prediction equation on a second group of individuals similar to the first group.

curvilinear relationship A relationship between two variables best represented graphically by a curved line.

data analysis The methods of manipulating and analyzing the collected data to reveal relevant information.

data collection plan Detailed procedure for acquiring the information needed to attack the research problem.

data-collecting instruments The tools or procedures used by the researcher to collect relevant data pertaining to the research problem.

data reduction A process of investigating and transforming raw data, often using a coding technique, in order to make sense of and identify themes within the data; part of data analysis in qualitative research.

deductive analysis Examination of a phenomenon by going from broad ideas to specific application.

deductive reasoning Thinking that proceeds from a general assumption to a specific logical conclusion.

definition of terms Explanation of important terms as they are used in a research study.

degrees of freedom A value associated with a statistical test which is used when finding a table value of the statistical test.

delimitations Characteristics specified by the investigator that define the scope of the research study, in effect, "fencing it in."

Delphi technique A method of data collection using questioning techniques to obtain a consensus from a defined group of individuals on a specific issue.

dependability A form of reliability associated with qualitative research.

dependent variable The variable that is expected to change as a result of the independent variable; it is the variable that is observed or measured in a study.

descriptive questions Type of research question that seeks to describe phenomena or characteristics of a particular group of subjects.

descriptive research Research that attempts to systematically describe specific characteristics or conditions related to a subject group.

descriptive statistic Statistic used to describe characteristics of a group.

designs The ways a research study may be conducted.

difference questions Type of research question that seeks to determine if there are differences between or within groups or conditions.

directional hypothesis Type of research hypothesis that is posited when the researcher has reason to believe that a particular relationship or difference exists between groups of subjects.

discrete scores Scores that are limited to a specific number of values.

discussion section Section of a research report containing a nontechnical explanation or interpretation of the results, culminating with the researcher's conclusions.

distilling The process of narrowing an initial research question to a specific problem that is amenable to investigation.

double-blind study A study in which participants and those conducting the study are unaware of the purpose of the study and group membership of participants.

effect size An estimate of the practical difference between two means; used in meta-analysis as a standard unit of measurement.

element The basic unit from which data or information is collected; normally the research participant.

essence Core meaning of an experience.

ethics Moral principles that define one's values in terms of acceptable behaviors.

ethnographical research Research that describes and interprets a cultural or social group.

expected frequency The frequency hypothesized or expected for an answer in a chi-square test.

experiment-wise error rate Probability of making a type I error somewhere in all the two-group comparisons conducted.

experimental research Type of research in which an independent variable is manipulated to observe the effect on a dependent variable for the purpose of determining a cause-and-effect relationship.

ex post facto research See **causal-comparative research.**

external criticism Method used in historical research to determine the authenticity, genuineness, and validity of the source of data.

external validity Validity of generalizing the findings in a research study to other groups and situations.

extraneous variable Error-producing variable that could negatively affect the results of a research study if not adequately controlled.

factorial design A two-way ANOVA design with rows representing a classification or treatment and columns representing a treatment.

fishbowl technique Simple random sampling technique by which the names of all members of a population are placed in a container (such as a fishbowl) and then randomly drawn from the container one at a time.

45 C.F.R. 46 Specific federal law, referred to as the **Common Rule,** that establishes regulations governing research involving human participants in the United States.

focus group interview An interviewing technique where a group of participants are interviewed together.

frequency polygon A line graph of scores and their frequencies.

good test A test for which acceptable objectivity, reliability, and validity of the data have been determined; also described by the *test is good*.

grounded theory Derivation of a theory from the views of the participants in a study; develops theories that are "grounded" in real-world experiences.

halo effect The tendency to let initial impressions influence future ratings or scores of a participant.

Helsinki Declaration Ethical guidelines defined by the World Medical Association for medical research involving human participants.

histogram A bar graph of scores and their frequencies.

historical research Type of research involving an exploration of past events and phenomena in order to provide a better understanding of present events and help anticipate future occurrences.

hypothesis A tentative explanation or prediction of the eventual outcome of a research problem.

impact factor Computed index of the quality of a scholarly journal based upon the frequency with which a journal's articles are cited by other researchers.

imperfect induction Conclusion derived through inductive reasoning based on the observations of a small number of members of a population.

independent variable The experimental or treatment variable in a study; it is the variable that is purposively manipulated or selected by the researcher in order to determine its effect on some observed phenomenon; it is antecedent to the dependent variable.

induction Thinking method that proceeds from the specific to the general; basic principle of scientific inquiry in which information gained through observations of a small number of cases lead to generalized conclusions.

inferential statistics Statistics used in the process of making inference from a sample to a population.

informed consent Explicit statement informing potential research participants of the purposes, procedures, risks, and benefits of a research project; provides an acknowledgment that participation is done so voluntarily.

Institutional Review Board (IRB) Local committee established by an institution whose purpose is to ensure the protection of human participants involved in research activities.

instrumentation Portion of the methods section of a research report describing the measuring instrument or equipment, such as a questionnaire, test, or inventory, used to collect data from the research participants.

internal consistency reliability Consistency of test scores within a single day.

internal criticism Method used in historical research to assess the meaning and accuracy of the source of data.

internal validity Validity of the findings within or internal to the research study.

interval scores Scores that have a common unit of measurement between each score, but do not have a true zero point.

interview Face-to-face interaction (individual or group), telephone interaction (individual or group), or chat room discussion.

interview prompts Interpretive type questions used to seek more information or detail from the participant during an interview; also called interview probes.

intraclass correlation coefficient A correlation coefficient calculated as an estimate of objectivity and reliability.

introduction section The introductory portion of a research report that provides background information and develops the rationale for conducting the study.

justice Ethical principle requiring that the benefits and burdens of research be fairly distributed, thus impacting upon the selection of research participants.

kappa coefficient Another estimate of the reliability of dichotomous data.

Kuder-Richardson A correlation coefficient calculated as an estimate of reliability.

leptokurtic curve A curve that is more sharply peaked than a normal curve, indicating an extremely homogeneous group.

life histories Studies that cover the lives of individuals or that result from one or more individuals providing stories about their lives. Also known as *narrative research* or *biographical research*.

Likert scale A type of scaling technique by which respondents are presented with a series of statements and asked to indicate the degree to which they agree or disagree.

limitations Aspects of a research study that the investigator cannot control, that represent weaknesses to the study, and that may negatively affect the results.

line of best fit A straight line that represents the trend or relationship in the data; also known as the *regresson line*.

linear relationship A relationship between two variables best represented graphically by a straight line.

logical validity evidence A statement based on knowledge that a test measures an attribute and yields scores that can be validly interpreted.

longitudinal approach Method by which a group is measured and observed for years.

matched pairs design A form of selective manipulation by which participants are matched to gain control.

mean A measure of central tendency, used with interval or ratio data, that is the sum of the scores divided by the number of scores.

mean square (MS) value Values used in ANOVA to calculate an F statistic.

measurement techniques Methods for collecting information in which participants are directly tested or measured on the characteristics of interest; may include physical measures, cognitive measures, and affective measures.

median A measure of central tendency used with ordinal data that indicates the middle score.

meta-analysis A research approach involving the reanalysis of the results from a large number of research studies.

metasearch engine Website that uses multiple search engines simultaneously to perform an Internet search.

methods section Section of a research report that describes the research participants, instrumentation, and procedures for data collection.

mixed methods research Combination of both quantitative and qualitative research methods or combination of different types of qualitative research methods.

mode A measure of central tendency used with nominal data that indicates the score most frequently received.

modified kappa A third estimate of the reliability of dichotomous data.

multiple prediction Prediction of an individual's score on a measure based on the individual's scores on several other measures.

multiple-choice item Question for which responses are provided and the participant selects the most appropriate response(s).

multistage sampling A type of cluster sampling technique which involves the successive selection of clusters within clusters and/or elements within clusters.

multivariate statistic Statistic for which each participant contributes multiple scores to the data analysis.

multivariate tests Tests for which each participant contributes multiple scores to the data analysis.

Nazi experimentation Medical experiments conducted by German scientists during World War II, that subjected unwilling participants to extreme cruelty and inhuman treatment.

nominal scores Scores that cannot be hierarchically ordered.

nondirectional hypothesis Type of research hypothesis that is posited when the researcher has no reason to believe that a difference or relationship exists in any direction.

nonparametric statistic Statistic that has no requirement of interval data and normal distribution.

nonparametric tests Statistical tests that do not assume interval data and normal distribution of the scores.

nonprobability sampling A sampling technique such as convenience sampling in which random processes are not used and the probability of selecting a given sampling unit from the population is not known.

nonreferred journal Type of scholarly journal in which the manuscripts are not evaluated by external reviewers, although they may be appraised by the journal editor.

nonsignificant Value of the statistical test does not warrant rejection of the null hypothesis; differences among groups are sampling error.

norm-referenced standards Standards to rank-order individuals from best to worst.

normal curve A symmetrical curve centered around a point with a defined base to height ratio, indicating a balanced distribution; also called a *bell-shaped curve*.

null (statistical) hypothesis Hypothesis used for statistical testing purposes that proposes that there is no difference between comparison groups or no relationship between variables; hypothesis stating that the independent variable has "no effect" on the dependent variable.

Nuremberg Code Basic principles of ethical conduct that govern research involving human participants that were developed as a result of Nuremburg trials of German scientists.

objectivity The degree to which multiple scorers agree on the values of collected measures or scores; also called *rater reliability*.

objectivity coefficient A correlation coefficient indicating the relationship between the scores of the scorers.

observation techniques Methods for collecting information in which subjects are observed by the researcher, either directly or indirectly, and relevant data recorded.

observed frequency The frequency in the sample for an answer in a chi-square test.

odds ratio An estimate of relative risk.

one-group *t* test A statistical test used with one sample.

one-way (goodness of fit) chi-square tests A nonparametric statistical test using frequencies arranged in columns.

one-way ANOVA A statistical analysis used with two, or more, independent groups.

open-ended item Question for which no potential response is provided; participants respond however they choose.

ordinal scores Scores that do not have a common unit of measurement between each score, but are ordered from high to low.

outlier An extremely high or low score that does not seem typical for the group tested.

parameters Values or quantities calculated using information obtained from a population.

parametric statistic Statistic that requires interval data and a normal distribution.

parametric tests Statistical tests that assume interval data and normal distribution of scores.

participant observation An observational technique in which the researcher or observer participates in the setting and in the same activities as the people being observed.

per-comparison error rate Probability of making a type I error in a single two-group comparison.

percent agreement An estimate of the reliability of dichotomous data.

percentiles or percentile ranks A descriptive value that indicates the percentage of participants below a designated score; used in norm referenced standards.

perfect induction Conclusion derived through inductive reasoning based on the observations of all members of a population.

phenomenological research Identifies the "essence" or core of human experience.

phi A correlation coefficient calculated as an estimate of validity for dichotomous data.

physical manipulation Method of gaining control by the researcher physically controlling the research surroundings.

placebo A treatment that can have no effect on any dependent variable of participants in a control group.

plagiarism The presentation of ideas or the work of others as one's own, the absence of proper credit.

platykurtic curve A curve that is less sharply peaked than a normal curve, indicating an extremely heterogeneous group.

polynomial regression A regression model which does not assume a linear relationship; a curvilinear correlation coefficient is computed.

population An entire group or aggregate of people or elements of interest from which a sample will be selected.

prediction Estimation of a person's score on one measure based on the individual's score on one or more other measures.

preexperimental designs Designs that have poor control often due to no random sampling.

preliminary items Front matter of a thesis or dissertation that includes items such as a title page, approval page, acknowledgments page, table of contents, list of tables and figures, and an abstract; introductory material in a published research report; may include title, author, institution, acknowledgments, and abstract.

primary source material Original sources in historical research.

privacy The capacity of individuals to control when and under what conditions others will have access to their behaviors, beliefs, and values.

probability sampling A sampling technique based upon random processes in which the probability of selecting each participant or element is known.

procedures Portion of the methods section of a research report that includes a description of data collection procedures, experimental treatments, and how they were administered; a step-by-step description of how the study was conducted.

purpose statement A specific statement expressing the researcher's intent or goal for conducting the study; normally indicates the variables or phenomenon of interest and information regarding the participants and setting of the study.

qualitative research Research based upon nonnumerical data obtained in natural settings through extensive observations and interviews whose primary aim is the interpretation of phenomena and the discovery of meaning.

quantitative research Research involving the collection of numerical data in order to describe phenomena, investigate relationships between variables, and explore cause-and-effect relationships of phenomena of interest.

quasi-experimental design An acceptable design but with some loss of control due to lack of random sampling.

questioning techniques Methods for collecting information in which the subjects are asked to respond to questions posed by the researcher; may include self-report questionnaires, personal or group interviews, or telephone interviews.

random assignment Technique of using random processes to assign research participants to treatment conditions or comparison groups.

random blocks ANOVA A statistical analysis where participants similar in terms of a variable are placed together in a block and then randomly assigned to treatment groups.

random selection Technique of using random processes for the selection of a sample that is thought to be representative of the population of interest.

range A measure of variability that is the difference between the highest and lowest score.

rank order correlation coefficient *See* **rho.**

rater reliability *See* **objectivity.**

ratio scores Scores that have a common unit of measurement between each score and a true zero point.

real difference Difference among groups means because the groups are different and not due to sampling error.

recommendations Portion of a research report, often included in the discussion section, in which the researcher presents suggestions for professional practice and/or further research based upon the findings of the current research study.

refereed (peer-reviewed) journal Type of scholarly journal in which the manuscripts undergo a careful evaluation by the editor and expert reviewers in the field.

references Lists of all books, journal articles, or other sources cited by the author in a research report.

reflexivity Systematic reflection on how personal assumptions, biases, and values shape a study.

regression The statistical model used to predict performance on one variable from another.

related research Scientific reports of previous research related to the problem area being studied.

relationship questions Type of research question that seeks to investigate the relationship or association between two or more variables.

relative risk Likelihood that a group with a risk factor will have a health characteristic in comparison to a group without a risk factor; see also **odds ratio.**

reliability Degree to which a measure is consistent and unchanged over a short period of time.

reliability coefficient A correlation coefficient indicating the relationship between the repeated measures or scores of a test.

repeated measures A two dependent groups *t*-test design where participants are tested before and after a treatment.

repeated measures ANOVA A statistical analysis where each participant is measured on two or more occasions.

representative sample A sample or subgroup of a population that is similar to the population on the characteristics of interest.

research A systematic attempt to find solutions to a problem or to answer a question.

research approaches General procedures that a researcher may take in investigating the problem of interest; may include historical, descriptive, qualitative, or experimental methods.

research hypothesis A tentative explanation or prediction of the eventual outcome of a research problem; normally this is the outcome expected by the investigator.

research participants People participating in a research study; portion of the methods section of a research report used to present information about the people being studied.

research process Procedure founded upon the scientific method for investigating research problems that involve systematic progression through a series of necessary steps.

research proposal Document presenting a researchable problem and a plan of attack and protocol for investigating the problem; often required by a potential funding agency or thesis/dissertation committee.

research question The central focus of the research effort that serves as the basis for the research problem and provides direction for the entire process.

research report A scientific paper completed at the culmination of a research project in which the results of the investigation are presented to others.

respect for persons Ethical principle proclaiming respect for individuals involved as participants in research studies.

results section Section of a research report where the researcher reports the results of the data collection efforts as well as the outcomes of the various data analysis procedures.

reviews Comprehensive discourse or essay that provides a synthesis of the research and conceptual literature on a particular topic.

rho A value indicating the degree of relationship between two sets of ranks; also known as *Spearman's rho* and *rank order correlation coefficient.*

sample A subgroup of a population of interest from which data are collected.

sample size The number of elements or research participants in a sample selected for scientific study.

sampling The process whereby a small proportion or subgroup of a population of interest is selected for scientific study.

sampling error Difference among group means because the samples are not 100 percent representative of a population; the extent to which sample values (statistics) deviate from those that would be obtained from the entire population (parameter).

sampling frame The accessible population or collection of elements from which the sample is drawn.

sampling unit The element or group of elements (cluster) that is selected during the sampling process.

scaling techniques Methods for measuring the degree to which a subject values or exhibits a concept or characteristic of interest; uses a graded response format that assigns values to the strength or intensity of one's responses.

scattergram A graph that shows the relationship between two variables.

scholarly journals A primary source of literature that provides the firsthand reporting of research studies that serves to building the knowledge base in a field.

scientific method A way of solving problems and acquiring knowledge that involves both deductive and induction reasoning in a systematic approach to obtaining data.

scientific misconduct The fabrication, falsification, plagiarism, or other practices that seriously deviate from those commonly accepted by the scientific community for proposing, conducting, or reporting research.

search engines Websites that perform automated searches of Internet databases for specific information based upon specification of a key word or words.

secondary source material Secondhand sources in historical research.

selective manipulation Method of gaining control by selectively manipulating certain participants or situations.

semantic differential scale A type of scaling technique in which respondents are asked to make judgments about a concept of interest using a continuum consisting of bipolar adjectives.

semistructured interview Interview for which each participant is asked the same general questions.

significant Value of the statistical test that warrants rejection of the null hypothesis; differences among groups are real differences.

simple effects tests Tests to compare the column means for each row or the row means for each column in a two-way ANOVA design.

simple frequency distribution An ordered listing of the scores and their frequencies.

simple prediction Prediction of an individual's score on a measure based on the individual's score on another measure.

simple random sample A type of probability sample in which every element in the population has an equal chance of being selected and the selection of one element does not interfere with the selection chances of any other element (i.e., equal and independent).

single-blind study A study in which participants are unaware of the purpose of the research study and their role in the study.

situational ethics Ethical paradigm that proposes that no general rules can be applied to all situations and that ethics are situational specific.

skewed curve An asymmetrical curve, indicating an unbalanced distribution.

slope Angle of the graphed prediction line; rate of change in the predicted score with a change in the predictor score.

Spearman's rho *See* **rho.**

stability reliability Consistency of test scores across several days.

standard deviation A measure of variability that indicates the spread of the scores around the mean.

standard error of measurement An estimate of the amount of measurement error to expect in the score of any person in a group.

standard error of prediction The standard deviation for the errors of prediction; an index of the accuracy of a prediction equation.

standard scores Scores that are used to change scores from different tests to a common unit of measurement.

statistical hypothesis Hypothesis tested with a statistical test.

statistical power Probability of not making a type II error.

statistical techniques Method of gaining control if other control techniques are not possible.

statistics Values or quantities calculated using information obtained from a sample; used to estimate population information.

stratified random sampling A type of probability sampling in which the population is first divided into specific strata or subgroups and then a set number of research participants are randomly selected from each strata.

structured interview Interview for which each participant is asked the same specific questions.

structured questionnaire Type of measurement instrument that includes questions along with prescribed response alernatives from which the respondents must choose, such as yes-no or multiple-choice items; also called a *closed-ended questionnaire.*

subject directories Internet "yellow pages" that enable the user to peruse World Wide Web sources according to subject areas.

sums of squares (SS) Variability values in ANOVA.

supplementary items Back matter of a thesis or dissertation that includes items such as questionnaires, consent documents, instructions to research participants, diagrams of research settings, and tables of raw data.

syllogism A process of logical reasoning in which conclusions are based on a series of propositions or assumptions.

systematic sampling A type of probability sampling in which the sample is drawn by choosing every k_{th} element (research participant) from a listing of the population, where k is a constant representing the sampling interval.

table of random numbers A table (or book) consisting of numbers arranged in a random order that may be used to select a random sample or to assign research participants to groups.

test A data-gathering technique to obtain a set of scores.

test is good *See* **good test.**

theory A belief or assumption about the causal relationship between variables that serves to explain phenomena.

thesis format Traditional, generic format of a research report prepared by graduate students in which the body of the report is organized within specific chapters, such as introduction, review of literature, procedures or methods, results and discussion.

true experimental designs The best type of design because there is good control with sufficient random sampling.

Tuskegee Syphilis Study U.S. Public Health Service research study conducted in mid-1900s that is infamous for the maltreatment of the participants.

two dependent groups *t* test A statistical test used with two dependent groups or columns of scores.

two independent groups *t* test A statistical test used with two independent samples.

two-dimensional ANOVA Same as two-way ANOVA.

two-group comparisons Statistical techniques to compare groups two at a time following a significant *F* in ANOVA. Also called *multiple comparisons* and *a posteriori comparisons*.

two-way (contingency table) chi-square tests Nonparametric statistical test using frequencies arranged in rows and columns.

two-way ANOVA An ANOVA design with rows and columns.

type I error Rejection of a true null hypothesis.

type II error Acceptance or nonrejection of a false null hypothesis.

univariate statistic Statistic for which each participant contributes one score to the data analysis.

univariate tests Tests for which each participant contributes one score to the data analysis.

unstructured interview Interview for which no questions have been prepared for a participant; just a conversation.

unstructured questionnaire Type of measurement instrument that includes questions for which the response alternatives are not listed and respondents will answer freely in their own words; also called an *open-ended questionnaire*.

validity The degree to which interpretations of test scores or measures derived from a measuring instrument lead to correct conclusions.

variability A descriptive value that describes the data in terms of their spread or heterogeneity.

variable A characteristic, trait, or attribute of a person or thing that can take on more than one value and can be classified or measured.

variance A measure of variability that is the square of the standard deviation.

variate The score adjusted in ANCOVA.

verification Method for testing interpretations for plausibility, sturdiness, or confirmability.

working bibliography An annotated listing of all literature sources that are pertinent to the research problem being studied.

y-intercept The point where the graphed prediction line crosses the *Y*-axis; the value of the predicted score when the predictor score is zero.

z score A standard score with mean 0 and standard deviation 1.0.

References

Agbuga, B., Xiang, P., and McBride, R. (2010). Achievement goals and their relations to children's disruptive behaviors in an after-school physical activity program. *Journal of Teaching in Physical Education, 29*(3), 278–294.

Alreck, P. L., and Settle, R. B. (2004). *The survey research handbook* (3rd ed.). Chicago, IL: Irwin.

Alward, E. C. (1996). *Research paper, step-by-step*. Westhampton, MA: Pine Island Press.

American College of Sports Medicine (1999). Policy statement regarding the use of human subjects and informed consent. *Medicine and Science in Sports and Exercise, 31*(7), vi.

American Educational Research Association (1999). *Standards for educational and psychological testing*. Washington, DC: Author.

American Educational Research Association (2011). *Ethical standards of the American Educational Research Association*. Retrieved September 12, 2011, from http://www.aera.net/aboutaera/?id=222.

American Psychological Association (2010). *Publication manual of the American Psychological Association* (6th ed.). Washington, DC: Author.

American Psychological Association (2010). Ethical principles of psychologists and code of conduct. Retrieved September 12, 2011, from http://www.apa.org/ethics/code/index.aspx.

American Sociological Association (1999). *Code of ethics*. Washington, DC: Author.

Amis, J. (2005). Interviewing for case study research. In D. L. Andrews, D. S. Mason, and M. L. Silk (Eds.), *Qualitative methods in sports studies* (pp. 104–138). Oxford: Berg Publishers.

Amorose, A. J., and Horn, T. S. (2000). Intrinsic motivation: Relationships with collegiate athletes' gender, scholarship status, and perceptions of their coaches' behavior. *Journal of Sports and Exercise Psychology, 22*(1), 63–84.

Araki, K. (2000). The effect of color on a controlled accuracy task. Master's thesis, University of Northern Iowa, Cedar Falls.

Arthur, W., Bennett, W., and Huffcutt, A. I. (2001). *Conducting meta-analysis using SAS*. Mahwah, NJ: Lawrence Erlbaum Associates.

Ary, D., Jacobs, L. C., and Sorensen, C. (2010). *Introduction to research in education* (8th ed.). Belmont, CA: Wadsworth.

Babbie, E. (1990). *Survey research methods* (2nd ed.). Belmont, CA: Wadsworth.

Babbie, E. (2004). *The practice of social research* (10th ed.). Belmont, CA: Wadsworth.

Bandura, A. (1986). *Social foundations of thought and action: A social-cognitive theory.* Englewood Cliffs, NJ: Prentice-Hall.

Baumgartner, T. A. (1969). Stability of physical performance scores. *Research Quarterly, 40,* 257–261.

Baumgartner, T. A., Jackson, A. S., Mahar, M. T., and Rowe, D. A. (2007). *Measurement for evaluation in physical education and exercise science* (8th ed.). New York: McGraw-Hill.

Baumgartner, T. A., Oh, S., Chung, H., and Hales, P. (2002). Objectivity, reliability, and validity for a revised push-up test protocol. *Measurement in Physical Education and Exercise Science, 6*(4), 225–242.

Bax, L., Yu, L., Ikeda, N., Tsuruta, H., and Moons, K. (2006). Development and validation of MIX: Comprehensive free software for meta-analysis of causal research data. *BMC Medical Research Methodology, 6*(50), www.biomedcentral.com/1471-228816/50.

Beets, M. W., and Pitetti, K. H. (2004). A comparison of shuttle-run performance between midwestern youth and their national and international counterparts. *Pediatric Exercise Science, 16*(2), 94–112.

Behlendorf, B., MacRae, P. G., and Vos Strache, C. (1999). Children's perceptions of physical activity for adults: Competence and appropriateness. *Journal of Aging and Physical Activity, 7*(4), 354–373.

Berg, B. L. (2004). *Qualitative research methods for the social sciences* (5th ed.). Boston, MA: Pearson.

Berryman, J. W. (1995). *Out of many, one: A history of the American College of Sports Medicine.* Champaign, IL: Human Kinetics.

Best, J. W., and Kahn, J. V. (2005). *Research in education* (10th ed.). Boston, MA: Allyn & Bacon.

Bian, W. (1999). Physical activity patterns among physical education major students in selected institutions of China and the United States. Master's thesis, University of Northern Iowa, Cedar Falls.

Billings, D. (2002). The female athlete triad. Master's thesis, University of Northern Iowa, Cedar Falls.

Bookwalter, C. W., and Bookwalter, K. W. (1959). Library techniques. In M. G. Scott (Ed.), *Research methods in health, physical education, and recreation* (pp. 20–38). Washington, DC: American Association for Health, Physical Education, and Recreation.

Borg, G. (1962). *Physical performance and perceived exertion.* Studia Psychologica et Paedagogica. Series altera, Investigationes XI. Lund: Gleerup.

Bradburn, N. M., Sudman, S., and Wansink, B. (2004). *Asking questions: The definitive guide to questionnaire design—for market research, political polls, and social and health questionnaires.* San Francisco, CA: Wiley.

Brown, W. J., Mishra, G., Lee, C., and Bauman, A. (2000). Leisure time physical activity in Australian women: Relationship with well being and symptoms. *Research Quarterly for Exercise and Sport, 71*(3), 206–216.

Brustad, R. J. (1993). Who will go out and play? Parental and psychological influences on children's attraction to physical activity. *Pediatric Exercise Science, 5,* 210–223.

Bukowski, B. J., and Stinson, A. D. (2000). Physical educators' perceptions of block scheduling in secondary school physical education. *Journal of Physical Education, Recreation, and Dance, 71*(1), 53–57.

Campbell, D., and Stanley, J. (1963). *Experimental and quasi-experimental designs for research.* Chicago, IL: Rand McNally.

Cardinal, B. J. (2000). (Un)informed consent in sport science research? A comparison of forms written for two reading levels. *Research Quarterly for Exercise and Sport, 71*(3), 295–301.

Cardinal, B. J., Martin, J. J., and Sachs, M. L. (1996). Readability of written informed consent forms used in exercise and sport psychology research. *Research Quarterly for Exercise and Sport, 67,* 360–362.

Cardinal, B. J., and Thomas, J. R. (2005). The 75th anniversary of Research Quarterly for Exercise and Sport: An analysis of status and contributions. *Research Quarterly for Exercise and Sport, 76,* S122–S134.

Cerin, R., Leslie, E., Sugiyama, T., and Owen, N. (2010). Perceived barriers to leisure-time physical activity in adults: An ecological perspective. *Journal of Physical Activity and Health, 7,* 451–459.

Cheatham, C. C., Manon, A. D., Brown, J. D., and Bolster, D. R. (2000). Cardiovascular responses during prolonged exercise at ventilary threshold. *Medicine and Science in Sports and Exercise, 32*(3), 1080–1087.

Cohen, J. (1988). *Statistical power analysis for the behavioral sciences* (2nd ed.). Mahwah, NJ: Lawrence Erlbaum Associates.

Cohen, J., Cohen, P., West, S. G., and Aiken, L. S. (2003). *Applied multiple regression/correlation analysis for the behavioral sciences.* Mahwah, NJ: Lawrence Erlbaum Associates.

Collins, M. E. (1989). Body figure perceptions and preferences among preadolescent children. Doctoral dissertation, Indiana University, Bloomington.

Columna, L., Foley, J. T., and Lytle, R. K. (2010). Physical education teachers' and teacher candidates' attitudes toward cultural pluralism. *Journal of Teaching in Physical Education, 29*(3), 295–311.

Cone, J. D., and Foster, S. L. (2006). *Dissertations from start to finish* (2nd ed.). Washington, DC: American Psychological Association.

Cook, T. D., and Campbell, D. T. (1979). *Quasi-experimentation: Design and analysis issues for field settings.* Boston, MA: Houghton Mifflin.

Cooper, J. M., and Andrews, E. W. (1975). Rhythm as a linguistic art: Signs, symbols, sounds, and motions. *Quest, 23,* 68–74.

Corbin, J., and Strauss, A. (2008). *Basics of qualitative research* (3rd ed.). Los Angeles, CA: Sage Publications.

Craig, D. V. (2009). *Action research essentials.* San Francisco: John Wiley & Sons, Inc.

Creswell, J. W. (2007). *Qualitative inquiry and research design: Choosing among five traditions* (2nd ed.). Thousand Oaks, CA: Sage.

Creswell, J. W., and Miller, D. L. (2000). Determining validity in qualitative inquiry. *Theory into Practice, 39,* 121–131.

Crimi, K. (2007). Psychosocial correlates of physical activity in children and adolescents. Master's thesis, University of Northern Iowa, Cedar Falls.

Crocker, L., and Algina, J. (2008). *Introduction to classical and modern test theory.* Mason, Ohio: Cengage Learning.

Cronk, B. C., and West, J. L. (2002). Personality research on the Internet: A comparison of Web-based and traditional instruments in take-home and in-class settings. *Behavior Research Methods Instruments and Computers, 34,* 177–180.

Culver, D. M., Gilbert, W. D., and Trudel, P. (2003). A decade of qualitative research in sport psychology journals: 1990–1999. *The Sport Psychologist, 17,* 1–15.

Daley, E. M., McDermott, R. J., Brown, K. R. M., and Kittleson, M. J. (2003). Conducting Web-based survey research: A lesson in Internet design. *American Journal of Health Behavior, 27,* 116–124.

Darracott, S. H. (1995). Individual differences in variability and pattern of performance as a consideration in the selection of a representative score from multiple trial physical performance data. Doctoral dissertation, University of Georgia, Athens, GA.

Dattilo, A. M. (1992). Meta-analysis in nutrition and dietetics. In E. R. Monsen (Ed.), *Research: Successful approaches.* Chicago, IL: The American Dietetic Association.

Day, R. A., and Gastel, B. (2011). *How to write and publish a scientific paper* (7th ed.). Westport, CT: Greenwood Press.

Dees, R. (2003). *Writing the modern research paper* (4th ed.). Toronto: Pearson Education Canada.

Denzin, N. K., and Lincoln, Y. S. (2000). The discipline and practice of qualitative research. In E. G. Guba, Y. S. Lincoln, and N. K. Denzin (Eds.), *Handbook of qualitative research* (2nd ed.) (pp. 1–28). Thousand Oaks, CA: Sage.

Dillman, D. A. (1978). *Mail and telephone surveys: The total design method.* New York: John Wiley and Sons.

Dillman, D. A., Smyth, J. D., and Christian, L. M. (2008). *Internet, mail, and mixed-mode surveys: The tailored design method* (3rd ed.). New York: John Wiley and Sons.

Dishman, R. K., and Buckworth, J. (1996). Increasing physical activity: A quantitative synthesis. *Medicine and Science in Sport and Exercise, 28,* 706–719.

Dishman, R. K., Washburn, R. A., and Heath, G. W. (2004). *Physical activity epidemiology.* Champaign, IL: Human Kinetics.

Domangue, E., and Solmon, M. (2010). Motivational responses to fitness testing by award status and gender. *Research Quarterly for Exercise and Sport, 81,* 310–318.

Drew, C. J., Hardman, M. L., and Hosp, J. L. (2008). *Designing and conducting research in education* (2nd ed.). Needham Heights, MA: Allyn & Bacon.

Drowatzky, J. N. (1996). *Ethical decision making in physical activity research.* Champaign, IL: Human Kinetics.

Duda, J. L. (Ed.). (1998). *Advances in sport and exercise psychology measurement.* Morgantown, WV: Fitness Information Technology, Inc.

Eisenmann, J. C., Bartee, R. T., and Damori, K. D. (2004). Moderate to vigorous physical activity and weight status in rural university students. *Journal of Physical Activity and Health, 1*(3), 209–217.

Eisenmann, J. C., Sarzynski, M. A., Tucker, J., and Heelen, K. A. (2010). Maternal prepregnancy overweight and offspring fatness and blood pressure: Role of physical activity. *Pediatric Exercise Science, 22,* 369–378.

Engels, H. J., Zhu, W., and Moffat, R. J. (1998). An empirical evaluation of the prediction of maximal heart rate. *Research Quarterly for Exercise and Sport, 69*(1), 94–98.

Eshelman, M. (2010). Parental influence on children's physical activity according to community setting. Master's thesis, University of Northern Iowa, Cedar Falls.

Escamilla, R. F., et al. (2010). Cruciate ligament forces between stort-step and long-step lunge. *Medicine and Science in Sports and Exercise, 42,* 1932–1942.

Etnier, J. L., and Landers, D. M. (1998). Motor performance and motor learning as function of age and fitness. *Research Quarterly for Exercise and Sport, 69*(2), 139–146.

Faucette, N., Sallis, J. F., McKenzie, T., Alcaraz, J., Kolody, B., and Nugent, P. (1995). Comparison of fourth grade students' out-of-school physical activity levels and choices by gender: Project SPARK. *Journal of Health Education, 26*(2), S82–S89.

Fenton, L. T., and Pitter, R. (2010). Keeping the body in play: Pain, injury, and socialization in male rugby. *Research Quarterly for Exercise and Sport, 81,* 212–223.

Fey, M. A. (1998). Relationship between self-esteem, eating behaviors, and eating attitudes among female college swimmers. Master's thesis, University of Northern Iowa, Cedar Falls.

45 C.F.R. 46 (1991). Protection of human subjects. Code of Federal Regulations, Vol. 45, Part 46. Retrieved October 15, 2000, from the World Wide Web: ohrp.osophs.dhhs. gov/humansubjects/guidance/45.cfr.46.htm.

Fox, K. R., and Corbin, C. B. (1989). The Physical Self-Perception Profile: Development and preliminary validation. *Journal of Sport and Exercise Psychology, 11,* 408–430.

Frey, G. C. (2004). Comparison of physical activity levels between adults with and without mental retardation. *Journal of Physical Activity and Health, 1*(3), 235–245.

Gall, M. D., Gall, J. P., and Borg, W. R. (2003). *Education research: An introduction* (7th ed.). New York: Allyn and Bacon.

Gall, M. D., Gall, J. P., and Borg, W. R. (2010). *Applying educational research* (6th ed.). Boston, MA: Pearson.

Gay, L. R., Mills, G. E., and Airasian, P. (2008). *Educational research* (8th ed.). Upper Saddle River, NJ: Merrill.

Gibaldi, J. (2009). *MLA handbook: For writers of research papers* (7th ed.). New York: Modern Language Association.

Glaser, B. G., and Strauss, A. (1967). *The discovery of grounded theory: Strategies for qualitative research.* Chicago, IL: Aldine.

Glew, D. (2001). Effect of strength training and other activities on physical self-concept of females. Master's thesis, University of Northern Iowa, Cedar Falls.

Goliszek, A. (2003). *In the name of science: A history of secret programs, medical research and human experimentation.* New York: St. Martin's Press.

Gravetter, F. J., and Forzano, L. B. (2009). *Research methods for the behavioral sciences.* Belmont, CA: Wadsworth.

Gravetter, F. J., and Wallnau, L. B. (2008). *Statistics for the behavioral sciences* (8th ed.). Belmont, CA: Wadsworth Publishing.

Green, L., and Lewis, F. M. (1986). *Measurement and evaluation in health education and health promotion.* Mountain View, CA: Mayfield.

Green, S. B., and Salkind, N. J. (2005). *Using SPSS for Windows and Macintosh: Analyzing and understanding data* (4th ed.). Upper Saddle River, NJ: Prentice-Hall.

Greenbaum, T. L. (1998). *The handbook of focus group research.* Thousand Oaks, CA: Sage Publications.

Grosshans, I. R. (1975). Delbert Oberteuffer: His professional activities and contributions to the fields of health and physical education. Doctoral dissertation, Indiana University, Bloomington.

Guba, E. G. (1990). The alternative paradigm dialog. In E. G. Guba (Ed.), *The paradigm dialog* (pp. 17–27). Newbury Park, CA: Sage.

Hamdan, S. M., and Martinez, R. (2000). An exploration of ethnic/cultural violence perceptions among urban middle and high school students. *Journal of Health Education, 31*(4), 238–246.

Harley, A. E., Buckworth, J., Katz, M. L., Willis, S. K., Odoms-Young, A., and Heaney, C. A. (2009). Developing long-term physical participation: A grounded theory study with African American women. *Health Education Behavior, 36,* 97–112. DOI: 10.1177/1090198107306434.

Harris, M. B. (1998). *Basic statistics for behavioral science research* (2nd ed.). Boston Heights, MA: Allyn & Bacon.

Harter, S. (1982). The perceived competence subscale for children. *Child Development, 53,* 87–97.

Hashim, T. J. (1988). A health knowledge test for male college freshmen in Saudi Arabia. Doctoral dissertation, Indiana University, Bloomington.

Henderson, K. A. (2006). *Dimensions of choice: A qualitative approach to recreation, parks, and leisure research* (2nd ed.). State College, PA: Venture.

Hendrick, J. (1981). Biomechanical analysis of selected parameters in the field hockey drive. Doctoral dissertation, Indiana University, Bloomington.

Henry, G. M. (1974). The shooting accuracy of third grade students who practiced shooting at goals less than ten feet high. Doctoral dissertation, Indiana University, Bloomington.

Herring, M. P., O'Connor, P. J., and Dishman, R. K. (2010). The effects of exercise training on anxiety symptoms among patients: A systematic review. *Archives of Internal Medicine, 170*(4), 321–331.

Hess, D. (2004). Effects of trampoline training on balance in functionally unstable ankles. Master's thesis, University of Northern Iowa, Cedar Falls.

Holland, J. C. (1970). Heart rates of Indiana high school basketball officials as measured by electrocardiographic radio telemetry. Doctoral dissertation, Indiana University, Bloomington.

Holt, N. L., and Sparkes, A. C. (2001). An ethnographic study of cohesiveness in a college soccer team over a season. *Sports Psychologist, 15,* 237–259.

Huberty, C. J., and Olejnik, S. (2006). *Applied MANOVA and discriminant analysis* (2nd ed.). New York: John Wiley and Sons.

Houser, L. D., Metzler, M. W., Schempp, P. G., and Templin, T. J. (2009). *Historic traditions and future directions of research on teaching and teacher education in physical education.* Morgantown, WV: Fitness Information Technology.

Huberman, A. M., and Miles, M. B. (1998). Data management and analysis methods. In N. K. Denzin and Y. S. Lincoln (Eds.), *Collecting and interpreting qualitative materials* (pp. 179–210). Thousand Oaks, CA: Sage.

Huck, S. W. (2008). *Reading statistics and research* (5th ed.). Boston: Pearson.

Hult, J. S., and Trekell, M. (Eds.). (1991). *A century of women's basketball.* Reston, VA: American Alliance for Health, Physical Education, Recreation and Dance.

Interagency Research Animal Committee (1985). *U.S. government principles for utilization and care of vertebrate animals used in testing, research, and training.* Federal Register, May 20, 1985.

Isaac, S., and Michael, W. B. (1995). *Handbook in research and evaluation* (3rd ed.). San Diego: EdITS.

Johnson, B. J. (1993). *DSTAT 1.10 software for the meta-analytic review of research literature.* Mahwah, NJ: Lawrence Erlbaum Associates.

Jones, J. H. (1983). *Bad blood: The Tuskegee syphilis experiment.* New York: The Free Press.

Kandakai, T. L., and King, K. A. (1999). Perceived self-efficacy in performing lifesaving skills: An assessment of the American Red Cross's responding to emergencies course. *Journal of Health Education, 30*(4), 235–241.

Katz, D. L., Brunner, R. L., St. Jeor, S. T., Scott, B., Jekel, J. F., and Brownel, K. D. (1998). Dietary fat consumption in a cohort of American adults, 1985–1991: Covariates, secular trends, and compliance with guidelines. *American Journal of Health Promotion, 12*(6), 382–390.

Keppel, G., and Wickens, T. (2004). *Design and analysis: A researcher's handbook* (4th ed.). Englewood Cliffs, NJ: Prentice-Hall.

Kowalski, C. L., and Waldron, J. J. (2010). Looking the other way: Athletes' perceptions of coaches' responses to hazing. *International Journal of Sports Science and Coaching, 5,* 87–100.

Kerlinger, F. N. (1973). *Foundations of behavioral science research.* New York: Holt, Rinehart and Winston.

Kraemer, H. C., and Thiemann, S. (1987). *How many subjects?* Newbury Park, CA: Sage Publications.

Krane, V., and Baird, S. M. (2005). Using ethnography in sport psychology. *Journal of Applied Sport Psychology, 17,* 87–107.

Krane, V., Greenleaf, C. A., and Snow, J. (1997). Reaching for gold and the practice of glory: A motivational case study of an elite gymnast. *The Sport Psychologist, 11,* 53–71.

Krane, V., Ross, S. R., Miller, M., Rowse, J. L., Ganoe, K., Andrzejczyk, J. A., and Lucas, C. B. (2010). Power and focus: Self-representation of female college athletes. *Qualitative Research in Sport and Exercise, 2,* 175–195.

Krane, V., Waldron, J. J., Michalenok, J., and Stiles-Shipley, J. (2001). Body image concerns in female exercisers and athletes: A feminist cultural studies perspective. *Women in Sport and Physical Activity Journal, 10,* 17–54.

Krejcie, R. V., and Margan, D. W. (1970). Determining sample size for research activities. *Educational and Psychological Measurement, 30,* 607–610.

Kuhn, T. (1962). *The structure of scientific revolutions.* Chicago: University of Chicago Press.

Kuzma, J. W., and Bohnenblust, S. E. (2005). *Basic statistics for the health sciences* (5th ed.). New York: McGraw-Hill.

Kwon, S. (2006). Obesity in adolescents and its associations with physical activity and diet. Master's thesis, University of Northern Iowa, Cedar Falls.

Lambdin-Abraham, R. (2009). Parental influence on children's physical activity. Master's thesis, University of Northern Iowa, Cedar Falls.

Larose, T. L. (1998). *Ready, set, run! A student guide to SAS software for Microsoft Windows.* New York: McGraw-Hill.

Lawrence Erlbaum Associates (2011). Publications Catalog. Lawrence Erlbaum Associates, Inc. 10 Industrial Ave., Mahwah, NJ 07430-2262; www.erlbaum.com.

Lewis, P. C., Harrell, J. S., Deng, S., and Bradley, C. (1999). Smokeless tobacco use in adolescents: The cardiovascular health in children study. *Journal of School Health, 69*(8), 320–325.

Lincoln, Y. S., & Guba, E. G. (1985). *Naturalistic inquiry.* Beverly Hills, CA: Sage.

Lipsey, M. W. (1990). *Design sensitivity: Statistical power for experimental research.* Thousand Oaks, CA: Sage.

Lipsey, M. W., and Wilson, D. P. (2001). *Practical meta-analysis.* London: Sage.

Liu, Y. (2002). Analyzing RM ANOVA related data using SPSS 10. *Measurement in Physical Education and Exercise Science, 6*(1), 43–60.

Locke, L. F., Spirduso, W. W., and Silverman, S. J. (2007). *Proposals that work: A guide for planning dissertations and grant proposals* (5th ed.). Thousand Oaks, CA: Sage Publications.

LoVerde, M. E., Prochazka, A. V., and Byyny, R. L. (1989). Research consent forms: Continued unreadability and increasing length. *Journal of General Internal Medicine, 4,* 410–412.

Luedke, G. C. (1980). Range of motion as the focus of teaching the overhand throwing pattern to children. Doctoral dissertation, Indiana University, Bloomington.

Major, M. J. (1998). Effects of Special Olympics participation on self-esteem of adults with mental retardation. Master's thesis, University of Northern Iowa, Cedar Falls.

Marcus, B. H., and Simkin, L. R. (1994). The transtheoretical model: Applications to exercise behavior. *Medicine and Science in Sport and Exercise, 26*(11), 1400–1404.

Maxwell, S. E., and Delaney, H. D. (2004). *Designing experiments and analyzing data* (2nd ed.). Mahwah, NJ: Lawrence Erlbaum Associates.

McCracken, G. (1988). *The long interview.* Thousand Oaks, CA: Sage.

McCuen, G. E. (1998). *Human experimentation: When research is evil.* Hudson, WI: GEM Publications.

McDermott, R. J., and Sarvela, P. D. (1999). *Health education evaluation and measurement: A practitioner's perspective* (2nd ed.). New York: McGraw-Hill.

McKenzie, T. L., Marshall, S. J., Sallis, J. F., and Conway, T. L. (2000). Student activity levels, lesson context, and teacher behavior during middle school physical education. *Research Quarterly for Exercise and Sport, 71*(3), 249–259.

McMillan, J. H. (2008). *Educational research: fundamentals for the consumer* (5th ed.). Boston, MA: Allyn and Bacon.

Merriam, S. B. (1998). *Qualitative research and case study applications in education* (2nd ed.). San Francisco: Jossey-Bass.

Merriam, S. B. (2009). *Qualitative research: A guide to design and implementation.* San Francisco, CA: Jossey-Bass.

Miles, M. B., and Huberman, A. M. (1994). *Qualitative data analysis* (2nd ed.). Thousand Oaks, CA: Sage.

Mills, G. E. (2011). *Action research: A guide for the teacher researcher.* (4th ed.). New York: Pearson, Inc.

Mintah, J. K. (2001). Teacher's perceptions about the impact of authentic assessment use on students' skill achievement, motivation, and self-concept. Doctoral dissertation, University of Northern Iowa, Cedar Falls.

Monette, D. R., Sullivan, T. J., and DeJong, C. R. (2001). *Applied social research* (5th ed.). Belmont, CA: Wadsworth Publishing.

Moore, D. S. (2010). *The basic practice of statistics* (5th ed.). New York: Freeman.

Morrow, J. R., Krzewinski-Malone, J. A., Jackson, A. W., Bungum, T. J., and Fitzgerald, S. J. (2004). American adults' knowledge of exercise recommendations. *Research Quarterly for Exercise and Sport, 75,* 231–237.

Mull, S. S. (1991). The role of the health educator in development of self-esteem. *Journal of Health Education, 22*(6), 349–351.

Murphy, K. R., and Myars, B. (2003). *Statistical power analysis.* Mahwah, NJ: Lawrence Erlbaum Associates.

Musser, K. A. (2002). Psychosocial factors related to eating disorders among female college cheerleaders in Iowa. Master's thesis, University of Northern Iowa, Cedar Falls.

National Commission for the Protection of Human Subjects on Biomedical and Behavioral Research (1979). *The Belmont report: Ethical principles and guidelines for the protection of human subjects of research.* Washington, DC: U.S. Government Printing Office. Retrieved October 5, 2000, from the World Wide Web: ohrp.osophs.dhhs.gov/humansubjects/guidance/Belmont.htm.

National Science Foundation (2002). *Research misconduct.* Federal Register, March 18, 2002, 11936–11939.

Neutens, J. J., and Rubinson, L. (2002). *Research techniques for the health sciences* (3rd ed.). New York: Benjamin Cummings.

Nunnally, J. C. (1978). *Psychometric theory* (2nd ed.). New York: McGraw-Hill.

Nunnally, J. C., and Bernstein, I. H. (1994). *Psychometric theory* (3rd ed.). New York: McGraw-Hill.

Nuremberg Code (1949). *Reprinted in trials of war criminals before the Nuremberg military tribunals under control council law.* No. 10, Vol. 2, Washington, DC: U.S. Government Printing Office.

O'Neill, D. E. T., Thayer, R. E., Taylor, A. W., Dzialoznski, T. M., and Noble, E. G. (2000). Effects of short-term resistance training on muscle strength and morphology in the elderly. *Journal of Aging and Physical Activity, 8*(4), 312–324.

Office of Research Integrity (1999). Case Summaries, ORI Newsletter, 7(2), March 1999. Retrieved October 17, 2000, from the World Wide Web: ori.dhhs.gove/html/publications/newsletters_vol7no2.asp.

Ogletree, R. J. (1991). Selected factors related to help-seeking behavior in college women victims of sexual coercion. Doctoral dissertation, Indiana University, Bloomington.

Ogloff, J. R. P., and Otto, R. K. (1991). Are research participants truly informed? Readability of informed consent forms used in research. *Ethics and Behavior, 1,* 239–252.

Osgood, C. E., Suci, G. J., and Tannenbaum, P. H. (1957). *The measurement of meaning.* Champaign, IL: University of Illinois Press.

Ostrow, A. C. (Ed.). (2002). *Directory of psychological tests in the sport and exercise sciences* (2nd ed.). Morgantown, WV: Fitness Information Technology, Inc.

Papaioannou, A. (1998). Students' perceptions of the physical education class environment for boys and girls and the perceived motivational climate. *Research Quarterly for Exercise and Sport, 69*(3), 267–275.

Park, R. J. (2005). Of the greatest possible worth: The *Research Quarterly* in historical contexts. *Research Quarterly for Exercise and Sport, 76,* s5–s26.

Park, R. J. (2000). "Time given freely to worthwhile causes": Anna S. Espenschade's contributions to physical education. *Research Quarterly for Exercise and Sport, 71,* 95–115.

Pate, D. J. (1987). Sea kayak touring and self-concept of persons with low-level spinal cord injury. Unpublished research proposal, Indiana University, Bloomington.

Patton, M. Q. (2002). *Qualitative evaluation and research methods* (3rd ed.). Thousand Oaks, CA: Sage Publications.

Pavkov, T. W., and Pierce, K. A. (2007). *Ready, set, go! A student guide to SPSS 13.0 and 14.0 for Windows*. Boston, MA: McGraw-Hill.

Payne, V. G., and Morrow, J. R., Jr. (1993). Exercise and VO2max in children: A meta-analysis. *Research Quarterly for Exercise and Sport, 64,* 305–313.

Payne, V. G., Morrow, J. R., Jr., Johnson, L., and Dalton, S. N. (1997). Resistance training in children and youth: A meta-analysis. *Research Quarterly for Exercise and Sport, 68,* 80–88.

Pealer, L. N., and Weiler, R. M. (2000). Web-based health survey research: A primer. *American Journal of Health Behavior, 24,* 69–72.

Pedhazur, E. J. (1997). *Multiple regression in behavioral research: Explanation and prediction* (3rd ed.). New York: Harcourt Brace College Publishers.

Pelegrino, D. A. (1979). *Research methods for recreation and leisure: A theoretical and practical guide.* Dubuque, IA: Wm. C. Brown.

Peña, C. (1990). Needs assessment of Indiana convention and visitor bureaus. Master's thesis, Indiana University, Bloomington.

Phoenix, C. (2010). Seeing the world of physical culture: The potential of visual methods for qualitative research in sport and exercise. *Qualitative Research for Sport and Exercise, 2,* 93–108.

Pitney, W. A., and Parker, J. (2009). *Qualitative research in physical activity and the health professions.* Champaign, IL: Human Kinetics.

Poon, P. P. L., and Rodgers, W. M. (2000). Learning and remembering strategies of novice and advanced jazz dancers for skill level appropriate dance routines. *Research Quarterly for Exercise and Sport, 71*(2), 134–144.

Prochaska, J. O., and DiClemente, C. C. (1983). The stages and processes of self-change in smoking: Towards an integrative model of change. *Journal of Consulting and Clinical Psychology, 51,* 390–395.

Prohaska, T. R., and Rodgers, W. M. (2000). Sources of attrition in a church-based exercise program for older African-Americans. *American Journal of Health Promotion, 14*(6), 380–385.

Public Health Service (1989). Responsibilities of awardee and applicant institutions for dealing with and reporting possible misconduct in science. Federal Register, August 8, 1989, 32446–32451.

Public Health Service (2002). Public health policy on humane care and use of laboratory animals. Washington, DC: U.S. Department of Health and Human Services.

Raudsepp, L., Kais, K., and Hannus, A. (2004). Stability of physical self-perceptions during early adolescence. *Pediatric Exercise Science, 16*(2), 138–146.

Reverby, S. (2000). *Tuskegee's truths: Rethinking the Tuskegee syphilis study.* Chapel Hill, NC: University of North Carolina Press.

Richards, L., and Morse, J. M. (2007). *READMEFIRST for a user's guide to qualitative research* (2nd ed.). Thousand Oaks, CA: Sage.

Rikard, L., and Banville, D. (2010). Effective mentoring: Critical to the professional development of first year physical educators. *Journal of Teaching in Physical Education, 29,* 245–261.

Riva, G., Teruzzi, T., and Anolli, L. (2003). The use of the Internet in psychological research: Comparison of online and offline questionnaires. *CyberPsychology and Behavior, 6,* 73–80.

Rosenthal, R. (1991). *Meta-analytic procedures for social researchers* (rev. ed.). Thousand Oaks, CA: Sage.

Rosenthal, R., and DiMatteo, M. R. (2001). Meta-analysis: Recent developments in quantitative methods for literature reviews. *Annual Reviews Psychology, 52,* 29–82.

Rubin, H. J. (1983). *Applied social research.* Columbus, OH: Charles E. Merrill.

Sage Publications (2011). Publications Catalog. Sage Publications, Inc., 2455 Teller Road, Thousand Oaks, CA 91320-2218; www.sagepublications.com.

Slade, C., and Perrin, R. (2009). *Form and style: Thesis, reports, term papers* (13th ed.). Belmont, CA: Wadsworth Publishing.

SAS (1998). StatView Software (version 5). Cary, NC: SAS.

Schram, T. H. (2006). *Conceptualizing and proposing qualitative research* (2nd ed.). Upper Saddle River, NJ: Pearson/Merrill Prentice Hall.

Schwarzer, R. (1991). *Meta: Programs for secondary data analysis, 5.3.* Berlin: Free University of Berlin.

Siegel, S. (1956). *Nonparametric statistics for the behavioral sciences.* New York: McGraw-Hill.

Siegel, S., and Castellan, N. J. (1988). *Nonparametric statistics for the behavioral sciences* (2nd ed.). New York: McGraw-Hill.

Sherar, L. B., Cumming, S. P., Eisenmann, J. C., Baxter-Jones, A. D., & Malina, R. M. (2010). Adolescent biological maturity and physical activity: Biology meets behavior. *Pediatric Exercise Science, 22,* 332–349.

Silk, M. L., Andrews, D. L., and Mason, D. S. (2005). Encountering the field: Sport studies and qualitative research. In D. L. Andrews, D. S. Mason, and M. L. Silk (Eds.), *Qualitative methods in sport studies* (pp. 1–20). Oxford: Berg Publishers.

Sills, S. J., and Song, C. Y. (2002). Innovations in survey research: An application of Web-based surveys. *Social Science Computer Review, 20,* 22–30.

Simsek, Z., and Veiga, J. F. (2000). The electronic survey technique: An integration and assessment. *Organizational Research Methods, 3,* 93–115.

Skinner, J. S., Corbin, C. B., Landers, D. M., Martin, P. E., and Wells, C. L. (1989). *Future directions in exercise and sport science research.* Champaign, IL: Human Kinetics.

Sparkes, A. C., and Smith, B. (2002). Sport, spinal cord injury, embodied masculinities, and the dilemmas of narrative identity. *Men and Masculinities, 4,* 258–285.

Smith, B., and Sparkes, A. C. (2009). Narrative inquiry in sport and exercise psychology: What can it mean, and why might we do it? *Psychology of Sport and Exercise, 10,* 1–11.

Spencer, L. (1999). College freshmen smokers versus nonsmokers: Academic, social, and emotional expectations and attitudes towards college. *Journal of Health Education, 30*(5), 274–281.

Spitz, V. (2005). *Doctors from hell: The horrific account of Nazi experiments on humans.* Boulder, CO: Sentient Publications.

Strauss, A., Schatzman, L., Bucher, R., Ehrlich, D., and Sabshin, M. (1981). *Psychiatric ideologies and institutions.* New Brunswick, NJ: Transaction Books.

Stunkard, A. J., Sorenson, T., and Schulsinger, F. (1983). Use of Danish adoption register for the study of obesity and thinness. In S. S. Kety, L. P. Rowland, R. L. Sidman, and W. W. Matthysee (Eds.), *Genetics of neurological and psychiatric disorders.* New York: Raven.

Sudman, S., and Bradburn, N. M. (1988). *Asking questions: A practical guide to questionnaire design.* San Francisco: Jossey-Bass.

Sullivan, L. M. (2008). *Essentials of biostatistics in public health.* Sudbury, MA: Jones and Bartlett.

Sun, D. C. (1988). Fat loss in moderately obese women using two walking protocols. Unpublished research proposal, Indiana University, Bloomington.

Sun, J., and Chen, A. (2010). An examination of sixth graders self-determined motivation and learning in physical education. *Journal of Teaching in Physical Education, 26,* 262–277.

Telama, R., Yang, X., Laasko, L., and Vilkari, J. (1997). Physical activity in childhood and adolescence as a predictor of physical activity in young adulthood. *American Journal of Preventive Medicine, 13,* 317–323.

Thomas, D. Q., Bowdoin, B. A., Brown, D. D., and McCaw, S. T. (1998). Nasal strips and mouthpieces do not affect power output during anaerobic exercise. *Research Quarterly for Exercise and Sport, 69*(2), 201–204.

Thomas, J. R., and French, K. E. (1986). The use of meta-analysis in exercise and sport: A tutorial. *Research Quarterly for Exercise and Sport, 57,* 196–204.

Thomas, J. R., Nelson, J. K., and Silverman, S. J. (2005). *Research Methods in Physical Activity* (5th ed.). Champaign, IL: Human Kinetics.

Thomas, J. R., Nelson, J. K., and Magill, R. A. (1986). A case for an alternative format for the thesis/dissertation. *Quest, 38,* 116–124.

Thompson, P. D. (2004). Historical concepts of the athlete's heart. *Medicine and Science in Sport and Exercise, 36,* 363–370.

Thorndike, R. M., Cunningham, G. K., Thorndike, R. L., and Hagen, E. P. (1991). *Measurment and evaluation in psychology and education.* New York: Macmillan.

Tucker, L. A. (1986). The relationship of television viewing to physical fitness and obesity. *Adolescence, 21,* 797–806.

Tuckman, B. W. (1999). *Conducting educational research* (5th ed.). Orlando, FL: Harcourt Brace.

Turabian, K. L. (2007). *A manual for writers of term papers, theses, and dissertations* (7th ed.). Chicago: University of Chicago Press.

U.S. Department of Health and Human Services (1996). Physical activity and health: A report of the Surgeon General. Washington, DC: Author.

University of Chicago (2010). *The Chicago manual of style* (16th ed.). Chicago: Author.

Vander Werff, A. R. (2003). An evaluation of the effectiveness of the Fire P.A.L.S. program on fire and life safety knowledge and behavioral intent of selected elementary school students. Master's thesis, University of Northern Iowa, Cedar Falls.

Visker, T. L. (1986). Self-consciousness and physical self-efficacy in relationship to exercise adherence. Doctoral dissertation, Indiana University, Bloomington.

Vispoel, W. P. (2000). Computerized versus paper-and-pencil assessment of self-concept: Score comparability and respondent preferences. *Measurement and Evaluation in Counseling and Development, 33,* 130–143.

Vogt, M. (2001). Demographics, treatment approaches, experience and knowledge of certified substance abuse counselors in Iowa. Master's thesis, University of Northern Iowa, Cedar Falls.

Waldron, J. J., and Dieser, R. B. (2010). Perspectives of fitness and health in college men and women. *Journal of College Student Development, 51,* 65–78.

Waldron, J. J., and Kowalski, C. L. (2009). Crossing the line: Rites of passage, team aspects, and ambiguity of hazing. *Research Quarterly for Exercise and Sport, 80,* 291–302.

Waldron, J. J., Lynn, Q., and Krane, V. (2010). Duct tape, icy hot, and paddles: Male athlete hazing narratives. *Sport, Education, and Society, 16,* 111–125.

Wang, J. (2000). Leisure participation of urban Chinese adolescents. Master's thesis, University of Northern Iowa, Cedar Falls.

Weisberg, H. F., and Bowen, B. D. (1977). *An introduction to survey research and data analysis.* San Francisco: W. H. Freeman.

Weiss, M. R., McCullogh, P., Smith, A. L., and Berlant, A. R. (1998). Observational learning and the fearful child: Influence of peer models on swimming skill performance and psychological responses. *Research Quarterly for Exercise and Sport, 69*(4), 380–394.

Welk, G. J. (1999). The youth physical activity promotion model: A conceptual bridge between theory and practice. *Quest, 51,* 5–23.

Welk, G. J., Wood, K., and Morss, G. (2003). Parental influences on physical activity in children: An exploration of potential mechanisms. *Pediatric Exercise Science, 15,* 19–33.

Welschimer, K. J., and Harris, S. E. (1994). A survey of rural parents' attitudes toward sexuality education. *Journal of School Health, 64*(9), 347–351.

Wen, L. M., van der Ploeg, H. P., Kite, J., Cashmore, A., and Rissel, C. (2010). A validation study of assessing physical activity and sedentary behavior in children aged 3 to 5 years. *Pediatric Exercise Science, 22,* 408–420.

Weston, A. R., Mbambo, Z., and Myburgh, K. H. (2000). Running economy of African and Caucasian distance runners. *Medicine and Science in Sports and Exercise, 32*(6), 1130–1134.

Wiersma, W. (1991). *Research methods in education* (5th ed.). Boston, MA: Allyn & Bacon.

Wiggins, D. K. (1991). Prized performers, but frequently overlooked students: The involvement of black athletes in intercollegiate sports in predominantly white university campuses, 1890–1972. *Research Quarterly for Exercise and Sport, 62*(2), 164–177.

Winer, B. J., Brown, D. R., and Michels, K. N. (1991). *Statistical principles in experimental design* (3rd ed.). New York: McGraw-Hill.

Wood, T. M. (2006). Measurement basics: Introduction. In T. M. Wood and W. Zhu (Eds.), *Measurement theory and practice in kinesiology* (pp. 3–8). Champaign, IL: Human Kinetics.

Wrynn, A. (2003). Contesting the canon: Understanding the history of the evolving discipline of kinesiology. *Quest, 55,* 244–256.

Wrynn, A. (2005). A fine balance: Margret Bell—Physician and physical educator. *Research Quarterly for Exercise and Sport, 76*(2), 149–165.

Wyatt, H. R., et al. (2004). Using electronic step counters to increase lifestyle physical activity: Colorado on the move. *Journal of Physical Activity and Health, 1*(3), 181–190.

Zieff, S. G. (2006). The American "Alliance" of Health and Physical Education: Scholastic programs and professional organization. *Research Quarterly for Exercise and Sport, 77*(4), 437–450.

Index